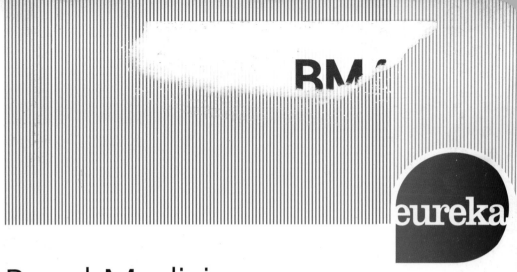

BMA

eureka

Renal Medicine

WITHDRAWN
FROM LIBRARY

BMA LIBRARY   BRITISH

WITH

D1352976

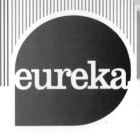

Renal Medicine

Stella Woodward BSc (Hons) MBBCh
MRCP
Core Medical Trainee
St George's University Hospitals NHS
Foundation Trust
London, UK

David Oliveira PhD FRCP
Professor of Renal Medicine
St George's, University of London
London, UK

Series Editors

Janine Henderson MRCPsych
MClinEd
MB BS Programme Director
Hull York Medical School
York, UK

David Oliveira PhD FRCP
Professor of Renal Medicine
St George's, University of London
London, UK

Stephen Parker BSc MS DipMedEd
FRCS
Consultant Breast and General
Paediatric Surgeon
St Mary's Hospital
Newport, UK

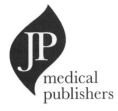

JP medical publishers

London • Philadelphia • New Delhi • Panama City

© 2017 JP Medical Ltd.

Published by JP Medical Ltd, 83 Victoria Street, London, SW1H 0HW, UK

Tel: +44 (0)20 3170 8910   Fax: +44 (0)20 3008 6180

Email: info@jpmedpub.com   www.jpmedpub.com, www.eurekamedicine.com

The rights of Stella Woodward and David Oliveira to be identified as the authors of this work have been asserted by them in accordance with the Copyright, Designs and Patents Act 1988.

All rights reserved. No part of this publication may be reproduced, stored or transmitted in any form or by any means, electronic, mechanical, photocopying, recording or otherwise, except as permitted by the UK Copyright, Designs and Patents Act 1988, without the prior permission in writing of the publishers. Permissions may be sought directly from JP Medical Ltd at the address printed above.

All brand names and product names used in this book are trade names, service marks, trademarks or registered trademarks of their respective owners. The publisher is not associated with any product or vendor mentioned in this book.

Medical knowledge and practice change constantly. This book is designed to provide accurate, authoritative information about the subject matter in question. However readers are advised to check the most current information available on procedures included and check information from the manufacturer of each product to be administered, to verify the recommended dose, formula, method and duration of administration, adverse effects and contraindications. It is the responsibility of the practitioner to take all appropriate safety precautions. Neither the publisher nor the authors assume any liability for any injury and/or damage to persons or property arising from or related to use of material in this book.

This book is sold on the understanding that the publisher is not engaged in providing professional medical services. If such advice or services are required, the services of a competent medical professional should be sought.

Every effort has been made where necessary to contact holders of copyright to obtain permission to reproduce copyright material. If any have been inadvertently overlooked, the publisher will be pleased to make the necessary arrangements at the first opportunity.

ISBN: 978-1-907816-95-6

British Library Cataloguing in Publication Data
A catalogue record for this book is available from the British Library

Library of Congress Cataloging in Publication Data
A catalog record for this book is available from the Library of Congress

Publisher:	Richard Furn
Development Editors:	Thomas Fletcher, Paul Mayhew, Alison Whitehouse
Editorial Assistants:	Katie Pattullo, Adam Rajah
Copy Editor:	Kim Howell
Graphic narratives:	James Pollitt
Cover design:	Forbes Design
Page design:	Designers Collective Ltd

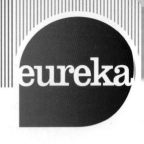

Series Editors' Foreword

Today's medical students need to know a great deal to be effective as tomorrow's doctors. This knowledge includes core science and clinical skills, from understanding biochemical pathways to communicating with patients. Modern medical school curricula integrate this teaching, thereby emphasising how learning in one area can support and reinforce another. At the same time students must acquire sound clinical reasoning skills, working with complex information to understand each individual's unique medical problems.

The *Eureka* series is designed to cover all aspects of today's medical curricula and reinforce this integrated approach. Each book can be used from first year through to qualification. Core biomedical principles are introduced but given relevant clinical context: the authors have always asked themselves, 'why does the aspiring clinician need to know this'?

Each clinical title in the series is grounded in the relevant core science, which is introduced at the start of each book. Each core science title integrates and emphasises clinical relevance throughout. Medical and surgical approaches are included to provide a complete and integrated view of the patient management options available to the clinician. Clinical insights highlight key facts and principles drawn from medical practice. Cases featuring unique graphic narratives are presented with clear explanations that show how experienced clinicians think, enabling students to develop their own clinical reasoning and decision making. Clinical SBAs help with exam revision while Starter questions are a unique learning tool designed to stimulate interest in the subject.

Having biomedical principles and clinical applications together in one book will make their connections more explicit and easier to remember. Alongside repeated exposure to patients and practice of clinical and communication skills, we hope *Eureka* will equip medical students for a lifetime of successful clinical practice.

Janine Henderson, David Oliveira, Stephen Parker

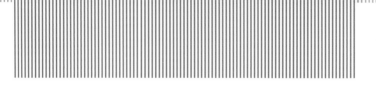

About the Series Editors

Janine Henderson is the MB BS undergraduate Programme Director at Hull York Medical School (HYMS). After medical school at the University of Oxford and clinical training in psychiatry, she combined her work as a consultant with postgraduate teaching roles, moving to the new Hull York Medical School in 2004. She has a particular interest in modern educational methods, curriculum design and clinical reasoning.

David Oliveira is Professor of Renal Medicine at St George's, University of London (SGUL), where he served as the MBBS Course Director between 2007 and 2013. Having trained at Cambridge University and the Westminster Hospital he obtained a PhD in cellular immunology and worked as a renal physician before being appointed as Foundation Chair of Renal Medicine at SGUL.

Stephen Parker is a Consultant Breast & General Paediatric Surgeon at St Mary's Hospital, Isle of Wight. He trained at St George's, University of London, and after service in the Royal Navy was appointed as Consultant Surgeon at University Hospital Coventry. He has a particular interest in e-learning and the use of multimedia platforms in medical education.

About the Authors

Stella Woodward is Core Medical Trainee at St George's Hospital, London with an interest in nephrology. She has taught medical students throughout her career and has written exam questions and clinical examination stations. She particularly enjoys the challenge of explaining complex subjects, such as renal physiology, in a concise, simple manner.

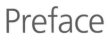

Preface

Renal medicine has a reputation as a difficult speciality: complex biochemistry and acid–base disorders, the mysteries of glomerular disease, challenging sick patients with acute kidney injury, and so on. Many problems, such as chronic kidney disease, are common and encountered in most clinical specialities, and contribute a considerable burden to health services.

Eureka Renal Medicine demystifies the subject by providing a thorough grounding in the core anatomical and physiological principles in chapter 1, followed by the key clinical skills required in chapter 2. Subsequent chapters explain approaches to the common problems that we have found helpful in clinical practice. In each chapter detailed cases explain how an experienced physician would approach a patient. Throughout the book boxes provide useful clinical tips, figures explain underlying pathology clearly and graphic narratives show real-life experiences. The final chapter consists of single best answer questions based on clinical reasoning, designed to test your knowledge and help you to revise.

We hope that this book, complemented by plenty of clinical experience, will help you acquire broadly applicable clinical skills (e.g. assessment of fluid balance, interpretation of biochemistry), and an appreciation of the wide scope of renal medicine.

Stella Woodward, David Oliveira
September 2016

Contents

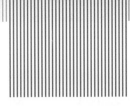

Glossary

1,25-$(OH)_2$D	1,25-dihydroxyvitamin D		ECF	extracellular fluid
25-(OH)D	25-hydroxyvitamin D		ECG	electrocardiogram or electrocardiography
AA	amino acid		ENaC	epithelial sodium channel
AA	amyloid A		ESRD	end stage renal disease
ABG	arterial blood gas			
ABPI	ankle–brachial pressure index		FGF-23	fibroblast growth factor 23
ABPM	ambulatory blood pressure monitoring			
ACE	angiotensin-converting enzyme		GBM	glomerular basement membrane
ACR	albumin:creatinine ratio		GCS	Glasgow coma scale score
ADH	antidiuretic hormone		GFR	glomerular filtration rate
ADPKD	autosomal dominant polycystic kidney disease		GI	gastrointestinal
			GP	general practitioner
AKI	acute kidney injury			
AKIN	Acute Kidney Injury Network		HBeAg	hepatitis B e-antigen
AL	amyloid light chain		HBPM	home blood pressure monitoring
ANA	antinuclear antibody		HLA	human leucocyte antigen
ANCA	antineutrophil cytoplasmic antibody		HR	heart rate
ANP	atrial natriuretic peptide		HTN	hypertension
AQP	aquaporin			
ARB	angiotensin II receptor blocker		IBD	inflammatory bowel disease
ARPKD	autosomal recessive polycystic kidney disease		Ig	immunoglobulin
			IV	intravenous
ATN	acute tubular necrosis			
ATP	adenosine triphophate		JVP	jugular venous pulse
BNP	brain natriuretic peptide		KDIGO	Kidney Disease: Improving Global Outcomes
BP	blood pressure			
CA	carbonic anhydrase		MAP	mean arterial pressure
c-ANCA	cytoplasmic antineutrophil cytoplasmic antibody		MG 3	mercaptoacetyltriglycine
			MR	mineralocorticoid receptor
CCF	congestive cardiac failure		MRI	magnetic resonance imaging
CKD	chronic kidney disease			
COPD	chronic obstructive pulmonary disease		NSAID	non-steroidal anti-inflammatory drug
CT	computerised tomography			
CTR	Cardiothoracic ratio		P_aCO_2	arterial partial pressure of carbon dioxide
CV	cardiovascular			
			p-ANCA	perinuclear antineutrophil cytoplasmic antibody
DBD	donation after brainstem death			
DCD	donation after circulatory death		P_aO_2	arterial partial pressure of oxygen
DCT	distal convoluted tubule		pco_2	partial pressure of carbon dioxide
DMSA	dimercaptosuccinic acid		PCR	protein:creatinine ratio
DTPA	diethylene triamine penta-acetic acid		po_2	partial pressure of oxygen

PTH	parathyroid hormone	SLE	systemic lupus erythematosus
P_vCO_2	venous partial pressure of carbon dioxide	TGF	transforming growth factor
P_vO_2	venous partial pressure of oxygen	TPN	total parenteral nutrition
RAAS	renin–angiotensin–aldosterone system	UO	urine output
RIFLE	Risk, Injury, Failure, Loss of kidney function, and End stage kidney disease	US	ultrasound
		USS	ultrasound scan
ROMK	renal outer medullary potassium channel	UTI	urinary tract infection
SCM	sternocleidomastoid muscle	VBG	venous blood gas
SGLT-2	sodium–glucose transporter 2		
SIADH	syndrome of inappropriate antidiuretic hormone secretion		

Acknowledgements

Figures 1.4, 1.5, 2.11, 2.16 and 2.19 are copyright of Sam Scott-Hunter and are reproduced from Tunstall R, Shah N. *Pocket Tutor Surface Anatomy.* London, JP Medical, 2012.

Figures 2.3, 2.14, 9.1 and 13.1 are reproduced from Morris P, Warriner D, Morton A. *Eureka Cardiovascular Medicine.* London, JP Medical, 2015.

Figure 2.11 is reproduced from Smith LJ, Quint J, Brown J. *Eureka Respiratory Medicine.* London, JP Medical, 2015.

Figure 2.16 is reproduced from Parker S. *Eureka General Surgery & Urology.* London, JP Medical, 2015.

Figure 7.1 is reproduced from Darby M, Edey A, Chandratreya L, Maskell N. *Pocket Tutor Chest X-Ray Interpretation.* London, JP Medical, 2012.

Figures 7.2 and 12.1 are reproduced from Oliveira D, Debasish B, Popoola J, MacPhee IAM, Shrivastava S, Jones D, Nelson S. *Pocket Tutor Renal Medicine.* London, JP Medical, 2013.

Chapter 1
First principles

Overview of the renal system

Starter questions

Answers to the following questions are on page 54.

1. What are the functional units of kidneys?
2. How is the kidney part of the endocrine (i.e. hormonal) system?

The renal system or urinary tract comprises two kidneys, two ureters, the bladder and the urethra (**Figures 1.1**). It has two divisions:

- The upper urinary tract: the kidneys, which produce urine
- The lower urinary tract: the ureters, through which urine passes to the bladder, which stores urine, and the urethra, through which urine passes during voiding

Each kidney contains >1 million nephrons, the functional units of the kidney. Each nephron is made up of:

- a glomerulus, a ball of capillaries in a capsule (the whole termed the renal corpuscle) which produces an ultrafiltrate (a filtrate produced by applying pressure across a semi-permeable membrane) from blood

- a tubule (consisting sequentially of proximal convoluted tubule, loop of Henle, distal convoluted tubule and collecting duct), which transports and modifies the filtrate before it is excreted as urine.

Thus the renal system:

- removes waste products
- regulates fluid balance, i.e. intake, retention and net loss from the body
- regulates the concentration of electrolytes in body fluids

The kidneys also have endocrine roles: they produce the hormones erythropoietin, responsible for formation of red blood cells, and renin, which regulates blood pressure; they also convert vitamin D to its active form, 1,25-dihydroxyvitamin D, which is required for calcium homeostasis and bone health.

Figure 1.1 The urinary tract.

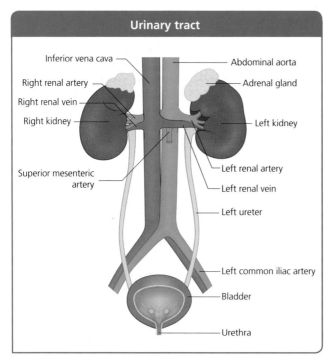

Urinary tract

- Inferior vena cava
- Abdominal aorta
- Right renal artery
- Adrenal gland
- Right renal vein
- Right kidney
- Left kidney
- Superior mesenteric artery
- Left renal artery
- Left renal vein
- Left ureter
- Left common iliac artery
- Bladder
- Urethra

Development of the renal system

Starter questions

Answers to the following questions are on page 54.

3. Does a fetus pass urine in the womb?
4. Why would a kidney be found in the pelvis?
5. Why might the kidney have more than one renal artery?

Embryonic development of the renal system occurs in several stages and is closely linked to development of the genital organs. Development begins at the end of the third week after conception. By week 16 the kidneys are functional and contribute to the formation of amniotic fluid. Development and maturation continue into postnatal life.

The kidneys and ureters develop from the mesoderm, the intermediate germ cell layer of the embryo (the other layers are the endoderm and ectoderm).

The bladder (apart from the trigone) and the urethra develop from the urogenital sinus, a structure that derives from the cloaca, which is a common opening for the renal, genital and gastrointestinal tracts. The cloaca is divided by the urogenital membrane into the urogenital sinus and the primitive rectum.

> Because renal and genital embryonic development are closely linked, malformations of the genital and renal tracts commonly occur together.

Embryonic stages of the kidney

There are three distinct stages to the development of the kidney, the pronephros, mesonephros, and the metanephros (**Figure 1.2**). These occur sequentially, although there is overlap with the next stage developing as the previous stage regresses. In addition, there are residual structures from each stage that contribute to the next.

Pronephros

The pronephros develops towards the head end of the embryo during week 4 of gestation. It soon regress, but leaves behind the pronephric duct which goes on to form the mesonephric duct.

Mesonephros

As the pronephros degenerates, the mesonephros forms in the lumbar region. It functions transiently, draining into the mesonephric (Wolffian) duct (previously the pronephric duct).

The mesonephros degenerates in turn, but the mesonephric duct persists. In both sexes, the portion of the duct that joins to the cloaca goes on to form the trigone of the bladder and an outgrowth from this distal portion of the mesonephric duct goes on to form the ureteric bud. In men, other parts of the mesonephric duct go on to form the ductal system of the reproductive tract; in women, the rest of the duct degenerates, leaving vestigial structures.

Metanephros

The metanephros arises in the sacral region and develops in to the definitive kidney. It is invaded by the developing ureteric bud, which divides repeatedly to form the collecting system of the kidney (ureters, renal pelvis, calyces and collecting ducts). The metanephros is induced to differentiate into glomeruli and renal tubules, which join up with the collecting ducts to form the complete nephron (**Table 1.1**).

Metanephros: development	
Section	Develops into
Proximal	Glomerular capsule
Middle	Proximal straight and convoluted tubules, descending limb of loop of Henle
Distal	Thick and thin ascending limbs of loop of Henle, distal convoluted tubule

Table 1.1 Development of the metanephros

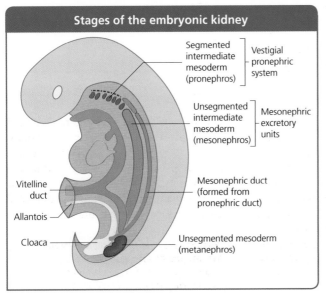

Stages of the embryonic kidney

- Segmented intermediate mesoderm (pronephros) — Vestigial pronephric system
- Unsegmented intermediate mesoderm (mesonephros) — Mesonephric excretory units
- Vitelline duct
- Allantois
- Cloaca
- Mesonephric duct (formed from pronephric duct)
- Unsegmented mesoderm (metanephros)

Figure 1.2 The three distinct stages of the embryonic kidney: the pronephros, mesonephros and metanephros.

Ascent of the kidneys

As the metanephros forms in the sacral region, the kidneys ascend to their adult position in the upper lumbar region. This occurs between the 6th and 9th week, during which the kidneys come to lie at the level of the 12th thoracic vertebra (T12), underneath the adrenal gland (**Figure 1.3**). As it ascends, the kidney is transiently supplied by blood vessels that originate from the aorta at progressively higher levels, until it receives its definitive blood supply from the lumbar aorta.

Congenital abnormalities are found in 3–4% of live births; urinary tract abnormalities account for 20–30% of these. Common abnormalities include pelvic kidney (1 in 2000–3000), in which the kidney fails to ascend and remains below the pelvic brim, and multiple renal vessels (20–30% of births), in which there is a persistence of some of the sequential arterial (or venous) vessels received during ascent of the kidney.

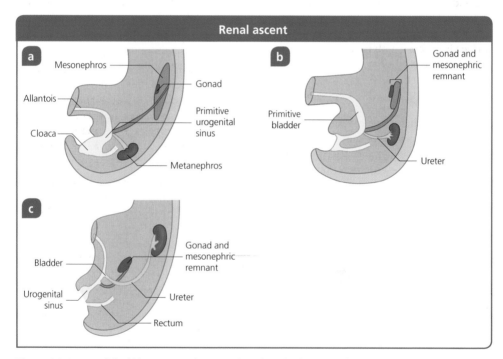

Renal ascent

a
- Mesonephros
- Allantois
- Cloaca
- Gonad
- Primitive urogenital sinus
- Metanephros

b
- Gonad and mesonephric remnant
- Primitive bladder
- Ureter

c
- Bladder
- Urogenital sinus
- Gonad and mesonephric remnant
- Ureter
- Rectum

Figure 1.3 Ascent of the kidneys occurs between the 6th and 9th weeks of embryonic development. (a) The adult kidney begins as the metanephros in the sacral region of the embryo. (b) As the embryo grows in length, the kidneys begin their ascent. (c) By the 9th week, the kidneys come to lie at the level of the 12th thoracic vertebra.

Structure of the kidney

Starter questions

Answers to the following questions are on page 54.

6. Why are all invasive procedures involving the kidney, such as a biopsy, so risky?

7. How does a long loop of Henle help a desert animal survive?

The kidneys are located on the posterior abdominal wall and are described as being retroperitoneal, because only their anterior surface is covered with peritoneum. They lie at the level of T11–T12 to L3 on either side of the lumbar vertebrae (**Figure 1.4**). The right kidney lies about 12 mm lower than the left, as the result of downward displacement by the liver.

Each kidney is bean-shaped with a medial indentation (hilum). The adult kidney is usually 10–14 cm long and 6 cm wide, depending on the individual. Both kidneys are surrounded by perirenal fat, which provides a protective cushion.

The anatomical relations of the kidney (**Figures 1.5** and **1.6**; see also **Figure 1.1**) are:

- Superior: adrenal glands
- Anterior to the right kidney: duodenum (second part), ascending colon and liver
- Anterior to the left kidney: stomach, pancreas, spleen and descending colon
- Posterior: diaphragm, quadratus lumborum, psoas, transversus abdominis, 12th rib, 12th subcostal nerve, and iliohypogastric and ilioinguinal nerves

Within the fibrous renal capsule there are two zones of tissue: the outer cortex and the inner medulla (**Figure 1.7**). The medullary

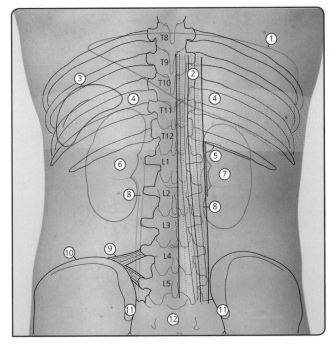

Figure 1.4 Surface anatomy and relations of the kidneys. ①, liver; ②, erector spinae muscle group; ③, spleen; ④, region of costodiaphragmatic recess (shaded white); ⑤, renal angle; ⑥, left kidney; ⑦, right kidney; ⑧, ureter; ⑨, iliolumbar ligament; ⑩, iliac crest; ⑪, posterior superior iliac spine; ⑫, sacrum.

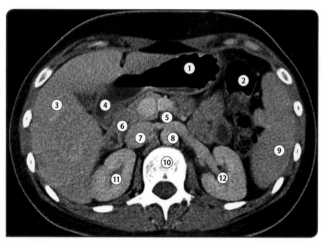

Figure 1.5 Axial CT scan of the abdomen at the level of the transpyloric plane (level of L1). ①, stomach; ②, transverse colon; ③, liver; ④, duodenum, firstpart; ⑤, superior mesenteric artery; ⑥, pancreas; ⑦, inferior vena cava; ⑧, aorta; ⑨, spleen; ⑩, L1 vertebra; ⑪, right kidney; ⑫, left kidney and hilum.

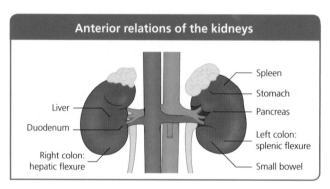

Anterior relations of the kidneys

Spleen

Stomach

Pancreas

Liver

Duodenum

Left colon: splenic flexure

Right colon: hepatic flexure

Small bowel

Figure 1.6 Anterior relations of the kidneys.

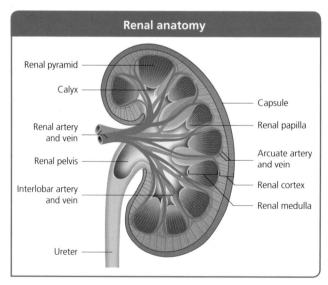

Renal anatomy

Renal pyramid

Calyx

Capsule

Renal artery and vein

Renal papilla

Renal pelvis

Arcuate artery and vein

Interlobar artery and vein

Renal cortex

Renal medulla

Ureter

Figure 1.7 Structure of the kidney. The kidney is organised as a group of pyramids facing inwards, and draining via the calyces into the renal pelvis. All vessels – renal artery, renal vein, ureter, lymphatics and nerves – pass through the medial hilum.

region is divided into triangular shaped areas of tissue, the pyramids; the apex of each of these pyramids is called a renal papilla. The hilum of each kidney contains the renal vein, renal artery and renal pelvis, in addition to lymphatics and nerves.

Vascular supply

Because their role is efficient filtration of the blood, the kidneys are highly vascular; they receive about 20% of cardiac output, roughly 1.1 L/min, which enables the entire blood volume (about 5.5 L) to be filtered 30–35 times a day. Blood is delivered to each kidney via a single renal artery, which enters the kidney at its hilum. In some people, multiple renal arteries are present; these arise directly from the aorta or branch off the existing renal artery.

Arterial circulation

After its entry at the hilum the renal artery branches progressively, first forming smaller arteries and then smaller arterioles until the capillary bed is reached (**Figure 1.8**). The order of branching of each renal artery is as follows:

- five segmental arteries
- interlobar arteries along the sides of the medullary pyramids
- arcuate arteries at the junction of the medulla and cortex
- cortical radiate arteries
- afferent arterioles
- glomerular capillary networks, where filtration occurs

Fluid moves out of the capillaries to enter the nephron as the glomerular filtrate, which

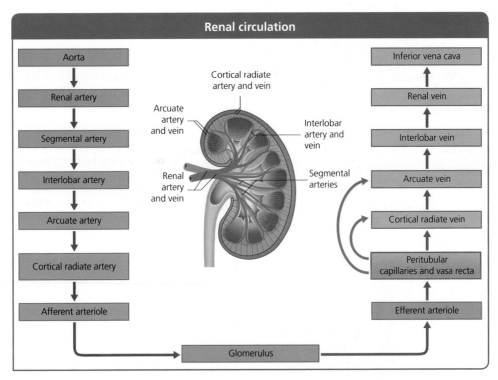

Figure 1.8 Renal circulation. The pink boxes show the successive divisions of the arterial supply from the aorta. The blue boxes show the successive joining of veins that eventually drain into the inferior vena cava. The red arrows show the direct passage of blood from arterioles to veins in the cortex: not all blood enters the deep medulla via the vasa recta (see **Figure 1.9**).

is processed by the kidney to eventually become urine. Blood remaining in the capillaries passes out of the glomerulus via the efferent arteriole.

The renal cortex is the most vascularised part of the kidney, receiving more than 90% of its blood supply. This enables a high glomerular filtration rate (GFR) to be maintained. Most cortical blood enters the medulla and the remainder supplies the renal capsule and adipose tissue. In the outer two thirds of the cortex, the efferent arterioles from the glomerulus form a capillary network (the peritubular capillaries) around the first part of the remaining tubule (the proximal convoluted tubule) (**Figure 1.9**).

Vasa recta

Juxtamedullary glomeruli, i.e. those in the inner third of the cortex, give rise to efferent arterioles that descend into the medulla and divide into hairpin-shaped capillaries and form the vasa recta, a capillary network surrounding the loops of Henle and collecting ducts (**Figure 1.9**). These capillaries have a role in the countercurrent exchange mechanism responsible for efficiently concentrating urine to preserve water (see page 22).

The vasa recta and peritubular capillaries drain into a series of venules and veins that eventually drain into the left and right renal veins and finally the inferior vena cava.

Venous drainage

This mirrors arterial supply, with a single renal vein draining into the vena cava from each kidney. The left renal vein is longer than the right and receives the left gonadal vein, the left adrenal vein and the left inferior phrenic vein. These drain separately into the inferior vena cava on the right side.

Nerve supply

The kidneys are innervated by the autonomic nervous system, the division of the peripheral nervous system that governs the functions of internal organs in the absence of conscious effort. Renal autonomic nerves regulate vasomotor tone, the level of muscular contraction in the walls of arterioles. Autonomic control of vasomotor tone also controls renal blood flow.

The kidney predominantly receives autonomic nerve supply via the sympathetic nervous system, the division of the autonomic nervous system that activates the body's 'fight or

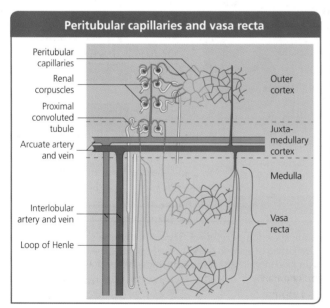

Peritubular capillaries and vasa recta

Peritubular capillaries

Renal corpuscles

Proximal convoluted tubule

Arcuate artery and vein

Interlobular artery and vein

Loop of Henle

Outer cortex

Juxta-medullary cortex

Medulla

Vasa recta

Figure 1.9 Peritubular capillaries and vasa recta. For simplicity only one juxtamedullary nephron is shown, its renal tubule descending deep into the medulla where the ascending and descending limbs of the loop of Henle are in close proximity to the vasa recta (as is the collecting duct). The tubules associated with cortical nephrons descend to the medulla near its junction with the cortex (not shown here).

flight' response. Each kidney is innervated via the renal plexus, which receives postganglionic fibres from the coeliac ganglia, aorticorenal ganglia and lower splanchnic nerves. The renal plexus is located around the renal artery and nerve fibres enter the kidney along its branches. These fibres make direct contact with renal blood vessels, renal tubules and juxtaglomerular cells. Increased sympathetic activity results in renal arterial vasoconstriction, and therefore decreased renal blood flow and decreased GFR, in addition to enhanced tubular Na^+ and water reabsorption, and stimulation of the renin–angiotensin–aldosterone system (RAAS; see page 35). Decreased sympathetic activity has the opposite effect. This system contributes to the homeostatic regulation of water and sodium balance and, in disease states, to pathological alterations to this balance.

In addition to autonomic innervation, the kidney contains afferent sensory nerve fibres located in the renal pelvis. Activation of these fibres results in reflex inhibition of sympathetic activity in the contralateral kidney, causing natriuresis and diuresis.

Lymphatic drainage

Plexuses of lymph vessels in the cortex drain into several trunks that follow the course of the renal vein and drain into aortic lymph nodes. Some protein is filtered from the blood in the glomerulus, but most is subsequently absorbed by the tubular cells and then returned to the blood via the lymphatic vessels. The lymphatic system also has a central role in the function of the immune system: lymph contains cellular debris and pathogens that are transported to lymph nodes where they encounter a high concentration of lymphocytes. Here, lymphocytes are activated by antigens and an adaptive immune response is initiated.

Microstructure: the nephron

The kidneys are composed of:

- the renal corpuscles (the filtration apparatus); collectively the corpuscle and tubule make up the nephron

- the renal tubules (the reabsorptive apparatus)
- the calyces and the renal pelvis (the collecting system). These structures drain into the ureter

The renal parenchyma, i.e. the functional tissue of the kidney, comprises of about 1 million nephrons, blood vessels and supporting structures such as fibroblasts (interstitial tissue). The nephron is a tube made up of simple epithelium, i.e. a single layer of epithelial cells; it is the functional unit of the kidney. Each nephron consists of two functional components: the renal corpuscle (**Figure 1.10**) and the renal tubule (**Figure 1.11**).

The majority of the renal corpuscles (about 85%), the proximal and distal convoluted tubules and part of the collecting tubules are situated in the outer cortex of the kidney. About 15% of renal corpuscles are in the juxtamedullary region, the deepest part of the cortex. These are associated with nephrons that have longer loops of Henle.

The descending limb and thin and thick ascending limbs of the loops of Henle, as well as the medullary collecting tubules and collecting ducts are situated in the medulla. The medulla is divided into dark, striated areas called pyramids, the apices of which are called papillae. Papillae project into the renal pelvis, which continues into the ureter.

> **The number of nephrons decreases over time.** This explains why renal function declines as an individual ages.

Renal corpuscle

The renal corpuscle is the site of initial filtration and comprises:

- Bowman's capsule, the cupped end of the renal tubule
- Bowman's space, the space between the glomerulus and Bowman's epithelium. Filtrate within it drains into the renal tubule
- the glomerulus, a network of blood vessels within the capsule. This term often refers to the whole renal corpuscle, not just the vessels

The renal corpuscle

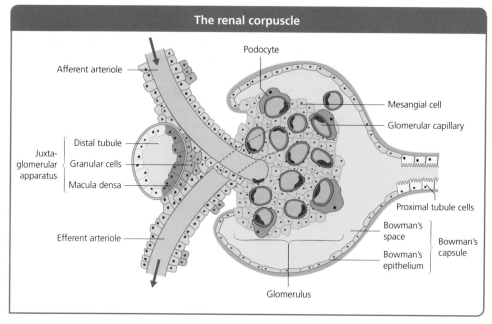

Figure 1.10 The renal corpuscle, often referred to as the glomerulus. The true glomerulus is the network of capillary vessels, which is fed by afferent and drained by efferent arterioles. The juxtaglomerular apparatus, which is involved in tubuloglomerular feedback (see page 18), is shown where the afferent arteriole and the distal tubule of the same nephron meet.

The nephron

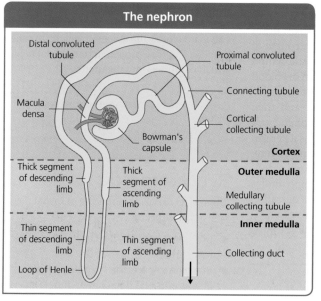

Figure 1.11 The nephron comprises the renal corpuscle and renal tubule; it culminates in the collecting duct, which drains into the renal pelvis. Each collecting duct receives fluid from several distal tubules.

The glomerular filtration membrane

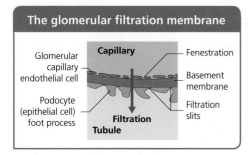

Glomerular capillary endothelial cell

Podocyte (epithelial cell) foot process

Capillary

Filtration Tubule

Fenestration

Basement membrane

Filtration slits

Figure 1.12 The glomerular filtration membrane

The process of filtration commences in the renal corpuscle, where plasma ultrafiltrate enters Bowman's space from the glomerulus. This process depends on the filtration membrane, which has three layers (**Figure 1.12**):

■ fenestrated endothelial cells of glomerular capillaries
■ the glomerular basement membrane, a continuous layer of connective tissue and glycoproteins
■ podocytes, the epithelial cells of the visceral layer of Bowman's capsule, named for their foot-like projections

Because of the fenestrations in the endothelium, the barrier to filtration principally consists of the basement membrane and podocytes. The basement membrane is made up of a number of macromolecules including type IV collagen, heparan sulphate and laminin, that provide a barrier to filtration based both on size and charge. The podocyte foot processes interdigitate on the outside of the basement membrane to form filtration slits 20–30 nm wide. The importance of proteins such as nephrin and podocin that

are expressed in the filtration slits is shown by the massive proteinuria that results from their genetic deficiency (see page 302).

Mesangial cells surround glomerular capillaries and have several functions, including:

■ structural support
■ secretion of extracellular matrix
■ phagocytic activity
■ secretions of prostaglandins

These cells can contract to help regulate blood flow through glomerular capillaries. The different glomerular cells and their functions are summarised in **Table 1.2**.

Renal tubule

The renal tubule is specialised for secretion and selective reabsorption. It is made up of the:

■ proximal convoluted tubule
■ loop of Henle
■ distal convoluted tubule
■ collecting duct

The epithelial cells of the renal tubule vary in structure along its length, reflecting the different functions of each segment (**Table 1.3**). The diameter of the tubule varies along its length, ranging from 15 µm to 60 µm.

Proximal convoluted tubule

The proximal convoluted tubule arises from the renal corpuscle and is roughly 15mm long. The wall of the tubule is made up of a single layer of interdigitating cuboidal cells (cube-shaped epithelial cells), connected by tight junctions at their apical (luminal) surfaces.

Glomerular cells and their functions	
Cell	**Function**
Mesangial cells	Structural support for glomerular capillary loop, secretion of extracellular matrix, secretion of prostaglandins, phagocytic activity, regulation of glomerular capillary blood flow through contractile property
Endothelial cells	Fenestrations (transcellular holes) allow free passage of filtrate
Podocytes	Specialised epithelial cells which form interdigitating foot processes. They contribute to the glomerular filtration barrier and stabilise glomerular architecture

Table 1.2 Cells of the glomerulus and their functions

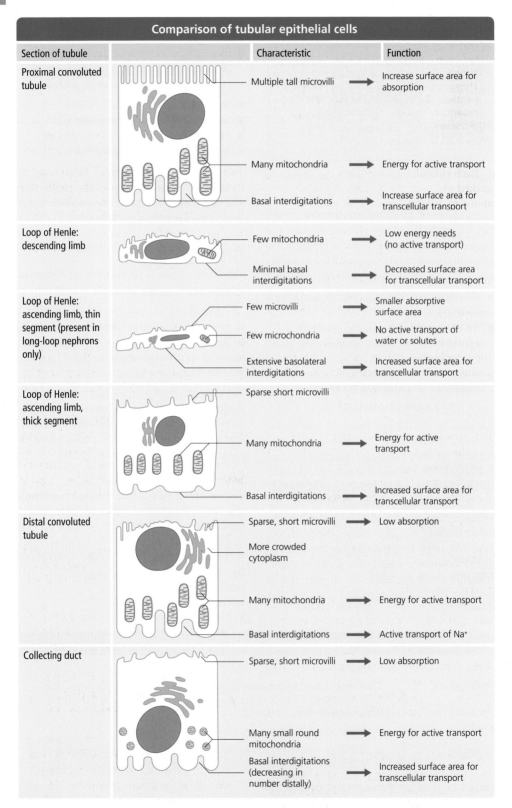

Comparison of tubular epithelial cells		
Section of tubule	**Characteristic**	**Function**
Proximal convoluted tubule	Multiple tall microvilli	Increase surface area for absorption
	Many mitochondria	Energy for active transport
	Basal interdigitations	Increase surface area for transcellular transport
Loop of Henle: descending limb	Few mitochondria	Low energy needs (no active transport)
	Minimal basal interdigitations	Decreased surface area for transcellular transport
Loop of Henle: ascending limb, thin segment (present in long-loop nephrons only)	Few microvilli	Smaller absorptive surface area
	Few microchondria	No active transport of water or solutes
	Extensive basolateral interdigitations	Increased surface area for transcellular transport
Loop of Henle: ascending limb, thick segment	Sparse short microvilli	
	Many mitochondria	Energy for active transport
	Basal interdigitations	Increased surface area for transcellular transport
Distal convoluted tubule	Sparse, short microvilli	Low absorption
	More crowded cytoplasm	
	Many mitochondria	Energy for active transport
	Basal interdigitations	Active transport of Na^+
Collecting duct	Sparse, short microvilli	Low absorption
	Many small round mitochondria	Energy for active transport
	Basal interdigitations (decreasing in number distally)	Increased surface area for transcellular transport

Table 1.3 Epithelial cells of the renal tubule, in order from proximal to distal

Tight junctions are protein complexes that form a semi-permeable barrier between neighbouring epithelial and endothelial cells at their apical surface. They regulate paracellular (intercellular) permeability, help maintain cellular polarity and play a role in cell signalling processes.

Each cuboidal cell is covered with densely packed microvilli on its luminal surface. The many microvilli of multiple adjacent cells make up the characteristic brush border of the proximal convoluted tubule. This is a specialised surface for transport; the microvilli increase the surface area over which solutes are exchanged by a factor of 200.

The basal aspect of each cell (the part of the cell adjacent to the basal lamina) is also adapted for transport. It contains invaginations of the cell membrane that increase its surface area. The cytoplasm is rich in mitochondria which provide the energy the cells need to actively transport substances across their membranes.

Loop of Henle

The proximal convoluted tubule continues into the U-shaped loop of Henle, which has a descending and an ascending limb. The limbs are divided into portions or segments. The thick segment of the descending limb (pars recta) is similar to that of the proximal convoluted tubule and it can be considered as an extension of this segment. The thick segment leads on to the thin segment of the descending limb, which is relatively metabolically inactive.

The thin segment of the ascending limb is also relatively inactive, whereas the thick segment is adapted for active transport of ions.

Nephrons in the juxtamedullary region, i.e. those closest to the medulla, have long loops of Henle that extend deep into the medulla. In contrast, cortical nephrons are entirely within the cortex or enter only the outer region of the medulla.

Juxtaglomerular apparatus

The juxtaglomerular apparatus is situated close to Bowman's capsule, where the distal convoluted tubule passes close to the capsule and its afferent and efferent arterioles (see Figure 1.10). It comprises:

- the macula densa: this is an area of specialised epithelial cells found only in this part of the distal convoluted tubule
- extraglomerular mesangial cells
- granular cells in the wall of the afferent arteriole: these are specialised smooth muscle cells containing secretory granules.

The granular cells synthesise renin, an enzyme involved in the control of aldosterone release from the adrenal cortex (see page 35). Thus the juxtaglomerular apparatus has a central role in sodium homeostasis and consequently fluid balance and blood pressure (see page 36).

Distal convoluted tubule

The loop of Henle continues into the distal convoluted tubule, which is around 5mm long and the shortest segment of the nephron. On the basal membrane, Na$^+$-K$^+$ ATPase pumps participate in active transport of Na$^+$ and potassium ions (K$^+$) across the basolateral membrane.

The late distal convoluted tubule (distal end), is functionally distinct from the 'early' distal convoluted tubule. It is sensitive to the actions of aldosterone due the the presence of aldosterone receptors and the 11-β hydroxysteroid dehydrogenase 2 enzyme, which prevents glucocorticoids from binding to this receptor.

Connecting tubule

The connecting tubule is a transitional region of the nephron between the distal convoluted tubule and collecting duct. It is lined with:

- cuboidal cells
- connecting tubule cells, which are flatter with a smooth apical surface and basolateral invaginations in which mitochondria are concentrated
- α and β intercalated cells, which contain many mitochondria and secrete H$^+$ and HCO$_3^-$, and therefore have a role in acid-base balance (Table 1.4)
- principal cells, which contain few mitochondria and regulate water, sodium and potassium balance under the control of antidiuretic hormone (ADH) and aldosterone (see page 36)

Collecting duct

The distal tubules of several nephrons merge into connecting tubules which each form a collecting duct up to 20mm in length. This is the final section of the nephron. It is lined with cuboidal cells, α and β intercalated cells and principal cells. Passing through the renal cortex and medulla, it opens at the tip of the renal papilla, where it drains filtrate into the renal pelvis. Each cortical collecting duct drains about six distal tubules.

Principal cells constitute about two thirds of cells within the epithelium of the cortical region of the collecting duct and become more abundant as the collecting duct passes into the medulla. They contain epithelial sodium channels and aquaporins, whose expression is controlled by aldosterone and ADH, respectively. These hormones are responsible for the control of plasma sodium and potassium concentrations, and extracellular fluid volume. As in the connecting tubule, α and β intercalated cells play a role in control of acid-base balance (**Table 1.4**).

Comparison of intercalated cells		
Cell	Function	Mechanism
α cells	Secrete H^+ into urine in exchange for K^+ Return bicarbonate to the circulation	Secrete H^+ into filtrate through apical H^+-ATPase and H^+/K^+ ATPase pumps Reabsorb HCO_3^- into the interstitium in exchange for Cl^- on the basolateral membrane via Cl^--HCO_3^- exchanger
β cells	Excrete bicarbonate Return H^+ to the blood	Apical Cl^--HCO_3^- exchanger secretes HCO_3^- into filtrate in exchange for Cl^- Basolateral H^+-ATPase pump transports H^+ to interstitium from where it reaches the circulation

Table 1.4 Intercalated cell types of the collecting duct

Function of the nephron

As the functional unit of the kidney, the nephron regulates plasma composition via the processes of filtration, reabsorption and secretion that are involved in the production of urine. Hydrostatic pressure within the glomerular capillaries forces plasma ultrafiltrate from blood through the capillary wall and into Bowman's space. This filtrate travels along the renal tubule, where its composition is altered by reabsorption and secretion of different substances.

Glomerular filtration

This is the first stage of urine production. Hydrostatic pressure within the glomerular capillaries forces plasma components through the capillary wall and into Bowman's space. During this passive process, known as ultrafiltration, small molecules pass through the filtration barrier and larger molecules (e.g. plasma proteins) remain in the capillary.

The maximum size of molecules able to pass through the filter is 70 kDa. Smaller proteins that are filtered are reabsorbed in the tubule. As a result little protein appears in normal urine (<0.2 gm/day, much of which is secreted by the tubule itself in the form of Tamm–Horsfall protein). Glucose, amino acids, Na^+ and K^+ are able to pass freely, but blood cells and platelets cannot. Passage through the filter also depends on electrical charge, because the negative charge of heparan sulphate in the basement membrane repels negatively charged molecules such as albumin.

> The presence of albumin in the urine (albuminuria) indicates a pathological process affecting the glomerular filter. Albumin has a molecular weight of 69 kDa and is negatively charged; only very small amounts pass through the healthy glomerular filter. Furthermore, in healthy individuals any albumin that passes through the filter is reabsorbed in the proximal convoluted tubule.

Glomerular filtration rate

The GFR is the rate at which fluid is filtered by the glomerulus from the blood into Bowman's space. This provides a useful indication of glomerular function and is used to detect renal damage. GFR is estimated by measuring the clearance of a substance that satisfies the following criteria:

- it has a steady blood concentration
- it is freely filtered, i.e. it passes unhindered across the glomerular filtration membrane, and
- it is neither reabsorbed nor secreted by cells of the renal tubule

The GFR is expressed as the amount of substance in the urine that came from a calculable volume of blood over time. It can be determined by applying the following formula to calculate the renal clearance of a substance:

$$C_y = \frac{U_y \times V}{P_y}$$

where:

- C_y is the renal clearance of substance 'y' in mL/min, i.e. the volume of plasma from which a substance is removed by the kidneys in one minute. This is the GFR
- U_y is the urine concentration of substance 'y' (mg/mL)
- V is the rate of urine flow (mL/min)
- P_y is the plasma concentration of substance 'y' (mg/mL plasma)

Extrinsic substances such as the plant polysaccharide inulin meet these criteria because all inulin filtered by the glomerulus is excreted in the urine. However, techniques to administer and measure inulin clearance are complicated, so it is not used in clinical practice and creatinine clearance is used instead.

Creatinine is produced during muscle metabolism and is filtered freely and without modification by the kidney. A small amount is secreted by the renal tubules; thus creatinine clearance overestimates GFR by 10–20%. In clinical practice creatinine concentration is combined in an equation with other variables such as age, gender and ethnic origin to produce an estimated GFR (eGFR). This is reasonably accurate, provided that muscle mass and muscle metabolism remain constant.

Factors affecting GFR

The factors with the greatest effect on GFR are:

- differences in hydrostatic pressure and oncotic pressure between tubule and capillaries (Starling's forces)
- renal blood flow and perfusion pressure
- surface area available for ultrafiltration (can be altered by changes in mesangial cell contractility; decreases as nephrons are lost due to age or disease)

Hydrostatic and oncotic pressure differences

The GFR is affected by Starling's forces, which determine the movement of fluid across capillary membranes (**Figure 1.13**):

- Hydrostatic pressure in the capillary, which is the pressure exerted by a fluid in a confined space
- The hydrostatic pressure within the interstitium surrounding the capillary
- Oncotic pressure within the capillary (the osmotic pressure exerted by plasma proteins)
- Oncotic pressure in the interstitium

The greater the positive difference between the hydrostatic pressure in the capillary and the interstitium, the more fluid moves from the capillary to the interstitium. A negative pressure difference between the capillary and the interstitium favours the movement of fluid from the interstitium to the capillary. Oncotic pressure opposes hydrostatic pressure. In a capillary bed, hydrostatic pressure exceeds colloid oncotic pressure at the arteriole end as narrowing of the vessel creates resistance to flow. If the capillary pressure exceeds the plasma oncotic pressure, the net filtration pressure is positive and fluid is forced out of the capillary. At the venous end, oncotic pressure exceeds hydrostatic pressure and enables net movement of fluid back into the capillaries (**Figure 1.14**).

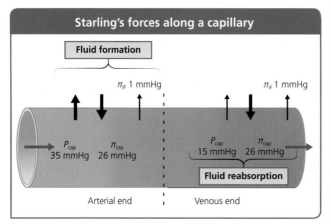

Figure 1.13 Starling's forces along the length of a capillary. Fluid is secreted at the arterial end and reabsorbed at the venous end as hydrostatic pressure decreases. Hydrostatic pressure at the arterial end of the capillary (P_{cap}) is around 35 mmHg and at the venous end of the capillary is 15 mmHg. Interstitial hydrostatic pressure is so small and variable that in practice it is assumed to be 0 mmHg. Along the capillary, the oncotic pressure (π_{cap}) of plasma is 26 mmHg and that of the interstitial fluid is 1 mmHg. Net filtration pressure is the difference between pressure driving fluid from the capillary and pressure opposing filtration, which can be expressed as $(P_{cap} - P_{int}) - (\pi_{cap} - \pi_{int})$. At the arterial end, this is around 10 mmHg, which favours filtration and at the venous end, it is around -10 mmHg which favours reabsorption of fluid. In the glomerulus, these figures are slightly different: the significant loss of fluid and impermeablity of the filtration membrane to protein means that glomerular capillary oncotic pressure increases along its length.

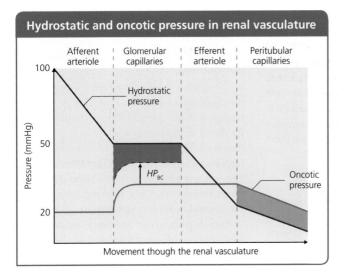

Hydrostatic and oncotic pressure in renal vasculature

Figure 1.14 Changes in hydrostatic and oncotic pressure through the renal vasculature. Glomerular ultrafiltration (dark blue shaded area) represents fluid leaving the capillaries, and tubular reabsorption of fluid (red shaded area) is fluid returning to the capillaries. Resistance in the efferent arterioles keeps pressure high in the glomerular capillaries and low in the peritubular capillaries, thereby favouring reabsorption. HP_{BC}, hydrostatic pressure in Bowman's capsule.

Renal blood flow and perfusion pressure

The kidneys receive about 20% of resting cardiac output, a blood supply of approximately 1200 mL/min. Renal plasma flow accounts for about 660 mL/min of this and about 120 mL/min (the GFR) is filtered from the blood into the nephron. About 1% of the filtrate (1.2 mL/min) is excreted as urine.

Renal blood flow is determined by the renal perfusion pressure (the difference in pressure between the renal artery and vein) and total renal vascular resistance (the sum of resistance in the arteries, arterioles, capillaries and veins) and is expressed as:

blood flow = perfusion pressure/vascular resistance

Blood flow increases when perfusion pressure rises and vascular resistance falls, and decreases when perfusion pressure falls and vascular resistance rises.

The relative cross-sectional area of the glomerular capillaries is much larger than that of a non-glomerular capillary bed, so there is less resistance to flow. Hydrostatic pressure decreases less along the length of a glomerular capillary, because a more constant pressure is maintained by efferent arterioles acting as secondary resistance vessels. As a result, glomerular hydrostatic pressure is maintained at about 50–55 mmHg. This is higher than the combined hydrostatic pressure within Bowman's capsule (15 mmHg) and the colloid oncotic pressure

within the capillary (30 mmHg). Fluid is reabsorbed into the peritubular capillaries when colloid oncotic pressure increases and hydrostatic pressure is low. The dilutional effect of reabsorption of fluid results in a decrease in colloid oncotic pressure.

> The kidneys have a rich blood supply; they receive a large proportion (about 20%) of cardiac output. Therefore they are particularly vulnerable to bleeding. This must be borne in mind when performing invasive procedures such as a percutaneous renal biopsy; the procedure can damage blood vessels and cause significant bleeding.

Regulation of glomerular filtration

Renal blood flow and GFR remain fairly constant, despite changes in systemic blood pressure, because of two autoregulatory mechanisms affecting the afferent and efferent arterioles:

- In the **myogenic mechanism**, autoregulation occurs when smooth muscle in the wall of blood vessels responds to pressure changes within the vessel wall
- In the **tubuloglomerular feedback mechanism**, tubular flow rate affects the tone of renal blood vessels

Renal autoregulation occurs over a wide range of perfusion pressures (90–200 mmHg). If perfusion pressure exceeds the limit of autoregulation, blood flow becomes proportional to perfusion pressure, resulting in an increase in renal blood flow and GFR with increasing perfusion pressure. Conversely, if perfusion pressure decreases below the autoregulatory threshold, renal blood flow and GFR decrease.

Myogenic mechanism

Increased blood pressure results in increased renal perfusion pressure and increased blood flow to the kidney. This stimulates stretch receptors in smooth muscle fibres within the wall of the afferent arteriole, causing them to constrict and therefore increase resistance to flow within the glomerulus (**Figure 1.15**). As a result, renal blood flow and GFR remain constant despite an increase in perfusion pressure.

Conversely, if blood pressure, and therefore renal perfusion pressure, decrease, the afferent arteriole dilates. This results in increased renal blood flow and increased GFR.

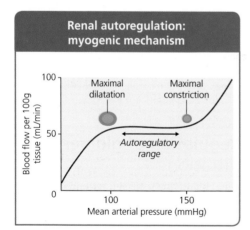

Figure 1.15 Regulation of renal blood flow: the myogenic mechanism. An increase in mean arterial pressure (MAP) increases pressure in the afferent arteriole, thereby stretching it. This stimulates stretch receptors, leading to reflex constriction and a decrease in pressure in the glomerular capillaries. The inverse occurs when MAP decreases. In this way, a constant glomerular pressure is maintained.

Tubuloglomerular feedback mechanism

This mechanism has a more significant effect on GFR than the myogenic mechanism. It is a negative feedback system; a regulatory mechanism in which a stimulus prompts a response that counteracts it (**Figure 1.16**). Its three components are the macula densa (the sensor), the granular (also known as juxtaglomerular) cells (the integrator) and the afferent and efferent arterioles (the effectors); these components are referred to jointly as the juxtaglomerular apparatus.

Tubuloglomerular feedback enables autoregulation of renal blood flow, and subsequently GFR, in response to information concerning the rate of fluid flow in the distal convoluted tubule. The mechanism keeps GFR and distal tubular fluid flow rate constant.

Macula densa

The cells of the macula densa sense the tubular fluid flow rate (which is directly proportional to the GFR) by detecting the rate of movement of Na^+ and chloride ions (Cl^-) into cells through the Na^+-K^+-$2Cl^-$ (NKCC2) cotransporter on the luminal membrane. Low tubular flow rate triggers a signalling cascade which:

- induces dilation of the afferent arterioles directly
- activates the RAAS by stimulating the secretion of the hormone renin from granular cells, which in turn generates angiotensin II (see page 36); angiotensin II then causes vasoconstriction of the efferent arterioles

Conversely, when the macula densa senses increased tubular fluid flow flow, afferent arteriolar tone is increased.

The RAAS is also central to the control of blood pressure throughout the body (see page 35).

Afferent and efferent arterioles

Decreased renal blood flow leads to relaxation of afferent arterioles and constriction of efferent arterioles via the mechanisms above

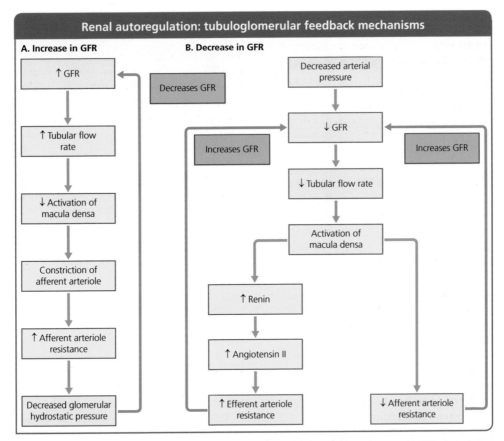

Figure 1.16 Regulation of renal blood flow: tubuloglomerular feedback. (a) An increase in GFR results in an increased rate of tubular flow. This deactivates the macula densa resulting in constriction of the afferent arteriole, a decrease in glomerular hydrostatic pressure and a compensatory decrease in GFR. (b) A fall in GFR results in a decreased tubular flow rate. This results in activation of the macula densa which dilates the afferent arteriole, and, as a result of renin and angiotensin II release, constricts the efferent arteriole. The overall effect is a rise in GFR. GFR, glomerular filtration rate. Red arrow, negative feedback.

to increase flow and glomerular hydrostatic pressure. This increases filtration within the glomerulus, thereby increasing GFR. The resultant increase in delivery of filtrate to the distal convoluted tubule corrects the initial decrease in flow rate through it.

Renal tubular function

The renal tubules contribute significantly to the control of body fluid balance (page 32), osmolality (see page 38) and electrolyte concentrations (see page 34) by controlling reabsorption and secretion of Na^+, K^+, calcium ions (Ca^{2+}), phosphate, magnesium ions (Mg^{2+}), Cl^- and bicarbonate, as well

as, eventually, excretion of certain solutes and water. Different sections of the tubule have specialised functions, which are summarised in **Table 1.5** and discussed in the subsections below.

Water and solutes can pass from the filtrate into the blood, or vice versa. The following processes occur:

- Reabsorption is the movement of water or solutes from the filtrate, via the tubular epithelium and interstitium, into the blood
- Secretion is the movement of substances from the peritubular capillaries into the tubular lumen. This occurs predominantly across tubular cells via active transport,

Functions of sections of the nephron

Section	Function
Glomerulus	Filtration of blood to form filtrate
Proximal convoluted tubule	Reabsorption of 65% of Na^+ and water, and most glucose, amino acids, bicarbonate and phosphate
Loop of Henle	Concentration of urine via the countercurrent exchange mechanism
Distal convoluted tubule	Reabsorption of Na^+ and Ca^{2+} Reabsorption and secretion of K^+ and H^+
Collecting duct	Principal cells: ■ ADH-mediated water reabsorption ■ Aldosterone-mediated Na^+ reabsorption ■ Secretion of K^+ and H^+ Intercalated cells: ■ Control of acid–base balance ■ K^+ excretion

ADH, antidiuretic hormone.

Table 1.5 Functions of sections of the nephron

but also occurs passively through intercellular spaces (the paracellular route; this also applies to reabsorption)
■ Excretion is the removal of waste products from the blood and is the end result of filtration and secretion

Most reabsorption and secretion depends directly or indirectly on the movement of Na^+ (**Figure 1.17**). The Na^+ gradient is the 'energy bank' of tubular transport; it is exploited to reabsorb other ions and molecules, such as glucose and amino acids. The Na^+ gradient is created by Na^+-K^+ ATPase pumps on the basolateral sides of cells of the proximal tubule. Na^+–K^+ ATPase pumps Na^+ out of cells and into the interstitial fluid, and pumps K^+ into cells.

Tubular reabsorption

This is the movement of solutes out of the luminal filtrate and into tubular cells, then to the interstitium and into the peritubular capillaries. It can take place:

■ via tubular cells (the transcellular route)
■ between tubular cells (the paracellular route)

Paracellular transport occurs by passive diffusion or solvent drag, when solutes are transported with water, whereas transcellular transport is either active, requiring energy, or passive (**Table 1.6**). Most reabsorption of ions and valuable solutes occurs in the proximal convoluted tubule.

Water follows the movement of solutes along an osmotic gradient by the transcellular or paracellular route. Certain substances, such as Cl^-, remain in the tubule and subsequently move between cells down their concentration gradient.

Blood within peritubular capillaries is rich in plasma proteins, because these are not filtered at the glomerulus. Therefore the oncotic pressure within these capillaries is high. In contrast, hydrostatic pressure within these capillaries is low, because intravascular pressure is lost as blood passes through the efferent arterioles due to their narrow diameter and therefore high vascular resistance. The high oncotic pressure and low hydrostatic pressure result in the movement of fluid out of the peritubular interstitium and into capillaries, according to Starling's forces.

Tubular secretion

Tubular secretion is the movement of substances from blood in the peritubular capillaries into the tubular lumen. This occurs

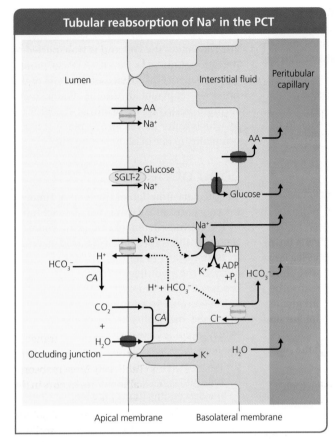

Tubular reabsorption of Na⁺ in the PCT

Figure 1.17 Tubular reabsorption of Na⁺ and its coupling to the transport of other substances in the proximal convoluted tubule (PCT). The active pumping out of Na⁺ basolaterally (into the interstitium) provides a driving force for Na⁺ entry on the apical (luminal) side, bringing other solutes with it. AA, amino acid; CA, carbonic anhydrase; SGLT-2, sodium–glucose transporter 2.

Tubular transport mechanisms

Mechanism	Example(s)
Across apical (luminal) surface of epithelial cells	
Passive diffusion through membrane lipids or tight junctions	Cl⁻ diffuses through tight junctions in the late proximal tubule
Facilitated diffusion by carrier proteins	Na⁺
Secondary active transport: symporter-mediated	Na⁺ is transported with other solutes (e.g. glucose and amino acids)
Secondary active transport: antiporter-mediated	H⁺ ions are exchanged for Na⁺ ions
Primary active transport	ATP-driven pumps actively transport Na⁺, K⁺, Ca²⁺, H⁺ and drug metabolites
Across basolateral surface of epithelial cells	
Passive diffusion through membrane lipids	Glucose
Facilitated diffusion through carrier proteins	Glucose, amino acids and other organic solutes
Secondary active transport: symporter-mediated	Bicarbonate and Na⁺, K⁺ and Cl⁻
Secondary active transport: antiporter-mediated	Na⁺ for Ca²⁺, and bicarbonate for Cl⁻
Primary active transport	Na⁺ via Na⁺–K⁺–ATPase. This generates an electrochemical gradient for Na⁺ reabsorption across the luminal membrane

Table 1.6 Mechanisms of tubular transport

predominantly by active transport and enables the elimination from the blood of ions such as H^+ and K^+, metabolites such as uric acid, ammonia and bile salts and drugs such as penicillin and salicylates.

> **Many drugs are actively secreted by kidney tubules** from the interstitium to tubular cells and into the urine, before they are excreted.

Proximal convoluted tubule

The multiple villi of the cuboidal cells lining the proximal convoluted tubule give it a large surface area for absorption. Here, two thirds of the filtered salt and water are reabsorbed into the blood, as well as almost all glucose and amino acids and some phosphate and bicarbonate.

The transport of Na^+ into cells of the proximal convoluted tubule occurs via:

- symporter membrane proteins, which absorb Na^+ together with glucose, phosphate, amino acids, sulphate and galactose

- antiporter membrane proteins, which absorb Na^+ in exchange for H^+

The Na^+ leaves the cell and is transported to the interstitium via Na^+–K^+ ATPase pumps on the basolateral surface of the cells of the proximal convoluted tubule. Water reabsorption is driven by osmosis, the process by which water moves form a place of lower osmolality to one of higher osmolality.

Loop of Henle

The primary function of the loop of Henle is the concentration of urine, which is achieved by the countercurrent exchange mechanism (**Figure 1.18**). Hypertonicity (raised osmolality with respect to normal interstitial osmolality) of the medullary interstitium is in part produced by the pumping of Na^+ from filtrate to interstitium. In addition, about half of the increased osmolality is produced by urea, which becomes concentrated in the inner medulla (see section below on urea handling). Thus osmolality within the medullary interstitium is greater than in the cortex.

The descending limb of the loop of Henle is impermeable to Na^+ but not to water. Therefore water moves freely out of this limb and into the interstitium, whereas Na^+ remains within

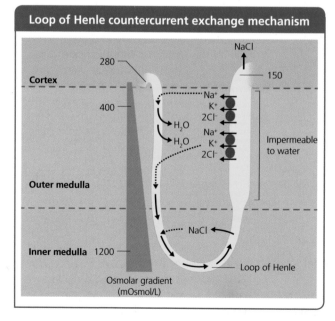

Figure 1.18 The loop of Henle countercurrent exchange mechanism. The loop of Henle maintains the hyperosmolar, extremely concentrated salt gradient in the inner medulla of the kidney. This gradient is used to concentrate the urine as much as possible as the filtrate subsequently passes through the collecting duct. Numbers represent concentrations in mOsm/kg H_2O.

the tubule. The ascending limb of the loop of Henle is impermeable to water but not to Na^+.

Descending limb

Fluid in the proximal convoluted tubule is isosmotic, i.e. of the same osmotic pressure, with the interstitium. Therefore fluid entering the descending limb of the loop of Henle is also isosmotic with the interstitium. However, in the thick ascending limb of the loop of Henle Na^+ is actively pumped out of the filtrate and into the interstitium by the Na^+–K^+–$2Cl^-$ cotransporter, a membrane protein that transports Na^+, K^+ and Cl^- into and out of cells, maintaining electroneutrality by transporting two positively charged ions (Na^+ and K^+) alongside two negatively charged chloride ions. Because each ion is moved in the same direction, this transporter is a symporter. Because the thick ascending limb is impermeable to water, water is unable to follow Na^+ to equilibrate the osmolality of the filtrate with that of the interstitium. As a result, the osmolality of the interstitium increases. This creates a differential osmolality between the fluid in the descending limb of the loop and the interstitium, with the osmolality of the interstitium being greater than that of the filtrate.

Because the descending limb is permeable to water, water leaves the filtrate and moves into the interstitium to equilibrate the osmolality of the interstitium and that of the descending limb. New filtrate with a lower osmolality is continuously delivered to the descending limb, and Na^+ is continuously pumped out of filtrate in the ascending limb. Therefore the osmolality of the filtrate reaching the bend of the loop of Henle (1400 mOsm/Kg H_2O) is much higher than that of the fluid entering it (300 mOsm/kg H_2O). The countercurrent exchange mechanism enables the osmotic gradient to increase the deeper the tubule lies in the medulla.

Ascending limb

This maintains a difference of 200 mOsm/kg H_2O between the tubular fluid and the interstitium along its length.

Because of the action of the Na^+–K^+–$2Cl^-$ cotransporter in the ascending limb, and its

impermeability to water, fluid leaving the loop of Henle is hypotonic (lower osmolality than the interstitium). Maintenance of this hypotonicity enables excess water to be excreted. The excretion of water is altered by the action of ADH (see page 38).

> **Diuretics are medications that promote urine production.** Furosemide, a loop diuretic, inhibits the Na^+–K^+–$2Cl^-$ cotransporter causing significant loss of Na^+ and therefore water via increased production of urine (diuresis), as well as loss of K^+, Ca^{2+} and Mg^{2+}. Thiazide diuretics such as bendroflumethiazide inhibit Na^+ reabsorption in the distal convoluted tubule, resulting in milder diuresis.

Vasa recta

The capillaries of the vasa recta are permeable to solutes and water (**Figure 1.19**). Descending capillaries passing through the medulla absorbs solutes from the interstitium, including Na^+, Cl^- and urea; water moves out of the capillary to the interstitium along an osmotic gradient. These effects produce an increasing osmolality of the blood.

At the bend of the vessel, the osmolality of capillary blood is equal to that of the interstitium (see **Figure 1.19**). As blood moves up the ascending capillaries, water moves in from the interstitium by osmosis, decreasing the osmolality of the blood. By the time blood drains from the vasa recta into the renal veins it is isosmotic with plasma, so has a similar osmolality to blood entering this capillary system. This prevents the medullary osmotic gradient from being 'washed out', which it would if the capillaries passed directly through.

Distal convoluted tubule

The distal convoluted tubule regulates the balance of Na^+ and K^+, as well as Ca^{2+}, within the body. Here, hormone-mediated reabsorption of Na^+ and Ca^{2+}, and secretion of K^+ occur. The distal convoluted tubule is also the site where the juxtaglomerular apparatus monitors filtrate composition as part of the tubuloglomerular feedback system.

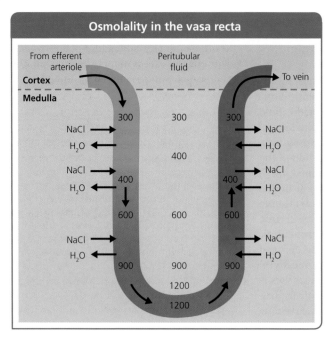

Figure 1.19 Osmolality in the vasa recta. Osmolality, shown in mOsm/kg H_2O, increases from the cortex to the deepest region of the medulla. The flow rate in the vasa recta is slow but sufficient to maintain adequate supply of oxygen and nutrients to the medulla, which diffuse freely between the descending and ascending limbs. One effect of this is that oxygen can bypass the deeper parts of the medulla, thereby increasing the risk of ischaemia and cell necrosis in these areas.

Collecting ducts

The final concentration of urine leaving the kidney is determined in the collecting ducts. Two functionally different parts of the collecting duct exist:

- the cortical collecting ducts
- the medullary collecting ducts (inner and outer)

Aldosterone and ADH induce reabsorption of salt and water by binding to receptors on the abundant principal cells of the medullary collecting ducts.

The cortical and medullary parts of the collecting duct are impermeable to Na^+. Within both parts, permeability to water is controlled by ADH, which causes intracellular water channels called aquaporins to fuse with the luminal membrane. The aquaporins mediate reabsorption of water from the luminal fluid, which is driven by the high interstitial osmolality established by the loop of Henle. This reabsorption of water results in a concentrated urine (net retention of water). Without ADH, collecting ducts have low permeability to water, so urine is not concentrated and the hypotonicity achieved at the top of the ascending limb is maintained (net excretion of water).

> **Deficiency of ADH secretion or resistance to ADH results in diabetes insipidus.** This is characterised by significant diuresis (urine production) and excessive thirst.

Water reabsorbed by the medullary collecting ducts passes to the interstitium and then to the vasa recta, enabling maintenance of the hypertonicity of the medullary interstitium. About 20% of glomerular filtrate reaches the distal nephron. However, only 5% enters the medullary collecting ducts because of water reabsorption in the cortical tubules.

Role of urea in the concentration of urine

Urea is $CO(NH_2)_2$. It is formed in the liver from ammonia, the toxic end-product of protein metabolism. As well as being excreted in urine it has a key role in concentrating urine in the loop of Henle. This role is based on differing permeability to urea in the different segments of the nephron.

Urea is freely filtered at the glomerulus, so its concentration is similar in blood plasma and in filtrate entering the proximal tubule. Subsequently its concentration increases along the proximal tubule as water is reabsorbed with sodium.

Although the thin limb of the loop of Henle is relatively permeable to urea, from the thick ascending limb to the inner medullary collecting duct the nephron is impermeable to urea. Combined with the ADH-dependent reabsorption of water in the collecting duct, this serves to raise urea concentration further by the time the filtrate reaches the medullary collecting duct.

From the medullary collecting duct a significant amount of urea is absorbed into the medullary interstitium via ADH-sensitive urea transporters. From there some of it diffuses into the thin descending limb of the loop of Henle and eventually returns to the medullary collecting duct, where it is reabsorbed.

This recycling results in concentration of urea within the medullary interstitium, which makes up about half (the other half is made up of sodium chloride) of the raised osmolality used to reabsorb water in the presence of ADH.

> **In pre-renal failure, tubular reabsorption of urea is enhanced.** This results in a disproportionate rise in serum urea concentration compared with creatinine concentration, at least early in the natural history of pre-renal acute kidney injury.

The lower urinary tract

Starter question

The answer to the following question is on on page 54.

8. Why are females more prone to urinary tract infections than males?

The bladder stores the urine it receives from the upper urinary tract via the ureters. It also allows the voluntary excretion of urine via the urethra at appropriate times. The tract comprises:

- the ureters
- the bladder
- the urethra
- the prostate gland (in men)

Ureters

The ureters are muscular tubes that connect the renal pelvis of each kidney to the bladder. They transport urine from the kidney to the bladder.

Macrostructure

Each ureter is 25–30 cm long and 6 mm wide. The ureters descend in the retroperitoneum, on the medial aspect of the psoas major muscle. They enter the bladder posteriorly and at an angle, which creates a valve to prevent backflow of urine to the kidneys; this is the vesicoureteric junction.

The three areas of anatomical narrowing within the ureter are common sites of blockage with ureteric stones. They are:

- the pelviureteric junction, the junction between the renal pelvis and the ureter
- the point at which the ureter crosses the iliac vessels
- the vesicoureteric junction, the junction between the ureter and the bladder

Vascular supply

As each ureter passes to the bladder, it is supplied by arterial branches from different vessels:

- renal arteries supply the superior portion
- the abdominal aorta, testicular and ovarian arteries and common iliac arteries supply the middle portion
- branches of the internal iliac arteries supply the inferior portion

These arterial branches divide to form longitudinal anastomoses around the ureter. Venous drainage of the ureters is paired with the corresponding arteries.

Nerve supply

The ureters are innervated by several nerve plexuses via nerves that follow the same path as blood vessels. Visceral efferent fibres derive from sympathetic and parasympathetic sources, and afferent fibres return to the spinal cord at T11–L2.

Because of the pattern of innervation of the ureter, ureteric pain is referred to cutaneous areas supplied by T11–L2 spinal cord levels. These areas include the posterolateral abdominal wall, the pubic region, the labia majora in females and the scrotum in males.

Lymphatic drainage

As with arterial blood supply, lymphatic drainage of the ureters changes along their course:

- the superior portion of each ureter drains into the lumbar lymph nodes
- the middle portion drains into nodes around the common iliac vessels
- the inferior portion drains into nodes around the external and internal iliac vessels

Microstructure

The wall of the ureter is made up of three layers:

- mucosa: the inner layer, comprises an avascular transitional epithelium (a stratified epithelium that can expand and contract; also lines the renal pelvis and calyces) and the connective tissue beneath it (lamina propria) containing blood vessels and nerves
- muscularis: the middle layer, consists of smooth muscle arranged in three layers: the inner longitudinal, middle circular and outer longitudinal layers
- adventitia: the fibrous coat that surrounds the ureter and provides a supporting outer layer

Successive waves of contraction (peristalsis) of the muscular layer propel urine towards the bladder.

Bladder

The bladder is a muscular chamber that lies in the pelvis behind the pubic bone (**Figure 1.20**). Its function is to store and, by contraction, void urine.

Macrostructure

In men, the prostate gland sits behind the bladder, whereas in women the vagina and uterus occupy this space. The body of the bladder tapers to the funnel-shaped bladder neck, which connects with the urethra. The smooth muscle at the junction of the bladder with the urethra forms the internal sphincter.

In the posterior wall of the bladder, above the bladder neck, is the trigone. This triangular area has a smooth mucosa, which contrasts with the folded mucosa (rugae) that lines the rest of the bladder. The ureters enter the bladder at the upper angles of the trigone. The apex marks the exit of the urethra.

Vascular supply

The bladder is supplied by branches of the internal iliac arteries. Venous drainage is via the internal iliac veins.

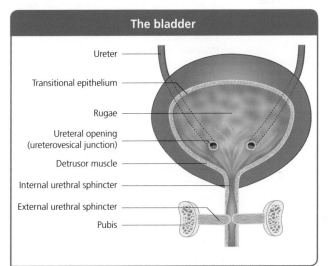

The bladder

Ureter

Transitional epithelium

Rugae

Ureteral opening
(ureterovesical junction)

Detrusor muscle

Internal urethral sphincter

External urethral sphincter

Pubis

Figure 1.20 The bladder. Micturition occurs as the detrusor muscle contracts and the internal urethral sphincter relaxes, enabling expulsion of urine. The process involves the central, somatic and autonomic nervous systems.

Nerve supply

The bladder is supplied by parasympathetic fibres from S2 to S4, which stimulate bladder emptying, penile vasodilation and erection. Its sympathetic supply arises from the T10–L3 nerve root segments. Sympathetic stimulation occurs in response to distension of the bladder as it fills with urine. This inhibits parasympathetic stimulation and therefore inhibits micturition by decreasing bladder tone. It also excites the muscle of the internal sphincter at the junction of the bladder neck and proximal urethra which causes its closure and allows the bladder to fill.

The bladder rests on the pelvic diaphragm, which is innervated by S2–S4 somatic motor neurones. These stimulate voluntary contraction of the external sphincter.

> **Alpha-blockers block sympathetic tone.** They can induce incontinence but also relieve bladder neck or urethral obstruction, for example in prostatic hypertrophy.

Lymphatic drainage

Lymphatic drainage of the bladder is to the common, external and internal iliac and sacral lymph nodes.

Microstructure

The bladder wall is made up of four principal layers:

- mucosa, the innermost layer, is composed of transitional epithelium (made up of cells whose appearance changes depending on the degree of stretch; when the bladder is stretched they appear as squamous cells and when it is relaxed, they appear as pseudostratified columnar cells) and connective tissue
- submucosa, beneath the mucosa, contains blood vessels and lymphatics, connective tissue and some adipose tissue
- muscularis, the smooth muscle layer also known as the detrusor muscle, is itself divided into three layers: the inner longitudinal, middle circular and outer longitudinal layers
- two types of tissue in the outer layer:
  - serosa: a covering of simple squamous epithelium derived from the peritoneum which overlies the upper region of the bladder
  - adventitia: connective tissue making up the outermost layer. This covers all other areas of the bladder

Contraction of the muscularis expels urine from the bladder through the urethra.

Urethra

The urethra is a tube, arising from the base of the bladder, that allows removal of urine from the body. The male and female urethras take different courses within the pelvis.

Macrostructure

The female urethra is short (4 cm) and passes through the pelvic floor into the perineum, before opening in the vestibule between the labia minora. The opening of the urethra lies anterior to the vaginal opening in the vestibule.

> **The relatively short length of the female urethra makes women more susceptible than men to urinary tract infections,** because bacteria are able to enter the urethra and move up to the bladder more readily.

The male urethra is significantly longer than the female urethra and follows a more complex course. It begins at the base of the bladder and passes inferiorly through the prostate. From the prostate, it passes through the deep perineal pouch and enters the root of the penis. When the penis is flaccid, the urethra makes a further bend inferiorly to the body of the penis. This bend disappears when the penis is erect.

The male urethra is divided into four parts (**Table 1.7**).

The male urethra	
Subsection	Features
Preprostatic part	1 cm long
	Extends from base of bladder to prostate
	Associated with internal urethral sphincter, which consists of smooth muscle and is under involuntary control
	Sphincter controls flow of urine by contracting around the urethral orifice and prevents retrograde movement of semen into the bladder during ejaculation
Prostatic part	3–4 cm long
	Surrounded by prostate
	Within the lumen, a midline fold of mucosa forms the urethral crest
	Prostatic ducts empty into the urethral sinuses either side of the urethral crest
	Halfway along its length, the urethral crest enlarges to form the seminal colliculus, a circular prominence where the ejaculatory ducts and prostatic utricle (a blind-ending pouch that is an embryonic remnant) join the urethra
Membranous part	Narrow, 1–2 cm long
	Passes through the urogenital diaphragm
	Surrounded by skeletal muscle, which forms the external urethral sphincter
Spongy urethra	Surrounded by penile erectile tissue (corpus spongiosum)
	Enlarged to form a bulb at the end of the penis (navicular fossa)
	Opens at external urethral orifice

Table 1.7 The male urethra

Vascular supply

The female urethra is supplied by the internal pudendal and vaginal arteries and drained by corresponding veins.

The proximal two parts of the male urethra are supplied by the prostatic branches of the inferior vesicular and middle rectal arteries.

Venous drainage of the proximal two parts of the male urethra is via the inferior vesicular and middle rectal veins. The distal two parts of the male urethra are supplied by branches of the internal pudendal artery and are drained by the internal pudendal veins.

Nerve supply

Innervation of the female urethra is via the pudendal nerve. The male urethra is supplied by branches of the pudendal nerves and the prostatic plexus. Afferent nerve fibres pass through the pelvic splanchnic nerves.

Lymphatic drainage

Lymph from the female urethra drains to the sacral and internal iliac lymph nodes. Lymph from the preprostatic, prostatic and membranous male urethra drains to the internal iliac lymph nodes, while the spongy urethra drains to the deep inguinal lymph nodes.

Microstructure

The wall of the urethra is made up of smooth muscle and lined with epithelial cells.

The female urethra is lined with stratified squamous epithelium and areas of pseudostratified columnar epithelium

The epithelium of the male urethra changes along its length; the prostatic urethra is lined with transitional epithelium, the membranous urethra with pseudostratified columnar epithelium, and the spongy urethra with pseudostratified columnar epithelium proximally and stratified squamous epithelium distally.

The opening between the bladder and the urethra is closed by two muscular sphincters: the internal and external sphincters. The internal sphincter is made up of smooth muscle fibres and is under involuntary control. Its resting tone keeps it closed. The external sphincter is formed from skeletal muscle supplied by the pudendal nerve. It is under voluntary control. Stimulation from higher centres in the central nervous system keeps the fibres of the external sphincter contracted and the sphincter therefore closed, except during voiding.

Functions of the lower urinary tract

The lower urinary tract conveys urine from the kidneys to the bladder, where it is stored until it can be excreted voluntarily via the urethra.

Passage of urine

Urine formed in the nephrons passes down the collecting ducts and into the renal pelvis. It exits the kidneys via the ureters, which deliver it to the bladder. Transport down the ureter is aided by peristaltic contraction of the muscular ureter wall and by gravity.

Storage of urine

As the bladder fills with urine, its folded wall expands and its tone relaxes to enable relatively large volumes of urine to be stored with minimal changes to pressure inside the bladder (intravesical pressure). This lasts until bladder volume reaches around 400 mL. Beyond 400 mL, intravesical pressure increases suddenly, which triggers the desire to void and the micturition reflex. The first sensation of bladder filling is normally felt when about 100–150 mL of urine is present in the bladder.

Micturition and continence

Micturition is the process of urination. It is an autonomic reflex under voluntary control in adults. Urinary continence is the voluntary control of urination.

As the bladder fills, stretch receptors within its wall are stimulated to activate sensory parasympathetic fibres. These relay information to the sacral spinal nerves, where it is integrated.

Parasympathetic motor neurones are subsequently activated and stimulate contraction of the detrusor muscle, which results in increased intravesical pressure and opening of the internal sphincter. Entry of urine into the urethra inhibits somatic motor neurones that supply the external sphincter via the pudendal nerve, which allows the sphincter to open and urine to flow out of the body.

> **Upper motor nerve lesions, such as those caused by stroke and spinal cord injuries, may result in loss of voluntary control of the bladder.** Depending on the site of the insult (e.g. brain, brainstem, spinal cord), upper motor neurone lesions affect the formation and transmission of signals from the brain responsible for descending inhibition to the detrusor muscle. This causes the bladder to become hyperreflexic, with more frequent contractions that void small amounts of urine.

Control of micturition

This is learned in early childhood. Sensory fibres in the bladder convey information concerning bladder fullness to higher centres in the thalamus and cerebral cortex. By inhibiting excitation of parasympathetic motor fibres to the bladder and strengthening contraction of the external sphincter, these higher centres are able to override the micturition reflex. When it is convenient to void, descending inhibition is removed and voluntary micturition occurs.

Fluid homeostasis and electrolyte balance

Starter questions

Answers to the following questions are on page 55.

9. What are the fluid compartments of the body?
10. How is sodium involved in the control of body fluid volume?

Body fluids exist within two compartments, the intracellular compartment and the extracellular compartment. Each compartment contains different concentrations of electrolytes. In healthy individuals, the volume and composition of body fluid are tightly controlled to ensure normal functioning of physiological processes. Water accounts for 60% of total body weight in adult men and 50% of total body weight in adult women.

The kidneys control body fluid homeostasis and the constituents of body fluid compartments through:

■ regulation of extracellular fluid volume
■ regulation of osmolality
■ regulation of ion concentrations

This is influenced by the following processes:

■ the renin–angiotensin–aldosterone system (RAAS), via renal production of renin and renal responses to angiotensin and aldosterone
■ the renal responses to atrial natriuretic peptide and brain natriuretic peptide
■ the renal response to ADH
■ the renal production of prostaglandins

Body fluid composition

Body fluid is divided into two compartments or spaces (**Table 1.8** and **Figure 1.21**):

■ intracellular compartment
■ extracellular compartment

These are separated by cell membranes, which control the movement of water and solutes between them. The extracellular compartment is subdivided into intravascular, interstitial and transcellular compartments or spaces.

Body fluid compartments			
Compartment	Definition	Contents	
Intracellular fluid	Body fluid inside cells	Tiny separate collections of fluid inside each cell	
Extracellular fluid	Body fluid outside cells	Intravascular fluid	Plasma, the fluid component of blood in which blood cells, proteins and solutes are suspended
		Interstitial fluid	Fluid outside the vascular system, within the interstices of all tissues. Bridges the intracellular and intravascular compartments and includes lymph
		Transcellular fluid	Fluid contained within epithelial-lined spaces (e.g. pericardial fluid, pleural fluid, peritoneal fluid, cerebrospinal fluid, synovial fluid), formed by transport activity of cells

Table 1.8 The two compartments of body fluid and their contents

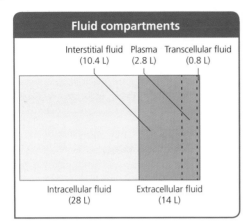

Fluid compartments

Interstitial fluid (10.4 L)   Plasma (2.8 L)   Transcellular fluid (0.8 L)

Intracellular fluid (28 L)   Extracellular fluid (14 L)

Figure 1.21 Fluid compartments of the body. Amounts are for a 70 kg man.

The kidneys regulate body fluid, osmolality and electrolyte concentration via tubular reabsorption and secretion of the major electrolytes: sodium (Na^+), potassium (K^+), calcium (Ca^{2+}), phosphate (PO_4^{3-}), magnesium (Mg^{2+}), chloride (Cl^-) and bicarbonate (HCO_3) (**Table 1.9**). By controlling the excretion of water and ions from the renal tubules, the kidneys regulate water balance and the osmolality of both plasma and urine. Plasma osmolality is maintained within a narrow range by several feedback mechanisms (see page 38).

The composition of intracellular and extracellular fluid differs greatly (**Table 1.10**). This reflects the selective permeability of cell membranes due to the action of transporter proteins and pumps, which transport solutes between the intracellular and extracellular spaces. Na^+ is the most abundant extracellular electrolyte, whereas K^+ is the most abundant intracellular electrolyte. The distribution of Na^+ and K^+ in each fluid compartment is maintained by the Na^+–K^+ ATPase pump present in all cell membranes.

Terms of solute concentration

Osmolality, osmolarity and tonicity are terms of solute concentration that often cause confusion, resulting in incorrect use.

Osmolality

Osmolality is an estimation of the solute concentration of plasma and is proportional to the number of particles per kilogram of solvent. It is expressed in milliosmoles (mOsm)/kg and is measured in clinical laboratories by using an osmometer. Normal plasma osmolality is 275–295 mOsm/kg.

> **Osmolality can be measured or calculated. The difference between the measured and calculated value, usually < 10 mmol/L, is called the osmolar gap. A greater gap indicates the presence of an exogenous osmotically active substance not included in the calculation, such as mannitol or ethanol, and may inform diagnoses, particularly in cases of substance abuse.**

Osmolarity

Osmolarity is also an estimation of the osmolar concentration of plasma but is proportional to the number of particles per litre of solution. It is affected by changes in water content, temperature and pressure. It is usually given as a calculated value, derived using the following equation (all concentrations in mmol/L):

$$\text{calculated osmolarity} = 2[Na^+] + 2[K^+] + [\text{glucose}] + [\text{urea}]$$

Tonicity

Tonicity is a measure of the osmotic pressure gradient or water potential, i.e. the potential for water to move from one area to another by osmosis, of two solutions separated by a semipermeable membrane.

Salt and water balance

Water balance is largely controlled by the movement of Na^+, because it is the main ion influencing osmosis. Control of water balance affects plasma volume and blood pressure.

	Biological ions: functions and sites of regulation	
Ion	Functions	Site of regulation
Na^+	Body fluid homeostasis Generation of action potentials in nerves and muscle Acid–base balance (Na^+/H^+ antiporters)	Gastrointestinal tract Kidney (proximal tubule, loop of Henle thick ascending limb, distal tubule, cortical collecting duct)
K^+	Generation of action potentials in nerves and muscle Acid–base balance Body fluid homeostasis and blood pressure	Gastrointestinal tract Kidney (proximal tubule, loop of Henle thick ascending limb, distal tubule, collecting duct)
Ca^{2+}	Structural integrity of bones and teeth Second messenger in cell signalling cascades Generation of action potentials Neurotransmitter release Initiation of muscle contraction Coenzyme for clotting factors	Parathyroid gland Bone Gastrointestinal tract Kidney (proximal tubule, loop of Henle thick ascending limb, distal tubule, collecting duct)
PO_4^{3-}	Energy metabolism Bone homeostasis Cell signal transduction Component of phospholipid cell membrane Component of nucleic acids	Gastrointestinal tract Bone Kidney (proximal tubule)
Mg^{2+}	Cell signalling pathways Cofactor for DNA and protein synthesis Energy metabolism Neuromuscular excitability Bone formation Cardiovascular tone	Gastrointestinal tract Kidney (proximal tubule, loop of Henle thick ascending limb, distal tubule) Bone
Cl^-	Body fluid homeostasis Transepithelial transport Component of stomach acid Regulation of electrical excitability Acid–base balance	Gastrointestinal tract Kidney (proximal tubule, loop of Henle, distal tubule, collecting duct)
HCO_3^-	Acid–base balance pH regulation in the gastrointestinal tract	Gastrointestinal tract Kidney (proximal tubule, loop of Henle thick ascending limb, intercalated cells of collecting duct) Lungs

Table 1.9 The main biological ions, their functions and key sites of regulation

Sodium

Sodium is the major extracellular cation and plays a key role in the regulation of the volume of extracellular fluid. Its other functions include generation of action potentials.

It has a significant effect on fluid osmolality and the volume of extracellular fluid. Homeostatic mechanisms based on ADH secretion, the RAAS and renal Na^+ handling maintain Na^+ within the normal range which is 133–146 mmol/L in plasma.

Composition of intracellular and extracellular fluid		
Electrolyte	Intracellular fluid concentration (mmol/L)*	Extracellular fluid concentration (mmol/L)*
Na^+	5–15	140
K^+	140	4
Ca^{2+}	0.0001	1
$PO_4{}^{3-}$	60	1
Mg^{2+}	2.7	0.5
Cl^-	4	100
HCO_3^-	10	25

*Concentration of ionised and therefore biologically active fraction.

Table 1.10 Concentrations of electrolytes in intracellular and extracellular fluid

Plasma is normally made up of 93% water, the remainder being proteins and lipids. Falsely low values for Na^+ concentration can be obtained when circulating levels of lipids or proteins are very high. In such cases, Na^+ concentration in the water phase is normal, as is plasma osmolality, but the measured value for Na^+ concentration will be low, because lipids and proteins are included in the volume from which the dissolved constituents of plasma are measured.

Renal control of sodium

The kidneys maintain Na^+ balance in the body by tightly regulating the amount of Na^+ they reabsorb and thereby controlling extracellular fluid volume.

- when there is a need to conserve Na^+, urinary Na^+ excretion is limited to a negligible amount
- when there is a need to lose Na^+, up to 300 mmol/L can be excreted in the urine

Na+ handling in the glomerulus

Sodium ions are freely filtered in the glomerulus, so the concentration of Na^+ in Bowman's capsule is equal to that in plasma. Nearly all filtered Na^+ is absorbed back into the circulation along the nephron.

Na+ handling in the proximal convoluted tubule

Most Na^+ reabsorption occurs in the proximal convoluted tubule. The Na^+–K^+ ATPase pumps Na^+ from the cells of the tubule into the interstitium to maintain a low concentration of Na^+ inside the cells. This drives the movement of Na^+ from the filtrate, along its concentration gradient, into the cells of the tubule via carrier molecules on the apical (luminal) membrane.

At the start of the proximal convoluted tubule, Na^+ is cotransported with other substances, such as amino acids and glucose, into tubular cells. Na^+ reabsorption and secretion is subsequently fine-tuned by the actions of aldosterone, which promotes Na^+ reabsorption, and natriuretic peptides, which promote Na^+ excretion, in the distal tubule and collecting ducts.

Na+ handling in the loop of Henle

The loop of Henle concentrates the urine in order to control osmolality. The descending loop is permeable to water but impermeable to salt, whereas the ascending loop is impermeable to water. This difference underlies the countercurrent exchange mechanism (see **Figure 1.18**).

Fluid leaving the ascending limb is hyposmolar compared with that entering it, and the osmolality of fluid at the 'U-bend' is higher than that of the fluid entering it. The interstitium around the limbs of the loop in the cortex has significantly lower osmolality than that of the tissue around the bend of the loop in the medulla. This enables the collecting ducts passing from cortex to medulla to extract as much water as possible under the influence of ADH.

Na⁺ handling in the distal convoluted tubule and collecting ducts

The distal convoluted tubule and collecting duct absorb about 10% of filtered Na⁺. This is regulated by the juxtaglomerular apparatus. When the sodium concentration of fluid in the distal tubule is low, macula densa cells stimulate the secretion of renin by the granular cells of the afferent arteriole, which ultimately results in secretion of aldosterone and increased reabsorption of sodium in the distal convoluted tubule and collecting duct (see below).

Renin–angiotensin–aldosterone system

The RAAS maintains Na⁺ balance and thereby fluid balance and blood pressure (**Figure 1.22**).

Renin

Renin is an enzyme that is synthesised and stored in the juxtaglomerular apparatus of the kidneys (see page 13). It is released by renal granular cells when a decrease in plasma

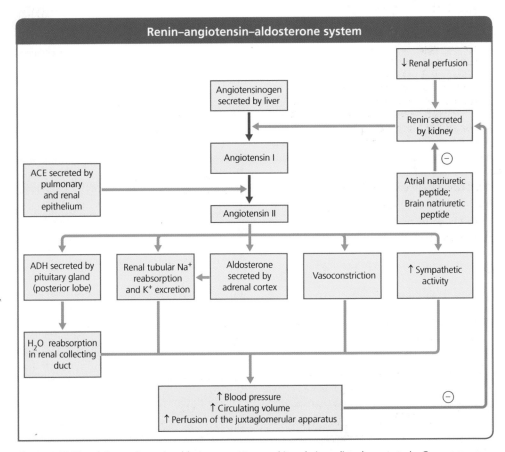

Renin–angiotensin–aldosterone system

Figure 1.22 The renin–angiotensin–aldosterone system and its role in sodium homeostasis. Green arrows show a positive effect; red arrows show an inhibitory effect. ACE, angiotensin-converting enzyme; ADH, antidiuretic hormone

Na$^+$ or fluid losses result in a decrease in extracellular fluid volume. This decrease in volume is sensed by three mechanisms:

■ **Peripheral baroreceptors in the carotid arteries** sense the decrease in extracellular fluid volume, resulting in increased sympathetic activity; the stimulation of sympathetic nerves activates β-adrenergic receptors on granular cells of the juxtaglomerular apparatus, causing them to increase their release of renin
■ **Macula densa cells** sense a decrease in Na$^+$ concentration in the distal convoluted tubule and secrete prostaglandin, which stimulates the release of renin from granular cells
■ **Granular cells** in afferent arterioles detect that their wall tension is decreasing as a result of decreased extracellular fluid volume and renal perfusion. They also release renin

Angiotensin II

Renin acts to restore extracellular fluid volume by cleaving angiotensinogen (an α2-globulin produced by the liver) in the circulation to produce angiotensin I. In the lungs, angiotensin-converting enzyme (ACE) converts angiotensin I to angiotensin II. Angiotensin II has the following effects (see **Figure 1.22**):
■ stimulation of ADH secretion by the posterior pituitary gland
■ increased Na$^+$ reabsorption in the proximal convoluted tubule
■ stimulation of aldosterone release by the zona glomerulosa, the outermost layer of the adrenal cortex
■ vasoconstriction of renal arterioles (greater in the efferent arterioles than in the afferent arterioles)
■ increased sympathetic activity

As well as catalysing the conversion of angiotensin I to angiotensin II, ACE cleaves and inactivates bradykinin, a potent vasodilator. Therefore the overall effect of this enzyme is systemic vasoconstriction. Inhibition of ACE or angiotensin II is the mode of action for many antihypertensive drugs.

Two classes of drug commonly used to treat hypertension block RAAS pathways. ACE inhibitors inhibit the conversion of angiotensin I to angiotensin II. Angiotensin II receptor blockers prevent angiotensin II from binding to angiotensin II receptors on blood vessel walls. Therefore these drugs cause systemic vasodilation, thereby lowering blood pressure.

Aldosterone

Aldosterone is synthesised in the zona glomerulosa of the adrenal cortex in response to (**Figure 1.23**):

■ release of angiotensin II
■ decreased plasma Na$^+$ concentration or circulating volume, which results in aldosterone release directly from the adrenal cortex and via the RAAS
■ increase in K$^+$ concentration, which stimulates direct release from the adrenal cortex

Its overall effect is an increase in plasma Na$^+$ concentration and blood pressure, and a decrease in plasma K$^+$ concentration. Aldosterone acts on the principal and intercalated cells of the late distal convoluted tubule and collecting duct (**Table 1.11**). It stimulates the synthesis of sodium channels which are inserted in the apical membrane of principal cells, as well as the synthesis of Na$^+$-K$^+$ ATPase pumps which are inserted in the basolateral membrane (**Figure 1.24**). This increase in the number of sodium channels promotes sodium reabsorption: sodium moves though the apical sodium channels and the principal cells along its concentration gradient and is actively transported to the interstitial fluid by the basolateral Na$^+$-K$^+$ ATPase pump. As sodium is exchanged for potassium, increased activity of this pump also increases intracellular potassium, which subsequently passes into tubular fluid down its concentration gradient. In the intercalated cells, aldosterone promotes excretion of H$^+$ by upregulating the apical H$^+$ pump and Na-H$^+$ cotransporter. These move H$^+$ from the intercalated cell into the filtrate (**Table 1.11**).

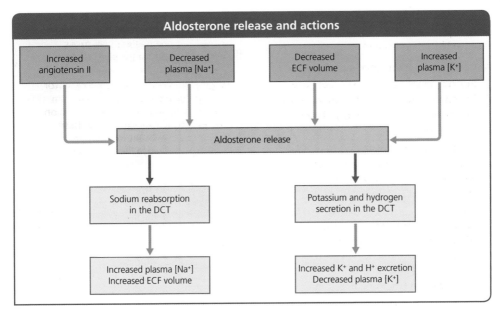

Figure 1.23 Release and actions of aldosterone. Aldosterone release is stimulated by angiotensin II, a fall in plasma Na^+ concentration, decreased extracellular fluid volume and increased plasma K^+ concentration. It causes reabsorption of Na^+ and increased ECF volume as well as excretion of K^+ and H^+ and a fall in plasma K^+ concentration. DCT, distal convoluted tubule; ECF, extracellular fluid.

Aldosterone: actions on late distal convoluted tubule cells		
Cell	Action	Effect
Principal cells	Increases activity of the basolateral Na^+–K^+ ATPase pump*	Overall reabsorption of Na^+, and as a result water, into the blood and excretion of K^+
	Up-regulation of apical Na^+ channels, increasing permeability to Na^+	Movement of Na^+ from filtrate into principal cells
	Up-regulation of apical K^+ channels	Movement of K^+ from principal cells into filtrate
Intercalated cells	Up-regulation of the H^+ pump on the apical membrane, which uses ATP to move H^+ from the intercalated cell and into the filtrate	Facilitation of excretion of H^+
	Up-regulation of the H^+–Na^+ cotransporter on the apical membrane, which moves Na^+ from the filtrate into the intercalated cell in exchange for H^+	Absorption of Na^+ and excretion of H^+

*The Na^+–K^+ ATPase pump transports three Na^+ ions out of the cell and into the interstitium and two K^+ ions into the cell from the interstitium.

Table 1.11 Actions of aldosterone on the apical (luminal) and basolateral (interstitial) membranes of cells of the late distal convoluted tubule

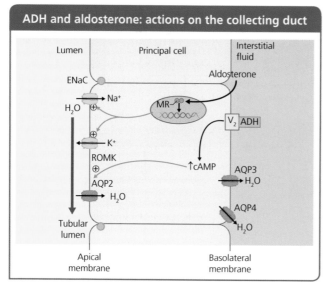

Figure 1.24 Actions of antidiuretic hormone (ADH) and aldosterone on principal cells of the collecting duct. ADH binds to V_2 receptors on the basolateral membrane, which leads to an increase in vesicular transport of aquaporin (AQP)-2 channels to the apical (luminal) membrane, thereby allowing water to flow out of the fluid in the lumen and into the tubular cell. Water leaves the cells of the collecting duct basolaterally via AQP3 and AQP4 channels, which are permanently present in the membrane. Aldosterone, a steroid hormone, binds intracellular mineralocorticoid receptors (MR) to increase the number and activity of basolateral Na^+–K^+ ATPase pumps (not shown) and apical Na^+ and K^+ channels, thereby increasing Na^+ reabsorption and K^+ secretion, respectively. ENaC, epithelial Na^+ channel; ROMK, renal outer medullary K^+ channel.

> Excess production of aldosterone (for example, due to an aldosterone-secreting benign adrenal tumour in Conn's syndrome) results in hypertension and hypokalaemia. This reflects the increased reabsorption of sodium (and therefore water) and secretion of potassium in the distal tubule.

Atrial and brain natriuretic peptides

Atrial natriuretic peptide and brain natriuretic peptide are small proteins secreted in response to stretch of cardiac myocytes as a consequence of increased extracellular fluid volume. Both cause peripheral vasodilation and increase renal excretion of Na^+ and water (**Table 1.12**).

The overall effect of natriuretic peptides is:

- natriuresis (increased urinary Na^+ excretion)
- diuresis (increased fluid excretion)
- reduction in blood volume, arterial pressure, central venous pressure and cardiac output

Antidiuretic hormone

Antidiuretic hormone, also known as vasopressin, is a nonapeptide hormone synthesised in the magnocellular neurones within the hypothalamus. It is produced as a large precursor molecule, preproantidiuretic hormone, and is transported to the posterior pituitary gland. Here, it is stored in neurosecretory granules as proantidiuretic hormone until its release as ADH.

Release of antidiuretic hormone

The release of ADH is triggered by:

- an increase in plasma osmolality, detected by osmoreceptor cells in the hypothalamus
- a decrease in blood volume, detected by stretch receptors in the walls of the atria and large veins
- hypotension, detected by arterial baroreceptors
- nausea and vomiting, stress, hypoxia and pain

Actions of ANP and BNP	
Effect	Mechanism
Peripheral vasodilation	Direct effect on peripheral vasculature, resulting in venous and arterial dilation
	Decreased renin secretion in the juxtaglomerular apparatus and subsequent decrease in angiotensin II and therefore inhibition of its vasoconstricting effect
Increased excretion of Na^+ and water	Inhibition of the $Na^+–K^+$ ATPase pump and closure of Na^+ channels in the collecting ducts, resulting in decreased Na^+ reabsorption in the renal tubules
	Increased glomerular filtration rate, via mesangial cell relaxation and vasodilation of the afferent arterioles
	Decreased renin secretion and therefore decreased aldosterone release, resulting in decreased reabsorption of Na^+ and water

Table 1.12 The effects of atrial natriuretic peptide (ANP) and brain natriuretic peptide (BNP)

Actions of antidiuretic hormone

Antidiuretic hormone has the following effects (see **Figure 1.24**):

- a decrease in water excretion, mediated by V_2 receptors in the basolateral membrane of cells of the collecting duct which promote fusion of intracellular water channels (aquaporins) with the luminal membrane, thereby rendering it permeable to water
- vasoconstriction, mediated by V_1 receptors on blood vessels

Release of ADH is affected by a number of drugs. It is increased by morphine, barbiturates, thiazide diuretics, cyclophosphamide and tricyclic antidepressants. It is decreased by alcohol and phenytoin.

Drugs that potentiate ADH release can cause hyponatraemia due to excess water reabsorption in the collecting duct whereas those that inhibit the release of ADH can cause an inappropriate diuresis.

Aquaporins

Aquaporins are integral membrane proteins that form channels for the transfer of water. More than 10 isoforms have been identified in mammalian cells; they are expressed differently in different cell types and tissues within the body. For example, Aquaporin-1 is expressed in the proximal tubule, blood vessels, the eye and the ear, and aquaporin-2 is present in the collecting duct. Aquaporin-2 responds to ADH. Water moves through these channels and into the cell across an osmotic gradient and enters the circulation via the basolateral membrane, which is freely permeable to water.

Lithium (used for treating some psychiatric conditions) down-regulates aquaporin-2. This results in loss of water, and is an acquired form of nephrogenic diabetes insipidus.

Prostaglandins and other eicosanoids

Eicosanoids are biologically active products of arachidonic acid metabolism and include prostaglandins, thromboxane and leukotrienes. They are regarded as local hormones because they affect cells in close proximity to their site of formation. In the kidney, the significant eicosanoids are prostaglandins and thromboxane (**Table 1.13**). Renal prostaglandins act to protect the kidneys during states of physiological stress. They maintain blood pressure and preserve renal function in states of volume depletion and have an antihypertensive effect in response to ingestion of large amounts of dietary salt. Whereas prostaglandins have a vasodilatory effect,

Actions of renal eicosanoids	
Eicosanoid	Action
Prostaglandin E_2	Vasodilation
	Increased excretion of water and Na^+ by the collecting tubules
	Protection of medullary tubular cells from hypoxia when volume of extracellular fluid decreases
Prostaglandin I_2 (prostacyclin)	Vasodilation
	Renin release
Thromboxane A_2	Vasoconstriction: synthesised in response to renal damage, and limits blood flow to a poorly functioning kidney

Table 1.13 Eicosanoids produced in the kidney and their actions

thromboxane A_2 is a vasoconstrictor and is synthesised in response to repeated renal damage to limit blood flow to a diseased kidney. Eicosanoids are synthesised in the renal arterioles and glomeruli, medullary intersitial cells and epithelial cells of the collecting duct. Synthesis of prostaglandin E_2 is stimulated by conditions associated with low renal perfusion pressure, elevated renin activity and increased sympathetic output. Prostaglandin I_2 is synthesised in response to a decrease in renal perfusion, renal ischaemia and renal parenchymal injury.

> **Prostaglandins dilate afferent arterioles, thereby increasing renal blood flow.** Non-steroidal anti-inflammatory drugs such as ibuprofen block prostaglandin production by blocking the cyclo-oxygenase enzyme. The loss of the effects of prostaglandins can cause decreased renal perfusion and therefore worsen renal failure in patients with chronic kidney disease.

Tubular transport of other solutes

In addition to the transport of Na^+, the kidneys play a central role in the reabsorption and secretion of other ions including calcium, phosphate, potassium and magnesium. Common sequelae of impaired renal function therefore include abnormalities in the balance of these ions in the body.

Calcium and phosphate

Calcium is the most abundant mineral in the body and has key roles in cellular function. Over 99% of total body calcium is stored as hydroxyapatite in bone. Less than 1% is located in the intracellular and extracellular compartments. Calcium in plasma exists in three states:

- free ionised calcium, Ca^{2+} (50%)
- protein-bound (40%)
- anion-bound (10%)

Calcium concentrations are tightly maintained in plasma between 2.1 and 2.5 mmol/L (normal range includes both free and bound ion). Only free ionised calcium is physiologically active, and its concentrations are controlled by homeostatic mechanisms. Ca^{2+} has many functions, including control of excitable tissues, neurotransmitter release and cell signalling.

Phosphate salts are an essential structural component of bones and teeth; 80% of total body phosphate is in bone, 20% is in the intracellular fluid and <0.1% is in the extracellular fluid. Plasma concentrations are maintained between 0.8 and 1.2 mmol/L. Plasma phosphate is mainly in the inorganic form as PO_4. This exists in three fractions, ionic (55%), in complexes with Na^+, Ca^{2+} and Mg^{2+} (35%) and protein-bound (10%).

Both calcium and phosphate enter the plasma from dietary sources (via absorption in the gut) and from bone, and are lost from the plasma via the kidneys or by reabsorption into bone. Although only a small fraction of total body calcium and phosphate is present in the plasma, the plasma concentrations of ionised calcium and inorganic phosphate are under hormonal control by parathyroid hormone, 1,25-dihydroxyvitamin D and calcitonin.

Homeostasis

Calcium homeostasis is controlled primarily by parathyroid hormone and vitamin D (active form, 1,25-dihydroxyvitamin D) (**Figure 1.25**). Calcitonin, a peptide hormone produced by the parafollicular cells (or C-cells) of the thyroid gland, plays a minor role (see page 43).

Of the Ca^{2+} filtered by the kidney, 98% is reabsorbed in the proximal convoluted tubules via the paracellular route. This process is linked to the movement of Na^+ by passive diffusion. Fine-tuning of Ca^{2+} reabsorption occurs actively against an electrochemical gradient in the distal convoluted tubule and collecting duct.

Vitamin D

This is not a single entity but a group of fat-soluble secosteroids (compounds derived from steroids, in which ring cleavage has occurred). They are obtained from dietary sources or produced by the action of ultraviolet light on the skin, which is the major source. In humans,

the most relevant compounds are vitamin D_3 (cholecalciferol) and vitamin D_2 (ergocalciferol): cholecalciferol is synthesised in the skin and found in fish whereas ergocalciferol is found in plant sources.

Vitamin D has to undergo two hydroxylations, one in the liver and other in the kidney, in order to become metabolically active. It then increases calcium concentration via its effects on the gut, skeleton and kidney (**Figure 1.26**).

Patients with renal disease have decreased activity of 1α-hydroxylase and are therefore unable to activate vitamin D. They require treatment with vitamin D analogues such as alfacalcidol, an analogue already hydroxylated at the 1α position.

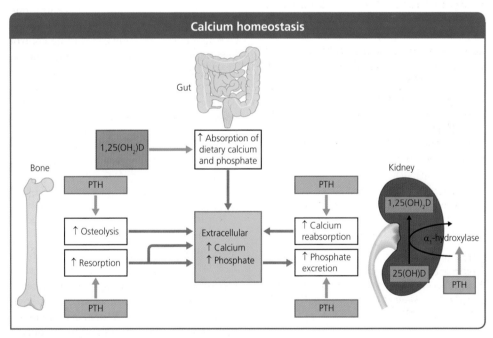

Calcium homeostasis

Figure 1.25 Calcium homeostasis. A decrease in serum calcium concentration is detected by the calcium receptor on chief cells of the parathyroid gland. This stimulates secretion of PTH by the parathyroid gland. PTH acts on the kidney to increase calcium reabsorption and phosphate secretion and on the bone to increase resorption which results in release of calcium into the plasma. PTH also increases synthesis of the metabolically active 1,25-dihydroxyvitamin D which increases calcium and phosphate reabsorption in the gut. 1,25-(OH)$_2$D, 1,25-dihydroxyvitamin D; 25-(OH)D, 25-hydroxyvitamin D; PTH, parathyroid hormone.

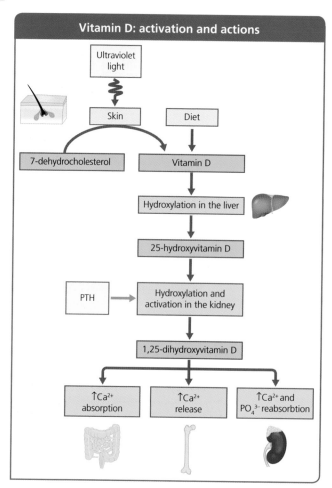

Vitamin D: activation and actions

Figure 1.26 Vitamin D: activation and action. Vitamin D, from the diet or synthesised in the skin, is activated in two steps via the liver and kidney to the metabolite 1,25-dihydroxyvitamin D. PTH, parathyroid hormone.

Parathyroid hormone

This peptide hormone is synthesised by chief cells in the parathyroid gland. It controls the active reabsorption of Ca^{2+} via Ca^{2+}-sensing receptors in the parathyroid gland which monitor the concentration of Ca^{2+} ions in the extracellular fluid. A decrease in the plasma concentration of Ca^{2+} ions stimulates increased synthesis of parathyroid hormone. Conversely, high concentrations of plasma Ca^{2+} inhibit its synthesis. Parathyroid hormone:

- stimulates active reabsorption of Ca^{2+} in the distal convoluted tubule and collecting duct
- stimulates renal synthesis of 1α-hydroxylase, which catalyses the conversion of 25-hydroxyvitamin D to its active form, 1,25-dihydroxyvitamin D; this promotes increased intestinal Ca^{2+} absorption and increased bone resorption to release Ca^{2+}
- decreases reabsorption of phosphate and bicarbonate in the proximal convoluted tubule
- stimulates osteoclast activity, resulting in increased bone resorption

Oversecretion of parathyroid hormone by the parathyroid gland, for example in cases of parathyroid hyperplasia or parathyroid adenoma, results in hypercalcaemia and hypophosphataemia. These electrolyte abnormalities result from increased renal reabsorption of calcium, increased renal conversion of 25-hyroxyvitamin D to 1,25-dihydroxyvitamin D, decreased renal reabsorption of phosphate and increased bone resorption.

Vitamin D acts directly on the parathyroid gland to suppress release of parathyroid hormone by decreasing transcription of the parathyroid hormone gene.

Calcitonin

This peptide hormone is produced by the parafollicular cells of the thyroid gland. These are neuroendocrine cells situated adjacent to thryroid follicles. It opposes the actions of parathyroid hormone by decreasing Ca^{2+} release from bone, thereby contributing to a decrease in the concentration of Ca^{2+} in the extracellular fluid.

Renal regulation of phosphate

After being freely filtered in the glomerulus, 80% of phosphate is reabsorbed in the proximal convoluted tubule and 20% is excreted in the urine. Phosphate is reabsorbed with Na^+ at the apical (luminal) membrane of the cells of the tubule. An increase in plasma phosphate concentration results in increased phosphate filtration and excretion as the phosphate transport capacity of the tubules is exceeded. A decrease in GFR results in increased plasma phosphate concentration. This occurs because compensatory mechanisms associated with an increase in plasma phosphate (e.g. decreased production of 1,25-dihydroxyvitamin D, which normally acts to decrease intestinal phosphate absorption) fail and suppression of phosphate reabsorption by the remaining nephrons is insufficient to balance phosphate intake.

Hyperphosphataemia is common in chronic kidney disease and results from decreased GFR. It is a common cause of troublesome itching. It is managed by limiting dietary intake of phosphate and by regular use of phosphate binders, which bind phosphate in the gastrointestinal tract and prevent its absorption.

Potassium

Potassium is the major intracellular cation; 98% of total body K^+ is found in the intracellular fluid (150 mmol/L) and 2% in extracellular fluid (4–5 mmol/L). K^+ has a number of physiological functions:

- generation of action potentials for the conduction of nerve impulses
- skeletal and smooth muscle contraction
- cardiac muscle contraction

The Na^+–K^+ ATPase pump maintains a low concentration of extracellular K^+ and a high concentration of intracellular K^+ in all cells. Its activity is influenced by acid–base balance, the hormones insulin and glucagon, and circulating catecholamines (**Table 1.14**).

The influence of insulin and β-adrenergic activity on the Na^+–K^+ ATPase pump is used clinically in the treatment of hyperkalaemia. Insulin, infused together with glucose to prevent hypoglycaemia, and $β_2$ agonists (e.g. salbutamol) are used to drive K^+ into cells.

Factors affecting Na^+–K^+ ATPase pump activity	
Factor	Effect
Acid–base balance	
Alkalosis	Secretion of intracellular H^+ in exchange for absorption of K^+ across cell membranes, resulting in hypokalaemia
Acidosis	Absorption of extracellular H^+ and secretion of K^+ from cells into the extracellular compartment, resulting in hyperkalaemia
Hormones	
Insulin	Movement of K^+ into cells as a result of direct action on the pump
Glucagon	Impairment of K^+ entry into cells
Catecholamines	
α-Adrenergic activity	Decreased intracellular uptake of K^+
β-Adrenergic activity	Increased intracellular uptake of K^+

Table 1.14 Factors affecting the activity of cell membrane Na^+–K^+ ATPase pumps

Tubular transport of K^+

Potassium is freely filtered by the glomerulus and 89-90% is reabsorbed in the proximal convoluted tubule. The late distal convoluted tubule and cortical collecting duct are the main sites of K^+ secretion into the urine. The amount of K^+ excreted in the urine varies greatly depending on dietary intake, acid–base status and aldosterone activity.

Potassium activates the RAAS, so it has a direct effect on aldosterone release.

■ An increase in plasma K^+ concentration stimulates aldosterone secretion, which promotes the secretion of K^+ into the filtrate
■ A decrease in plasma K^+ concentration suppresses aldosterone release, which decreases the secretion of K^+, so more is retained

Tubular transport of Na^+, which is closely linked to the transport of K^+, is discussed on page 33.

Magnesium

Magnesium is the fourth most abundant cation in the body. It is a cofactor for enzyme processes requiring ATP and many enzymes involved in nucleic acid metabolism. It also regulates K^+ and Ca^{2+} channels in cell membranes and facilitates cell adhesion to substrates. It is vital for the structural function of proteins, multiple enzyme complexes and mitochondria.

Most magnesium is sequestered in bone and about 1% is in extracellular fluid. Plasma concentrations are maintained between 0.7 and 1.2 mmol/L and are affected by dietary intake, renal handling and gastrointestinal absorption. About 30% of circulating magnesium is protein-bound.

Tubular transport of Mg^{2+}

Ionised magnesium is filtered in the glomerulus. A small amount is reabsorbed in the proximal convoluted tubule, but most is reabsorbed in the thick ascending limb of the loop of Henle. Ca^{2+}/Mg^{2+}-sensing receptors located in the basolateral membrane of cells in the thick ascending limb and distal convoluted tubule play a key role in magnesium homeostasis.

■ When Mg^{2+} or Ca^{2+} levels are low, the receptors stimulate cotransporters, resulting in increased Mg^{2+} and Ca^{2+} absorption
■ When Mg^{2+} or Ca^{2+} levels are high, Mg^{2+} and Ca^{2+} reabsorption is inhibited

Acid–base balance

Starter questions

Answers to the following questions are on page 55.

11. Why must excess acid be excreted?
12. How are the potassium concentration and acid-base balance of the blood related?

An acid is a substance that raises the H^+ ion concentration in a solution, usually by dissociating to release H^+ ions. A base is a substance that combines with H^+ ions. The term 'alkali' is often used synonymously with base, but more specifically means a base soluble in water.

There is net formation of H^+ ions in the body:

- Acids are consumed in the diet directly or indirectly as a product of metabolism of protein-rich food
- Acids are constantly produced as by-products of metabolism

For example in cellular respiration, the production of cellular energy from the breakdown of glucose generates carbon dioxide (CO_2). In solution, CO_2 combines with water to form the weak acid carbonic acid (H_2CO_3). If this accumulated body fluids would become acidic, which would cause changes in protein structure and interfere with protein function.

Excess acid is largely excreted in the urine, but there are also buffering systems that ensure fluid remains at the optimal pH. These systems also buffer the excess acid or alkali generated in pathological conditions

Acidosis is an excess of acid in the blood. Alkalosis is an excess of alkali. Both have metabolic causes and respiratory causes. They are discussed in detail in Chapter 8.

pH

pH measures the acidity of an aqueous solution; it is the negative logarithm, to base 10, of H^+ concentration.

- The lower the pH, the more H^+ ions are present: increasing acidity
- The higher the pH, the fewer H^+ are present: increasing alkalinity

Acidity has a significant effect on the structure and function of proteins; the pH of body fluid must therefore be tightly controlled for normal cell and metabolic function to be maintained. pH also affects the ionisation of certain molecules, which can be the difference between biological activity or inactivity, or even destructive activity.

Control of acid–base balance

Acid-base balance within the human body is tightly regulated to enable optimal function of biochemical and enzymatic process. Blood pH is maintained at 7.35–7.45, the range in which enzymes function optimally. The corresponding normal concentration of H^+ is 35–45 nmol/L.

Blood acid–base balance is measured by running arterial or venous blood samples through a blood gas analyser. Blood pH < 7.35 indicates acidaemia; > 7.45 indicates alkalaemia.

Buffering systems

A buffer is a solution containing substances that resist changes in pH when an acid or a base is added. Many buffers consist of a mixture of a weak acid with a conjugate base. A weak acid is only partly dissociated in solution (as opposed to a strong acid which is completely dissociated). A conjugate base is the anion that is generated when a weak acid dissociates. The reaction that takes place is represented as:

$$H^+ + A^- \text{ (conjugate base)} \rightleftharpoons HA \text{ (weak acid)}$$

Buffering in different fluids

The body has a significant buffering capacity due to several different buffering systems. They operate in the blood, intracellular fluid, urine and bone, and are vital for maintaining the pH of intracellular and extracellular fluid. The systems include the following (**Table 1.15**):

- bicarbonate
- phosphate
- proteins
- haemoglobin
- bone
- ammonium

In the blood, bicarbonate in plasma and haemoglobin in red blood cells contribute most to the buffering capacity. Buffering within the interstitium depends on bicarbonate and intracellular buffering is due to proteins and phosphates. The kidneys maintain the acid-base balance and buffering through the excretion of acid and the reabsorption of bicarbonate. Eighty-five to ninety per cent of filtered bicarbonate is reabsorbed in the proximal tubule; the remainder is reabsorbed by cells of the ascending limb of the loop of Henle and by the intercalated cells of the distal tubule and collecting duct. From here, it enters the circulation. The kidneys are also responsible for the production of urinary buffers, ammonium and hydrogen phosphate, which enable the excretion of hydrogen ions. Ammonium is predominantly produced in the proximal tubular cells and the excretion of ammonium is a means of removing acid from the body when systemic acidosis is present. The hydrogen phosphate buffer system depends on the amount of phosphate filtered and excreted by the kidneys, which depends on diet and parathyroid hormone activity. Unlike ammonium, its activity cannot be altered to respond to changes in acid-base balance.

Whereas the kidneys are responsible for the excretion of metabolic acids, the lungs enable excretion of carbon dioxide, the 'respiratory acid'.

The Henderson-Hasselbalch equation

This equation is used to determine the pH of a buffer system based on the concentrations of HA and A^-:

$$pH = pKa + \log_{10}([A^-]/[HA])$$

Ka is the acid dissociation constant, a measure of the tendency of a compound to dissociate. pKa is a related value calculated by using the following equation:

$$pKa = -\log_{10}(Ka)$$

For any weak acid:

$$pH \propto [A^-]/[HA]$$

Therefore changes in pH are proportional to the relative concentrations of a conjugate base and its acid.

Bicarbonate buffer system

This system, also known as the bicarbonate–carbonic anhydrase system, is the buffering system with the largest capacity in the body and operates in the extracellular fluid.

Carbon dioxide (CO_2), produced constantly by cellular respiration, combines with water to form carbonic acid (H_2CO_3). This weak acid dissociates into bicarbonate (HCO_3^-) and H^+, in a reaction catalysed by the enzyme carbonic anhydrase.

$$CO_2 + H_2O \rightleftharpoons H_2CO_3 \rightleftharpoons H^+ + HCO_3^-$$

When excess H^+ is added to the system, e.g. due to production of lactic acid in anaerobic metabolism or ketone bodies due to

Buffering systems			
Site	Buffering system	Mechanism	Effect
Interstitial fluid	Bicarbonate and carbonic anhydrase	HCO_3^- binds H^+ to form carbonic acid, which dissociates into CO_2 and H_2O CO_2 is excreted by the respiratory tract	Major extracellular buffer
	Phosphate	At normal pH monohydrogen phosphate accepts protons and dihydrogen phosphate is a proton donor	Minor effect: concentration in interstitium is low
	Proteins	Imidazole groups of histidine residues accept or donate H^+ to buffer changes in pH	Minor effect: concentration in interstitium is low
Blood	Bicarbonate and carbonic anhydrase	HCO_3^- binds H^+ to form carbonic acid, which dissociates into CO_2 and H_2O CO_2 is excreted by the respiratory tract.	Major extracellular buffer
	Proteins	Imidazole groups of histidine residues accept or donate H^+ to buffer changes in pH	Minor buffer in the blood Lower effect than haemoglobin
	Haemoglobin	Imidazole groups of histidine residues accept or donate H^+	Extracellular buffer Greater effect than plasma proteins due to its higher concentration and a greater number of histidine residues per molecule
Cells	Phosphate	Dihydrogen phosphate is a weak acid and donates protons. Monohydrogen phosphate, its conjugate base, accepts protons	Buffers changes in intracellular pH
	Proteins	Imidazole groups of histidine residues accept or donate H^+	Buffers changes in intracellular pH
Bone	Calcium carbonate	Released from bone due to a direct effect of H^+ on hydroxyapatite crystals and increased osteoclast activity	Buffers excess H^+ Greatest effect during chronic metabolic acidosis
	Anionic exchange	H^+ taken up by bone in exchange for Na^+ and K^+	Greatest effect during chronic metabolic acidosis
Urine	Ammonium	Formed in the proximal tubule (in a process which generates HCO_3^-) and recycled in the medullary interstitium. Secreted into the collecting tubule lumen as NH_3, where it accepts protons to become NH_4^+ and is excreted	Increases net acid excretion during systemic metabolic acidosis
	Phosphate	Dihydrogen phosphate is a weak acid and donates protons. Monohydrogen phosphate, its conjugate base, accepts protons	H^+ in the distal tubule combines with monohydrogen phosphate

Table 1.15 The buffering systems of the body. Major and minor refer to high- and low-capacity buffer systems, respectively

breakdown of fatty acids, it reacts with bicarbonate to form carbonic acid. This shifts the equilibrium to the left, which results in removal of H⁺. Conversely, reduction in acidity, i.e. removal of H⁺, shifts the equilibrium to the right, which results in dissociation of carbonic acid to release H⁺ and bicarbonate. When carbonic acid dissociates into water and carbon dioxide, the latter is removed by the lungs The system is summarised in **Figure 1.27**.

Bicarbonate buffer system and the lungs

The majority of buffer systems are most effective when their pKa is about the same as the target pH. However, this is not the case for the bicarbonate buffer system. In this system, the ability of the lungs to excrete carbon dioxide increases the buffering capacity of the system, enabling it to be effective across a wider pH range. In effect, it makes the 'closed' system of the body an 'open' one with the external environment.

Bicarbonate buffer system and the kidneys

In the kidney, the amount of HCO_3^- filtered in the glomerulus depends on the GFR and plasma bicarbonate concentration, and is usually between 4000 and 5000 mmol/day. Reabsorption of the vast majority of this filtered bicarbonate is vital for the maintenance of the bicarbonate buffer system.

Eighty-five per cent of filtered HCO_3^- is reabsorbed in the proximal tubule. The remaining 10–15% is reabsorbed in the thick ascending limb of the loop of Henle and 0–5% in the distal tubule.

Bicarbonate reabsorption in the proximal tubule and loop of Henle

Filtered HCO_3^- cannot cross the apical membrane of the proximal tubular cell, so it combines with H⁺ to form CO_2 and H_2O, catalysed by carbonic anhydrase. CO_2 diffuses freely in to the cell, where carbonic anhydrase again catalyses the formation of HCO_3^-. HCO_3^- crosses the basolateral membrane via the Na^+–HCO_3^- symporter which transfers 3 HCO_3^- for 1 Na^+. H⁺ is transported from the proximal tubule cell to the proximal tubule lumen via the Na^+-H⁺ antiporter and the H⁺-ATPase pump. The Na^+–K^+ ATPase pump on the basolateral membrane transports 3 Na^+ out of the proximal tubular cell and 2 K^+ in, which establishes the concentration gradient required for H⁺–Na^+ exchange at the apical membrane. The overall effect of these mechanisms is the reabsorption of one molecule of HCO_3^- and one molecule of Na^+ from the tubular lumen for every molecule of H⁺ secreted. H⁺ is consumed as it reacts with filtered bicarbonate in the tubular lumen so there is no net excretion of H⁺.

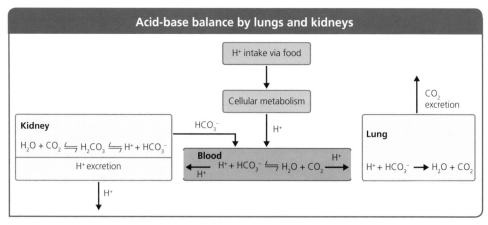

Figure 1.27 Acid–base balance by the lungs and kidneys. H⁺ ions are produced as a result of cellular metabolism. They are buffered by HCO_3^- and by proteins such as haemoglobin so that they can be carried in the blood. They are also buffered by ammonia and other substances and excreted in the kidney. The kidney also replaces the supply of bicarbonate. In the lungs H⁺ combines with HCO_3^- to produce CO_2 which is exhaled. The two excretion methods can be up or down regulated in response to changes in the overall acid–base balance.

The relative concentration of remaining HCO_3^- in the filtrate increases along the nephron as water is reabsorbed in the loop of Henle. The mechanism of HCO_3^- reabsorption in the loop of Henle is similar to that in the proximal tubule.

Bicarbonate reabsorption in the distal tubule

The mechanism of reabsorption of HCO_3^- by the intercalated cells of the distal tubule differs from the proximal tubule and loop of Henle. The intercalated cells secrete H^+ into the lumen via the H^+-ATPase pump. The acidification of tubular fluid promotes conversion of HCO_3^- to CO_2 and H_2O. CO_2 diffuses along its concentration gradient into the intercalated cell where carbonic acid is reformed in the presence of carbonic anhydrase. This dissociates into H^+ and HCO_3^-; H^+ is secreted via the ATP-dependent H^+ pump and HCO_3^- leaves the intercalated cell via the HCO_3^--Cl^- exchanger on the basolateral membrane (**Figure 1.28**). As the apical membrane of the distal tubule and collecting duct has low permeability to H^+, it remains in the tubular fluid and is excreted. pH of fluid in the distal tubule and collecting duct is around 4–5, much lower than elsewhere along the nephron. This mechanism of H^+ excretion removes only a small fraction of H^+; the remainder is excreted with phosphate and ammonium (see below).

Phosphate buffer system

Phosphates are buffers in the urine and the intracellular fluid. However, they do not contribute significantly to blood buffering, because their concentration is too low.

Monohydrogen phosphate and dihydrogen phosphate are the main phosphate ions acting as buffers in the human body. Within cells, they act as an effective buffer when the intracellular fluid is at a physiological pH, as their pKa lies within this range. At a physiological pH, dihydrogen phosphate acts as as weak acid and therefore donates protons and its conjugate base, monohydrogen phosphate, accepts protons to buffer changes in pH.

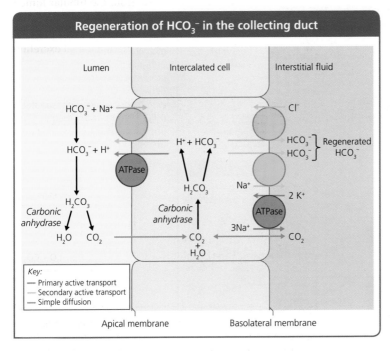

Key:
— Primary active transport
— Secondary active transport
— Simple diffusion

Figure 1.28
Regeneration of bicarbonate in cells of the collecting duct. Bicarbonate (HCO_3^-) is essential as a global pH buffer. Intercalated cells actively secrete H^+, which combines with bicarbonate in the filtrate to become carbonic acid (H_2CO_3). Carbonic anhydrase splits the carbonic acid into carbon dioxide and water. Carbon dioxide diffuses freely into the Intercalated cell, where carbonic anhydrase recombines it with water to form carbonic acid. This dissociates to form H^+, which is actively secreted, and bicarbonate, which is reabsorbed into blood via secondary transport or exchange with sodium or chloride ions respectively.

Monohydrogen phosphate is an effective buffer in urine.

Urine is acidified as intercalated cells of the distal convoluted tubule and collecting duct actively secrete H^+ via the H^+-ATPase pump (**Figure 1.29**). H^+ combines with monohydrogen phosphate to form dihydrogen phosphate in the cortical collecting ducts and is subsequently excreted in the urine.

Proteins as buffers

Proteins have significant buffering capacity in the intracellular fluid, but, because their concentration is lower, less capacity in the blood, interstitial fluid and cells. Different proteins are able to buffer H^+ to varying degrees through the binding of H^+ to imidazole groups of histidine residues.

Plasma proteins such as albumin are able to buffer H^+. However, their buffering capacity is less than that of haemoglobin, because of their lower concentration and the presence of fewer histidine residues. Intracellular proteins also contribute to buffering, particularly in the context of chronic acidosis, which occurs in chronic kidney disease (see page 167).

Haemoglobin as a buffer

Haemoglobin, contained within red blood cells, is a high-capacity blood buffer. Each molecule contains 38 histidine residues and is able to accept many H^+ ions. Deoxyhaemoblobin is a more effective buffer than oxyhaemoglobin, because oxygenation of haemoglobin increases dissociation of H^+ from haemoglobin.

Bone as a buffer

Bone contains carbonate and phosphate salts, which act as buffers during prolonged metabolic acidosis. There is uptake of excess H^+:

- in exchange for Ca^{2+}, Na^+ and K^+ on the bone surface
- when dissolution of bone mineral results in the release of buffering compounds such as sodium bicarbonate and calcium bicarbonate.

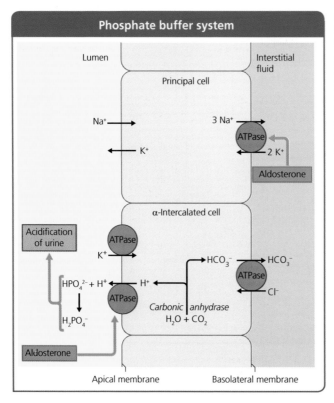

Figure 1.29 The phosphate buffer system. Hydrogen phosphate (HPO_4^{2-}) is freely filtered at the glomerulus and acts as a urinary buffer in the distal tubule. H^+ produced from the reaction between CO_2 and H_2O combines with monohydrogen phosphate (HPO_4^{2-}) to form dihydrogen phosphate ($H_2PO_4^{2-}$) which is excreted in the urine.

Chronic metabolic acidosis, as occurs in chronic kidney disease, can result in significant loss of bone mineral, which contributes to osteomalacia and osteopenia. Therefore acidosis must be controlled in renal patients. This may be achieved with oral sodium bicarbonate supplementation.

Bone disease resulting from chronic kidney disease (renal osteodystrophy) does not occur because of acidosis alone. Altered vitamin D and phosphate metabolism and secondary hyperparathyroidism contribute more significantly to loss of bone mineral.

Ammonium as a buffer

Ammonium (NH_4^+) is a high-capacity buffer because it is based on an essentially unlimited supply of ammonia (NH_3) derived from glutamine in the proximal tubular cells.

Ammoniagenesis in the proximal tubule

Deamination of glutamine by the enzyme glutaminase generates NH_4^+ and glutamate. Glutamate is then deaminated by the enzyme glutamate dehydrogenase to form NH_4^+ and α-ketoglutarate. The ammonium produced in these reactions is secreted into the lumen of the proximal convoluted tubule in exchange for Na^+. α-ketoglutarate is subsequently metabolised by the Krebs cycle, which generates HCO_3^-. This passes into the interstitum and then the plasma (**Figure 1.30**). This generation of bicarbonate is an important part of the process, helping to counteract systemic acidosis.

The ammonium ion passes down the tubule and is subsequently reabsorbed in the thick ascending limb of the loop of Henle. Because the environment within the tubular cell is less acidic than the tubular lumen, NH_4^+ reabsorbed in the ascending limb dissociates into ammonia (NH_3) and H^+. The luminal membrane of the thick ascending limb is impermeable to NH_3, so it is unable to diffuse back into the lumen. Instead, it diffuses across the basolateral membrane into the medullary interstitium. From the medullary interstitium, NH_3 enters the proximal tubular cells and the lumen of the proximal convoluted tubule, where it gains a H^+ ion to become NH_4^+. This NH_4^+ is then reabsorbed at the thick ascending limb and recycled in the medullary interstitium. The effect of this recycling is to create a concentration gradient of interstitial NH_3, with higher concentrations in the deeper medulla.

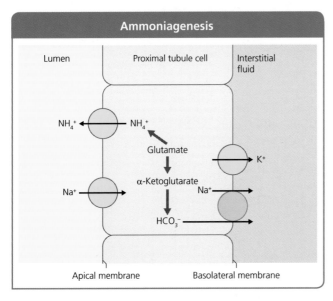

Ammoniagenesis

Lumen — Proximal tubule cell — Interstitial fluid

NH_4^+ ← NH_4^+

Glutamate

K$^+$

α-Ketoglutarate

Na^+ — Na^+

HCO_3^-

Apical membrane — Basolateral membrane

Figure 1.30 Ammoniagenesis in the proximal convoluted tubule. NH_4^+ and α-ketoglutarate are produced from glutamate. NH_4^+ is secreted in exchange for Na^+. α-ketoglutarate is metabolised in the Krebs cycle which generates HCO_3^-. This passes to the interstitium and then the plasma. Much of the NH_4^+ is reabsorbed in the loop of Henle and circulated to the medullary interstitium then pumped into the collecting tubule as NH_3. This takes up H^+ ions secreted by intercalated cells.

Ammonia buffering in the collecting duct

Because NH_3 is removed (as NH_4^+) in the loop of Henle, its concentration in fluid entering the distal convoluted tubule and collecting duct is low. Therefore there is a large concentration gradient to drive secretion of NH_3 from its high medullary interstitial concentration into the lumen of the collecting tubule. The collecting tubule lumen is permeable to NH_3 but not NH_4^+. NH_3 secreted into the collecting duct takes up H^+ secreted into filtrate by the intercalated cells to form NH_4^+. This NH_4^+ becomes trapped, because it is unable to diffuse back into the cell; it is subsequently excreted.

In the presence of metabolic acidosis, there is:

■ increased secretion of NH_4^+ by the proximal tubule
■ increased NH_4^+ reabsorption in the thick ascending limb of the loop of Henle
■ increased recycling of NH_3 to the medullary interstitium
■ increased diffusion of NH_3 into the collecting duct
■ As NH_3 combines with H^+, secretion of H^+ into urine by intercalated cells of the collecting duct decreases the concentration of NH_3 and facilitates its diffusion from the medullary interstitium into the collecting duct lumen along its concentration gradient. The overall result is excretion of an acid load as NH_3 binds and traps H^+ in the urine

Endocrine function of the kidney

Starter questions

The answer to the following question is on page 55.

13. Why might a patient with a chronic respiratory condition develop a raised haemoglobin?

In addition to being the target of hormones such as ADH, aldosterone and ANP, the kidneys are responsible for the production of several hormones with local and systemic roles:

- erythropoietin (see below)
- renin (see page 35)
- vitamin D (see page 41)
- eicosanoids (see page 39)
- endothelins (see below)

In addition to its endocrine role, the kidney also synthesises glucose.

Erythropoietin production

Erythropoietin is a glycoprotein that stimulates erythropoiesis (production of red blood cells) in the bone marrow, by inducing differentiation of bone marrow progenitor cells into erythroblasts (immature red blood cells). The kidney produces 80% of the body's erythropoietin; the remaining 20% is synthesised by the liver.

> **Decreased production of erythropoietin is common in chronic kidney disease and results in anaemia (low haemoglobin concentration).** This is treated with erythropoietin replacement, using erythropoietin produced from recombinant DNA administered as regular subcutaneous injections.

Production occurs in the peritubular fibroblasts of the renal cortex and is mediated by prostaglandins. The primary stimulus for synthesis and secretion of erythropoietin is hypoxia; however, it is enhanced by androgens, catecholamines (adrenaline and noradrenaline) binding to β_2 receptors and, in the context of haemorrhage, by angiotensin II.

Endothelin production

The endothelins are a family of peptides comprising endothelin 1 (ET-1), endothelin 2 (ET-2), endothelin 3 (ET-3) and endothelin 4 (ET-4) produced by vascular endothelial cells throughout the body. They exert various biological effects and most notably stimulate vasoconstriction and cell proliferation. They are synthesised from a propeptide, 'big endothelin', by endothelin-converting enzymes and act in an autocrine or paracrine fashion. ET-1 is the predominant isoform. Endothelins are produced in response to ADH, angiotensin II, thrombin, cytokines, reactive oxygen species and shearing forces, and are inhibited by prostacyclin, ANP and nitric oxide.

In the kidney, they are synthesised and secreted by the mesangial cells and afferent and efferent arterioles. ET-1 is involved in normal renal function by modulating GFR, solute and water reabsorption, and excretion of acid. It may also promote glomerular and tubulointerstitial fibrosis and dysfunction of the glomerular filtration barrier in the setting of CKD.

Production of glucose

The renal cortex contains glucose-6-phosphatase responsible for gluconeogenesis in which glucose is produced from lactate, glutamine and glycerol (as opposed to glycogen).

This process is regulated by insulin and catecholamines. After overnight fasting, renal gluconeogenesis contributes 20–25% of glucose released into the circulation; after prolonged fasting, this contribution may increase.

Normally all glucose filtered through the glomerulus is absorbed in the proximal convoluted tubule. Drugs that inhibit the transporter involved in this uptake therefore promote excretion of glucose and help control hyperglycaemia during diabetes.

Answers to starter questions

1. Nephrons are the functional units of kidneys. They consist of a filtering end, the glomerulus, where fluid is filtered from the blood into the start of the tubule, and a long section of tubule with cells that absorb and secrete substances into the filtrate. Each kidney contains over 1 million nephrons, which all empty filtrate into the renal pelvis as urine.

2. The kidneys have important endocrine roles in the regulation of blood pressure, red blood cell (RBC) formation and the activation of vitamin D. Renal peritubular fibroblasts cells produce erythropoietin, a hormone that stimulates RBC formation, and juxtaglomerular cells in the afferent arteriole produce renin, a hormone central to the regulation of blood pressure and sodium handling. The kidneys (along with the liver) also play an important role in the activation of vitamin D, which contributes to calcium homeostasis and bone health.

3. Amniotic fluid is initially produced by the placenta from maternal plasma. The fetus begins to make urine from as early as 8 weeks gestation and, around this time, the urethra also becomes patent. Fetal urine is excreted via the urinary tract into the amniotic fluid but does not contribute significantly to amniotic fluid until the second half of pregnancy. Fluid is in circulation as the fetus swallows and then excretes it.

4. Kidneys normally ascend in embryonic development, from the pelvis to the superior abdomen. This ascent is interrupted in 1 in 3000 births resulting in a pelvic kidney.

5. A kidney may have more than one artery due to the way renal vasculature develops. As it ascends, the kidney receives transient blood vessels originating at the aorta, from progressively higher levels. It is relatively common (i.e. up to 30% of births) for vessels to persist, resulting in an additional arterial supply.

6. Great care is required during invasive renal procedures because kidneys are so highly vascular in nature. Damage to a renal blood vessel can cause catastrophic bleeding, necessitating interventional radiological procedures, surgery, and even removal of the kidney.

7. In order to limit water loss, a desert animal must produce very concentrated urine. This is achieved with a long loop of Henle, which allows more water to be reabsorbed by the kidney tubule, and results in a very concentrated urine.

8. The female urethra is shorter than the male urethra, which provides bacteria with a shorter distance to travel to reach the bladder. It is also closer to the anus, and therefore faecal bacteria.

Answers *continued*

9. The body is made up of the two major compartments: the intracellular space and the extracellular space. The extracellular space is divided into the intravascular space (plasma), the interstitium (including lymph) and the transcellular space (e.g. pericardial and peritoneal fluid).

10. Sodium is the major determinant of plasma osmolality; the measure of osmoles of solute per kilogram of solvent (osmol/kg). As water follows sodium along an osmotic gradient, from low to high osmolality, when sodium is reabsorbed by the kidneys, water is too. This is how control of plasma sodium is closely linked to the control of blood volume and pressure.

11. Metabolism constantly generates acid as a by-product. If left unheeded, this alters the structure and function of macromolecules and disturbs cellular metabolism. pH also alters the degree of ionisation of weak acids and bases, which can affect many biochemical reactions. For example, the generation of ATP via the mitochondrial electron transfer chain is dependent upon a H^+ gradient. So pH must be tightly regulated, largely by the excretion of excess acid in urine and exhaled CO_2.

12. Acid–base and K^+ homeostasis are interconnected. Acidaemia is generally associated with hyperkalaemia and alkalaemia is associated with hypokalaemia. The effect of acid–base disturbances on K^+ homeostais is complex. This may result in part from K^+ shifts that occur when intracellular K^+ is exchanged for extracellular H^+ when acidosis is present, and when extracellular K^+ is exchanged for intracellular H^+ when alkalosis is present. Disorders of K^+ balance also affect acid–base balance. Hypokalaemia is associated with increased renal production of NH_3, resulting in increased acid excretion as NH_3 binds H^+ in the tubular lumen and NH_4^+ is excreted. Conversely, hyperkalaemia is associated with decreased NH_4^+ excretion due to decreased NH_3 synthesis in the proximal tubule, decreased NH_4^+ reabsorption in the ascending limb and decreased NH_3 concentration in the medullary interstitium. The overall effect is a reduction in acid secretion and metabolic acidaemia; normalising the K^+ concentration can correct this.

13. A patient with a chronic respiratory condition resulting in chronic hypoxia may develop secondary polycythaemia, an increase in haemoglobin. The hypoxia stimulates the release of erythropoietin, which in turn increases red blood cell production.

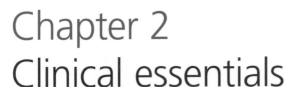
Chapter 2
Clinical essentials

Introduction

The effects of renal disease alter the function of other organ systems and physiological processes such as the cardiovascular system and bone metabolism, so renal patients present with problems related to many different systems. Unlike some organs, in which disease presents with symptoms specific to the organ, for example shortness of breath signalling disease of the respiratory system or diarrhoea signifying a gastrointestinal problem, renal disease tends to present with non-specific symptoms.

Renal medicine encompasses treatment of the primary cause of kidney disease in each case, as well as management of other medical problems in renal patients. Therefore it requires a secure understanding of, and skills in, general medicine.

Renal physicians work closely with vascular surgeons managing vascular access for haemodialysis patients, as well as with transplant surgeons when caring for transplant patients.

Common symptoms and how to take a history

Starter questions

Answers to the following questions are on page 132.

1. Why is a careful drug history required in assessing a patient for renal disease?
2. What causes tiredness in renal failure?
3. How can kidney disease cause difficulties in breathing?

Symptoms of renal disease tend to be non-specific and may not immediately point to a renal problem. This contrasts with, for example, symptoms of certain diseases of the respiratory system, which are likely to be specific, such as shortness of breath or cough.

- Chronic kidney disease (CKD) typically causes fatigue, anorexia (loss of appetite), nausea, shortness of breath and weight loss; however, many other symptoms may also be present
- Symptoms of acute kidney injury (AKI) are more likely to be related to:
  - the underlying cause, for example fever, shortness of breath and cough with pneumonia
  - associated complications, for example shortness of breath in cases of fluid overload

The non-specifc nature of clinical presentations of renal disease makes it a diagnosis of exclusion in many cases.

Taking a renal history

A patient's history comprises their current health problem, previous health problems, medication use, allergies, a family history, social history and a review of all body systems. The history is the foundation of a diagnosis and informs both the examination and subsequent investigations; it should at least produce a shortlist of potential diagnoses.

First introduce yourself, initially addressing the patient formally. Then seek their permission to take a history. Choose an area of privacy, such as a side room, for the interview, and ensure that there are no physical barriers (e.g. a desk) between you and the patient. Next, ask them if you can make notes as you proceed.

History taking requires active listening skills, both verbal and non-verbal.

Verbal listening skills include:

- acknowledging what the patient is saying, e.g. 'yes', 'I understand'
- paraphrasing what the patient has said, e.g. 'so, from what I understand, you've been feeling tired, occasionally breathless and have lost a little weight over the last 3 months'
- asking relevant questions, e.g. if the patient mentions shortness of breath, 'what makes you short of breath?'

Non-verbal listening skills include making eye contact throughout the consultation; clinician and patient should be at the same eye level. Adopt an open posture and pay attention to the patient's body language.

The structure of renal history taking is identical to that for other major organ systems and is organised as shown in **Table 2.1**.

Presenting complaint

The presenting complaint is the problem or symptom that prompted the patient to present, and is best ascertained by using open questions such as 'How can I help today?' The presenting complaint forms the basis of the clinical encounter, thereby enabling the

The renal history	
Component	**What to ask about and example question(s)**
Presenting complaint	The problem or symptom that has caused the patient to present ■ 'What has brought you here today?'
History of presenting complaint	Further detail concerning the presenting problem ■ 'When did this start?' ■ 'How has the symptom progressed?' ■ 'How is it affecting you?'
Past medical history	Other medical problems the patient has (or has had), for example hypertension, diabetes, previous stroke, or transient ischaemic attack or recurrent urinary tract infections ■ Do you have kidney problems?' ■ 'Are you on dialysis?' and if so, 'Haemodialysis or peritoneal dialysis?' ■ 'Any complications?' ■ 'Have you ever had a kidney transplant?'
Drug history	The patient's current and past use of medications, adherence to pharmacological therapy and any previous adverse drug reactions ■ Prescribed medications ■ Nephrotoxic drugs (including non-steroidal anti-inflammatory drugs specifically) ■ Over-the-counter medications ■ Herbal preparations ■ Recreational drugs ('have you ever used drugs recreationally?') ■ Drug allergies ■ Any recent changes to medications
Family history	Medical problems that run in the family* ■ 'Any family history of medical problems?' ■ 'Is there any family history of kidney disease?' (Consider asking specifically about polycystic kidney disease, Alport's syndrome and Fabry's disease)
Social history	Social, occupational, recreational and other aspects of the patient's personal life ■ Occupation ■ Domestic arrangements and relationships with others ■ Smoking ■ Alcohol consumption ■ Pets ■ Travel ('Have you had any recent trips abroad?' and if so, 'What did you do while you were there?')

*If a condition runs in the family, a family tree may be useful to show relationships between those affected.

Table 2.1 The renal history

clinician to ask relevant questions to elicit any further information that is required.

History of presenting complaint

The history of the presenting complaint leads on from the presenting complaint, and is usually elicited by asking both open and closed questions. In this part of the history, the patient's symptoms are explored, as well as their ideas, concerns and explanations.

For example, if the patient has pain, they might be questioned about the site, severity and character of the pain; how it affects their lifestyle; what they think it could be; and what they are most concerned about.

SOCRATES mnemonic

Pain is a common presenting symptom. It must be carefully characterised, for example by using the SOCRATES mnemonic (**Table 2.2**), to help differentiate underlying causes.

		The pain history	
Letter	Characteristic of pain	Example question(s)	Significance
S	Site	'Where is the pain?'	Flank pain suggests renal pathology
		'Can you point to where it is worst?'	Suprapubic pain suggests a bladder abnormality
O	Onset	'When did the pain start?'	Pain lasting for weeks or more may be caused by a tumour
		'Was is sudden or gradual?'	Sudden onset pain is more likely to be renal colic or other causes of ureteric obstruction e.g. a blood clot
			Gradual onset over hours to days is more likely to be the result of an infection
C	Character	'Can you describe the pain?'	Intermittent colicky pain suggests renal colic or other causes of ureteric obstruction
		'Is it sharp and stabbing, dull or throbbing?'	Dull, constant pain may suggest pyelonephritis or a renal tumour
		'Does it stay the same or does it change?'	
R	Radiation	'Does the pain move anywhere?'	Loin-to-groin radiation is typical of renal colic
A	Associated features	'Do you have any other symptoms with the pain?'	Vomiting may be associated with various causes of loin pain
		'Have you had any vomiting?	Fever, dysuria and frequency suggest infection
		'Have you had any fever?'	
		'Any pain or burning when you pass water?'	Haematuria is associated with stones, glomerular disease or a renal tumour
		'Are you passing water more or less often than usual?'	
		'Is there any blood in the urine?'	
T	Timing	'Is the pain constant or does it come and go?'	A short episode of pain is more likely to represent acute pathology
		If the pain is intermittent, 'How long do these episodes last for?' and 'How often do they occur?'	Frequent episodes of intermittent or constant pain over a long period suggest a chronic process
E	Exacerbating and relieving factors	'Does anything make the pain worse?'	Passing urine can exacerbate the pain associated with a urinary tract infection
		'Does anything make it better?'	Moving around may make renal colic better
S	Severity	'If you had to give the pain a mark out of 10, with 10 being the worst pain ever, what would you give it?'	Renal stone pain is often rated '10' and described as 'the worst pain ever'

Table 2.2 The pain history: the SOCRATES mnemonic

Past medical history

This checks what other medical problems the patient might have had. It is often necessary to be specific, by asking the patient directly whether they have ever had conditions such as hypertension, stroke, diabetes, deep vein thrombosis, pulmonary embolism, urinary tract infection (UTI) and epilepsy. These comorbidities may be related to the underlying diagnosis and must not be missed. For example, a patient seen in clinic with blood test results showing deranged renal function and who has a history of recurrent UTIs may have sustained chronic kidney damage as a result of these infections.

A good history taking is the foundation of patient assessment. 'Listen to your patient, (s)he is telling you the diagnosis.' (Sir William Osler, 1849–1919).

Drug history

The patient is asked whether they are taking any medications, and what medications they have taken in the past, including prescribed and over-the-counter medications. Patients are also asked specifically about any use of recreational drugs or herbal remedies; this information may not be volunteered otherwise. If the patient is taking any medications, enquire about their adherence and any adverse reactions.

By establishing a medication history, drug reactions or interactions that could be causing the symptoms can be identified and further insight can be gained into the patient's other medical conditions.

Family history

The patient is asked about medical problems that affect other members of their family.

Inherited renal conditions to ask about are polycystic kidney disease, Alport's disease and Fabry's disease. If a condition runs in the family, a pictorial family tree (genogram) is useful to record the patient's relationship with affected family members and illustrate patterns of inheritance (**Figure 2.1**).

Social history

The social history addresses the social, occupational and recreational aspects of a patient's life. It includes questions about what the patient's occupation is (or was), who they live with and whether they smoke or drink. The answers to these questions provide an understanding of the patient's symptoms in the context of their life and the level of social support they receive. They also provide information on habits that might affect their health and therefore make certain conditions more likely.

Common symptoms

A symptom is a disturbance that is a manifestation of a disease or disorder and is identifiable by patients. Many symptoms of renal disease are non-specific and do not

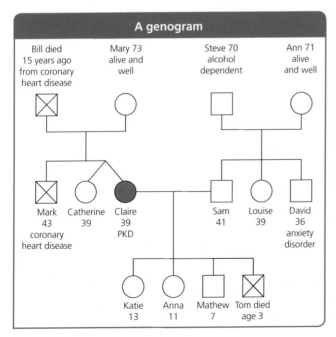

A genogram

| Bill died 15 years ago from coronary heart disease | Mary 73 alive and well | Steve 70 alcohol dependent | Ann 71 alive and well |

Mark 43 coronary heart disease   Catherine 39   Claire 39 PKD   Sam 41   Louise 39   David 36 anxiety disorder

Katie 13   Anna 11   Mathew 7   Tom died age 3

Figure 2.1 Example of a pictorial family tree (genogram). A genogram is used to record and interpret the patient's genetic relationships and the incidence of inherited disease among family members.

necessarily point towards renal pathology, for example tiredness, shortness of breath, nausea and loss of appetite, all of which could be caused by various other conditions. Renal disease is commonly asymptomatic; many cases of renal impairment are detected only incidentally, on the basis of blood test results.

Urinary abnormalities

These are abnormalities associated with passing urine. They generally result from problems in the lower urinary tract. However, some symptoms discussed in this section may result from a systemic process or an abnormality elsewhere in the urinary tract. Most urinary symptoms prompt a through abdominal examination, dipstick urinalysis, and sometimes imaging of the urinary tract.

Common urinary symptoms are discussed below. Questions to ask about urinary symptoms are listed in **Table 2.3**.

Dysuria

This is pain or a burning sensation on passing urine, and is caused by several pathologies affecting the bladder, urethra and other parts of the lower urinary tract. The most common cause is a UTI. Other causes are:

- interstitial cystitis, a condition characterised by chronic inflammation of the bladder wall
- urethral stricture, i.e. narrowing of the urethra
- bladder or urethral malignancy
- urethral or vaginal trauma
- prostatic, epididymal or testicular infection or inflammation
- compression from a pelvic mass

The patient is asked if they feel 'pain or burning on passing water'. It must be ascertained how long any symptoms have been present for, as well as any factors that improve or worsen the symptom.

Infective causes of dysuria, such as a UTI or a prostatic, epididymal or testicular infection, tend to develop quickly and resolve with the use of appropriate antibiotics. Dysuria

Questions for assessing urinary symptoms	
Symptom	Question(s)
Dysuria	'Have you had any pain or burning on passing water?'
Suprapubic pain	'Have you had any pain in the bladder area?'
Urinary frequency	'Have you found yourself needing to pass urine more frequently than normal?' If so, 'How many times a day are you going?'
Polyuria	'Are you passing more urine than normal?' If so, 'How much more?'
Oliguria	'Have you noticed passing less urine than normal?' If so, 'How many times a days are you going?'
Nocturia	'Do you get up at night to pass water?' If so, 'How many times?'
Hesitancy	'Have you had problems initiating your stream of urine?'
Terminal dribbling	'Have you had difficulty stopping the stream of urine after you have finished emptying your bladder?'
Urgency	'Have you found yourself needing to pass urine urgently or had any problems controlling your urinary system?'
Haematuria	'Have you noticed any blood in your urine?' If so, 'How much?' 'What colour is the urine?' 'Have you seen any clots?'

Table 2.3 Questions for assessing a patient with urinary symptoms

caused by a malignancy or stricture is likely to be more long-standing and will not improve significantly with antibiotics.

Suprapubic pain

This is pain in the area above the pubic bone and results from bladder abnormalities such as infection or urinary retention (inability to pass urine). Bladder infection or inflammation (cystitis) typically produces a burning type of pain. Urinary retention can cause severe pain in the suprapubic area.

Urinary frequency

This is the symptom of passing urine more frequently than normal. It may result from:

- production of too much urine, for example because of diabetes mellitus, diuretic use, excessive fluid intake or diabetes insipidus
- inability of the bladder to stretch, for example as a result of scarring after radiotherapy or post-infective fibrosis
- pathology within the bladder, for example a tumour, renal stones or a foreign body
- pressure on the bladder from surrounding structures, for example a gravid uterus or pelvic tumour
- instability of the detrusor muscle, which is responsible for bladder contraction, for example as a result of infection or a neurological condition such as multiple sclerosis

In cases of urinary frequency, in contrast to polyuria, the amount of urine passed may be small.

Different people pass urine more or less frequently than others, so what is normal for one patient may be abnormal for another. Therefore 'Have you been passing urine more frequently than normal?' is a more helpful initial question than 'How many times a day do you pass urine?' Be specific with language; for example, ask about 'passing urine' rather than 'going to the toilet', which could be interpreted as passing urine or opening the bowels.

Polyuria

This is the passage of abnormally large volumes of urine (> 3 L over 24 h in adults) with an associated increase in urinary frequency. It may result from:

- excessive fluid intake
- a primary renal abnormality resulting in an inability of the kidneys to concentrate urine
- cranial diabetes insipidus, in which production of antidiuretic hormone by the hypothalamus is impaired, resulting in failure of the kidneys to reabsorb water
- the use of drugs, for example diuretics, that increase the excretion of water by the kidneys

It is useful to try to determine the number of times a day the patient is passing urine. Asking the patient to keep a bladder diary in which they record how often they pass urine and how much they produce, helps with this.

As with any symptom, information about its duration is helpful. For example, polyuria that has been present for a day during which large amounts of fluid have been consumed is likely to be the result of excessive fluid intake.

Ask the patient whether they have started any new medications recently, because polyuria associated with starting diuretic therapy is likely to be drug-related.

Oliguria

This is the symptom of passing less urine than normal. In adults, this is less than 400 mL urine per day. It can be caused by AKI or CKD, in which the kidneys are unable to produce urine, or by an obstruction within the renal tract that prevents the passage of urine.

When asking a patient about oliguria, try to quantify the number of times urine is passed and the amount of urine passed in a 24-h period, as well as how long the symptom has been present. Oliguria that started suddenly is more likely to be the result of an acute obstruction within the renal tract, whereas a steady decline in the daily amount of urine passed over a longer period of time, e.g. weeks to months, is more likely to reflect a primary renal pathology.

Nocturia

Waking at night to pass urine may be caused by:

- fluid balance abnormalities as a result of excessive fluid intake, diabetes mellitus, diabetes insipidus, hypercalcaemia, primary renal disease or cardiac failure
- the use of drugs that increase urine output, for example diuretics
- neurological problems, including multiple sclerosis, that cause detrusor instability
- lower urinary tract pathology, such as bladder outflow irritation (as a consequence of prostatic or urethral disease), bladder overactivity, UTI, inflammation or malignancy

■ pressure from outside the bladder, for example in pregnancy

> **Nocturia is a common symptom of benign prostatic hyperplasia.** It can be a source of significant distress for patients and is strongly associated with poor quality-of-life ratings. It is a prominent cause of sleep disturbance and increases the likelihood of depression and time off work, as well as all-cause mortality.

Ask the patient, 'Do you get up in the night to pass water?' Discern what is normal for the individual; some people will say they always get up to pass urine one or twice every night and that this is normal for them, whereas for others this is pathological.

Hesitancy

This is a delay in starting or maintaining a stream of urine. It is most common in older men as a result of bladder outflow obstruction from an enlarged prostate, but it can also result from the use of drugs such as anticholinergics and tricyclic antidepressants, prostatic infection or inflammation, UTIs and neurological disorders.

Hesitancy is most likely to develop slowly over a period of months and the patient may not notice it at first. Therefore ask about this symptom specifically, with questions such as, 'Have you noticed any difficulty starting or maintaining a stream of urine?'

Terminal dribbling

Difficulty stopping the urinary stream after passing urine is most likely to result from sphincter problems or prostatic hypertrophy.

Urgency

This is the sudden urge to urinate such that delay is not possible, and may result in incontinence. It occurs because of irritation or inflammation of the bladder wall, for example as a result of a UTI, and is exacerbated by consumption of caffeine and fruit juice.

Haematuria

This is blood in the urine. It may be microscopic, and therefore not detectable by the naked eye, or visible to the patient. Blood may originate from any part of the urinary tract, so the causes of haematuria are numerous. They include:

■ UTI
■ urinary tract tumour
■ trauma
■ glomerulonephritis
■ renal stone disease
■ clotting abnormalities
■ surgery to the urinary tract
■ toxins, such as chemotherapy agents
■ uterine or vaginal bleeding

When assessing a patient with haematuria, clarify that the blood is definitely coming from the urine; this may require a vaginal or rectal examination to identify bleeding from the vagina or rectum, respectively. Additionally, microscopic haematuria may be the result of contamination of the urine with menstrual blood if the sample is provided by a female patient around the time of menstruation. Remember that certain foods, such as beetroot, turn urine pink.

Once it has been established that a patient has haematuria, determine the duration of the symptom, as well as the frequency with which it occurs, i.e. intermittently or with each urination. Long-standing haematuria, particularly if painless, is more likely to result from a malignancy, whereas haematuria with a more acute onset may result from a UTI or renal stone. Episodic episodes of haematuria also suggest renal stone disease.

Ask about medications; anticoagulants such as warfarin make haematuria more likely, and chemotherapeutic agents can cause bladder irritation resulting in haematuria. Exclude any recent infections, because post-infectious glomerulonephritis and immunoglobulin A nephropathy can cause haematuria.

A travel history is necessary when assessing a patient with haematuria, because schistosomiasis, a disease caused by parasitic worms, is a possible cause. In addition, a thorough occupational history should be taken, because certain occupational exposures (e.g. to paint components and polycyclic aromatic hydrocarbons) are associated with bladder cancer.

Frothy urine

Urine that appears frothy can occur under normal circumstances, for example as a result of rapid urination or the presence of cleaning products in the toilet. However, if persistent, it may indicate proteinuria and therefore nephrotic syndrome. It can also be caused by a UTI.

When assessing a patient for renal disease, ask whether they have noticed frothy urine, because they may not volunteer this information otherwise. It is necessary to monitor for frothy urine in patients with nephrotic syndrome, because its presence may indicate a relapse.

Loin pain

Loin pain is pain in the flank (**Figure 2.2**) and typically arises from the kidney. Renal stones are a common cause, but others are also considered (**Table 2.4**). These include pyelonephritis (infection of the kidney), obstruction of the ureter (e.g. as a result of a blood clot or papillary necrosis), kidney tumours and renal infarction.

Leg swelling

Leg swelling can represent leg oedema, i.e. swelling of the soft tissue of both legs as a consequence of accumulation of interstitial fluid (**Figure 2.3**). The swelling is typically 'dependent', i.e. it is influenced by gravity. In mobile people, it is therefore maximal around the feet and ankles and extends upwards. In patients who are bedbound, it collects around the sacrum.

If oedema is extensive, fluid may also accumulate in visceral cavities, for example in cases of pleural effusion or ascites, as well as in other body areas with loose skin, for example the periorbital and genital regions.

Causes of leg oedema include kidney, heart and liver failure (**Table 2.5** and **Figure 2.4**). **Table 2.6** summarises the key questions to ask when assessing a patient with limb oedema.

Symptoms of hypovolaemia

Hypovolaemia is a state of decreased circulating volume most commonly caused by a haemorrhage or dehydration. In renal medicine, it is most likely to be encountered as a cause of prerenal AKI, i.e. AKI due to decreased renal perfusion. Hypovolaemia in renal patients can also occur because of excess fluid removal during dialysis. Symptoms of hypovolaemia include thirst

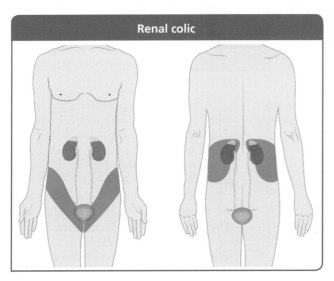

Renal colic

Figure 2.2 The referred 'loin-to-groin' loin or flank pain typically experienced with renal pain.

Causes of loin pain	
Cause	**Characteristics**
Renal stones	Sudden onset, severe pain that may radiate to the groin. The patient is often unable to lie still. On examination, there is tenderness over the renal angle. There may be invisible or visible haematuria.
Pyelonephritis	The patient is systemically unwell with pyrexia and, possibly, rigors. They may feel a dull ache. There may also be symptoms of dysuria and urinary frequency. There is tenderness at the renal angle. Dipstick urinalysis finds white blood cells and nitrites. Blood test results show leucocytosis and increased C-reactive protein.
Blood clots	Sudden ureteric obstruction and colicky pain similar to that of renal stones. Causes include renal biopsy, bleeding disorders, sickle cell disease and glomerulonephritis.
Papillary necrosis	Sloughed papillae can cause acute ureteric obstruction. This may occur with analgesic abuse, other causes of urinary tract obstruction, diabetes, renal transplant rejection and sickle cell disease.
Kidney tumours	Pain is likely to be gradual in onset, and there may be haematuria and a mass. Causes include renal cell carcinoma in adults and nephroblastoma (Wilms' tumour) in children.
Renal infarction	This causes loin pain on the affected side, which may be acute in onset and colicky (therefore indistinguishable from renal calculi), or more constant (similar to that of pyelonephritis). Risk factors include atrial fibrillation and older age.

Table 2.4 Causes of loin pain

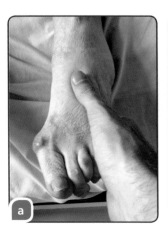
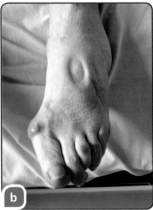

Figure 2.3 Assessing for pitting oedema of the lower limb. (a) A thumb or finger is pressed over the swelling for 5 seconds. (b) A pit is visible after removal.

as a result of osmoreceptor stimulation, and dizziness on standing, as a result of a sudden drop in blood pressure.

Uraemic symptoms

Uraemic symptoms comprise weakness, fatigue, generalised itching (pruritus), loss of appetite, nausea and vomiting (**Figure 2.5**). They are usually insidious and result from persistently increased levels of urea and other waste products in the blood.

The patient may not volunteer these symptoms, as complaints such as weakness and loss of appetite are easy to attribute to e.g. being stressed and are not recognised by the patient as symptoms of a disorder so it is necessary to ask about them directly.

Because these symptoms are so non-specific, the differential diagnosis is wide. It may include cardiac failure, liver failure, connective tissue diseases, malignancies, chronic infections and drug-related adverse effects.

Causes of leg oedema	
Cause	**Pathophysiology**
Renal failure	Increased hydrostatic pressure resulting from sodium and water retention and decreased oncotic pressure resulting from protein loss
Cardiac failure	Increased hydrostatic pressure resulting from pump failure, particularly in right heart failure
Liver cirrhosis	Decreased oncotic pressure resulting from hypoalbuminaemia and renal retention of sodium and water
Venous insufficiency	Increased hydrostatic pressure in veins, forcing fluid into the interstitium
Starvation, malabsorption, protein-losing enteropathy	Loss of protein, resulting in decreased oncotic pressure
Lymphoedema	Blockage of lymphatic channels, resulting in accumulation of interstitial fluid
Hypothyroidism (myxoedema)	Mucopolysaccharide deposition
Pregnancy	Increased hydrostatic pressure, resulting from water and sodium retention and lower limb venous congestion due to pressure exerted by the gravid uterus on the inferior vena cava and iliac veins
Deep vein thrombosis	Unilateral lower leg oedema (unless clinically apparent deep vein thrombosis affects both legs)

Table 2.5 Causes of leg oedema

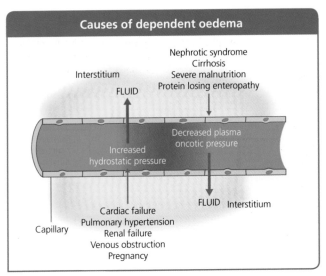

Figure 2.4 Causes of dependent oedema.

Key questions to ask are:

- 'Have you felt more tired than usual recently?'
- 'How is your appetite?'
- 'Have you had any nausea or vomiting?'
- 'Have you lost any weight recently?' If so, 'How much?' and 'Over what time period?'

Rash

Rashes, i.e. changes in the colour or texture of the skin, may be a sign of diseases with renal involvement. They are asked about when taking a renal history, and if present, inspected closely during the examination (see page 76).

Questions to ask the patient who has limb oedema	
Question	Significance
'When did it start?'	The swelling is likely to be gradual in onset, because most causes of limb oedema are chronic processes; more acute lower leg swelling may represent deep vein thrombosis
'How has it progressed?'	In mobile patients, dependent oedema starts around the feet and ankles and moves upwards
'Is it painful?'	Painful limb oedema suggests infection or deep venous thrombosis; dependent oedema can also be painful
'Have you felt breathless?'	Breathlessness suggests pulmonary oedema as a result of cardiac failure or renal insufficiency
'Do you feel short of breath when lying flat or wake up in the night short of breath?'	These symptoms (orthopnoea and paroxysmal nocturnal dyspnoea, respectively) suggest pulmonary oedema; they may indicate cardiac failure, or fluid overload as a consequence of renal failure

Table 2.6 Questions to ask the patient who has limb oedema

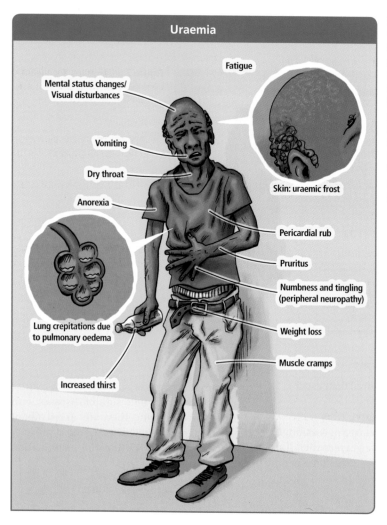

Figure 2.5 Clinical features of uraemia. Uraemic frost and neuropathy are very late signs that are rarely seen. Thirst is more common in patients on dialysis or who tend to lose sodium in the urine ('salt-wasting'), whereas oedema is seen in 'salt-retaining' patients.

Arthralgia

Arthralgia, i.e. joint pain, can occur in patients with connective tissue diseases (also known as autoimmune rheumatic diseases), such as vasculitis and systemic lupus erythematosus (SLE). Connective tissue diseases are chronic immune dysfunction or inflammatory disorders that can involve the kidneys either directly, with a targeted immune response, or indirectly, with deposition of inflammatory molecules.

Any joint may be affected, but arthralgia typically occurs in the small joints of the hands and feet. Pain in the large joints may be a symptom of Henoch–Schönlein purpura (see page 198).

Ear, nose and throat symptoms

These include ear pain, nasal blockage or discharge, and sinus pain. Such symptoms typically occur in granulomatosis with polyangiitis (previously called Wegener's granulomatosis), as a result of granulomatous disease of the ear, nose and throat mucosae. These symptoms may precede the onset of renal disease by years and need to be asked about specifically, because the patient might attribute them to a non-renal cause and not mention them.

Other possible causes of these symptoms include infections and ear, nose and throat malignancies. In cases of infection, an acute history is more likely. In cases of malignancy, the history is more chronic and systemic symptoms, such as weight loss, may be present.

Questions to ask the patient include:

- 'Have you had any ear problems recently or in the past?'
- 'Do you have any nasal congestion or discharge?'
- 'Have you ever had any sinus trouble?'

Eye symptoms

Eye pathology may occur in cases of connective tissue diseases that also cause renal disease, such as SLE and granulomatosis with polyangiitis. These conditions are associated with iritis, episcleritis or scleritis (**Table 2.7**).

Eye involvement in long-term conditions such as SLE can be episodic, so it is worth asking the following questions:

- 'Have you had red eyes?'
- 'Have you had any pain in your eyes, any blurred vision or any floating spots in your field of vision?'
- 'Have you found yourself more sensitive to light than normal?'

Connective tissue diseases: ophthalmological signs		
Sign	Definition	Symptoms
Iritis	Inflammation of the iris – a serious ocular condition	Redness, discomfort, headache, blurred vision, photophobia (light sensitivity) and floating spots in the field of vision
Episcleritis	Inflammation of the layer between the conjunctiva and the sclera – relatively benign and usually self-limiting	Redness of the eye, eye pain, photophobia and watering of the eye – less severe than scleritis
Scleritis	Inflammation of the sclera	Similar to those of episcleritis but often more severe and may be associated with decreased visual acuity

Table 2.7 Ophthalmological signs associated with connective tissue diseases

Common signs and how to examine a patient

Starter questions

Answers to the following questions are on page 132.

4. How does the renal examination vary from patient to patient?
5. Why might an examination of multiple systems be required in a renal patient?

Examination of the patient is usually carried out after the history and before investigations are arranged. The aim is to identify physical signs that support certain diagnoses and refute others. Potential diagnoses will have been suggested by the history, and the clinician has these in mind while examining the patient.

Many systemic diseases affect the kidneys, and renal disease causes abnormalities within other systems, for example when fluid overload resulting from a renal disorder causes pulmonary oedema. Therefore signs may be present in several different systems.

The renal examination starts with general inspection, which is followed by examination of each major system. The first to be examined is usually the cardiovascular system; next is the respiratory system, moving down to the abdomen, and finally the nervous system. An alternative approach is to base the examination around particular signs, specific to renal pathology, to be detected, elicited or excluded. This is the approach described in this section.

> In the context of an OSCE, the renal system is usually encountered within an abdominal examination station. In this setting, in addition to carrying out a full abdominal examination, look for features of fluid overload, dialysis access, transplantation scars and signs of connective tissue disease.

General inspection

Each clinical examination starts with an inspection of the patient and their surrounding area. If the patient is in a hospital bed, this is best done by standing at the foot of the bed, from where the patient and their surroundings are fully visible. If the patient is attending a clinic, the general inspection begins when they walk through the door. Traditionally, the examination starts with the patient supine, at a 45° angle.

> Before examining a patient, always explain what you are going to do before doing it, and ask for the patient's permission. Patients feel more at ease when they know what to expect during the examination.

> Ensure that the patient's dignity is maintained at all times by covering up parts of their body that are not being examined.

To avoid missing any diagnostic clues, the general inspection is approached systematically, for example looking at the patient from head to foot and then around their bed.

By making note of things that are immediately obvious, the clinician can deduce a large amount of useful information. The following questions are considered:

- Does the patient look well or unwell? (**Figure 2.6**)
- Are they comfortable or in pain?
- Are they attached to any monitoring equipment?
- Are there any drugs on the table next to the patient's bed?

Skin colour

Skin colour is assessed by looking at the patient, particularly their face. Pale skin suggests anaemia (low haemoglobin concentration), whereas a lemon-yellow tinge to the skin may represent uraemia. A clinically significant differential here is jaundice which indicates haemolysis, liver dysfunction or obstruction within the biliary tree. Look at the sclerae, they are yellow if jaundice is present but white if it is not.

Hands

Examination of the hands allows several signs to be sought. Ask the patient to hold their arms outstretched. This could show a postural tremor which may occur as a side effect of calcineurin inhibitors (e.g. tacrolimus in transplant patients). Then ask the patient to keep the arms outstretched and cock their wrists back; rapid jerking movements of the hands ('flapping tremor') can occur as a result of uraemia. White nails (leukonychia), a sign of hypoalbuminaemia, can occur in the nephrotic syndrome and koilonychia (spoon-shaped nails) is associated with iron-deficiency anaemia. Other finger nail changes are found in patients with vasculitis (see page 194). Fingertip pinpricks from capillary blood glucose monitoring are found in patients with diabetes (see page 79).

Scars, fistulae and catheters

Check for the presence of scars which provide evidence of previous surgery, biopsies or procedures for dialysis access (**Figure 2.7**).

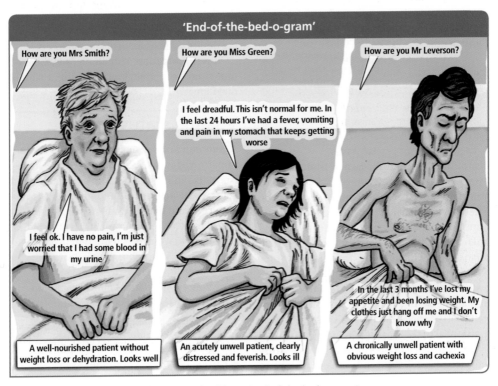

'End-of-the-bed-o-gram'

How are you Mrs Smith?

How are you Miss Green?

How are you Mr Leverson?

I feel dreadful. This isn't normal for me. In the last 24 hours I've had a fever, vomiting and pain in my stomach that keeps getting worse

I feel ok. I have no pain, I'm just worried that I had some blood in my urine

In the last 3 months I've lost my appetite and been losing weight. My clothes just hang off me and I don't know why

A well-nourished patient without weight loss or dehydration. Looks well

An acutely unwell patient, clearly distressed and feverish. Looks ill

A chronically unwell patient with obvious weight loss and cachexia

Figure 2.6 Initial impressions of a patient's health: an 'end-of-the-bed-o-gram'.

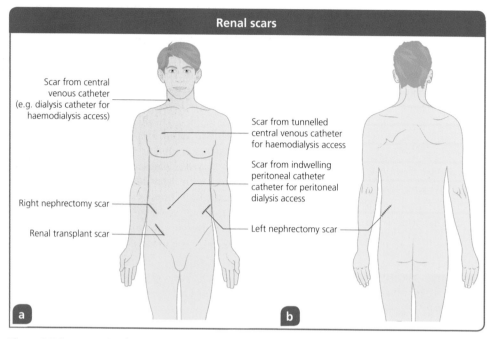

Figure 2.7 Scars associated with renal disease. (a) Anterior view. (b) Posterior view.

During an OSCE exam, systematically examine for scars, biopsies and dialysis access points to demonstrate an understanding that these provide important clues in differential diagnosis. In clinical practice, if the information is not easily accessible in the patient's notes this systematic approach will ensure signs are not missed.

Examine the neck for scars from central venous catheters, which may have been used for dialysis in the past. Inspect the anterior chest wall for scars from tunnelled dialysis lines. Transfer your attention to the abdomen and inspect for scars in the right or left iliac fossae, which may be from surgery for a kidney transplant. Ask the patient to sit forward, and inspect their back for large diagonal scars from a nephrectomy. Small scars anteriorly may be the former sites of entry of peritoneal dialysis catheters.

The presence of a peritoneal dialysis catheter (see **Figure 2.45**) indicates that the patient is or has been on peritoneal dialysis, or is soon to start on it. Therefore it shows that the patient has end–stage renal disease.

Catheters and fistulae created for dialysis are described in more detail on pages 116–117.

This information should, if possible, be drawn in the patient's notes using a simple diagram.

Volume status

A common and serious consequence of renal impairment is disturbance of volume status. Normally, to maintain a constant body fluid volume, the amount of fluid taken in is equal to the amount of fluid that is lost in urine, faeces, sweat, via the respiratory tract and vaginal secretions in women. A reduction in glomerular filtration rate (GFR) typically results in fluid overload, because the kidneys are unable to excrete excess water. Volume depletion can also occur in the context of renal impairment, for example as the cause of AKI.

Assessment of volume status is a key aspect of clinical assessment in renal medicine, and is carried out during both the history and the examination of the patient. As with any aspect of an examination, a systematic approach is used. Assessment usually begins with general inspection before moving up to the neck for the jugular venous pressure, then to relevant parts of the chest and down to the sacrum and legs to assess for oedema.

Inspection

Begin with a general inspection. Facial puffiness suggests fluid overload. If it is severe, the patient may be breathless at rest or receiving oxygen via nasal cannulae or a face mask. Feel the patient's skin to check its temperature; cool peripheries may be a sign of volume depletion.

Jugular venous pressure

Look for the jugular venous pressure waveform. This is an indirect measure of central venous pressure, because the internal jugular vein is connected to the right atrium, with no valves in between.

For this part of the examination, the patient sits at a 45° angle, with their head turned to the left. The internal jugular vein runs between the two heads of the sternocleidomastoid muscle, and the jugular venous pressure is visible as a double-waveform pulsation.

The level of the jugular venous pressure is measured as the vertical distance between the sternal angle and the top of the venous pulsation (**Figure 2.8**). Jugular venous pressure > 3 cm suggests that central venous pressure is increased and therefore indicates fluid overload. In contrast, if the patient has volume depletion, jugular venous pressure will not usually be visible, but it may be seen if the patient lies prone or if the hepatojugular reflex is assessed. This is done by first ensuring that the patient has no abdominal pain, then applying firm pressure to the right upper quadrant. A transient elevation in jugular venous pressure, of about 2 cm for a few seconds, is normal.

> If volume depletion is suspected, it may be helpful to compare the patient's blood pressure when lying and standing. A decrease of > 20 mmHg in systolic pressure within a minute of standing is a sign of hypovolaemia.

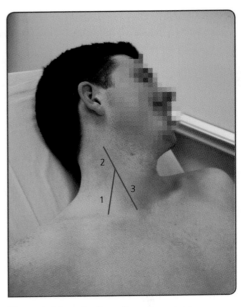

Figure 2.8 Examination of jugular venous pressure. The patient is positioned at a 45° angle with their head turned to the left. The internal jugular vein runs under the medial edge of the sternocleidomastoid muscle (SCM) ②. Look for a double-waveform pulsation; it is helpful to palpate the left carotid artery while doing so. ①, clavicular head of the SCM; ③, sternal head of the SCM.

Heart sounds

Listen with a stethoscope, with both the diaphragm and the bell, at the four valve areas (**Figure 2.9**). The diaphragm is best for detecting high pitch sounds, for example the murmurs of aortic and mitral regurgitation. The bell is better for low pitch sounds, for example the murmur of mitral stenosis.

While auscultating, palpate the carotid pulse to orient where sounds are occurring in the cardiac cycle.

Heart sounds reflect the valves shutting.

- S1 and S2 are normally the most obvious; they are audible as a 'lub-dub' sound, representing closure of the tricuspid and mitral (bicuspid) valve followed by that of the aortic and pulmonary valves
- S3 and S4 are 'added heart sounds' and can represent pathology (**Figure 2.10**)

In fluid overload, a third heart sound may be audible after the second heart sound, thereby producing a gallop rhythm. It is caused by

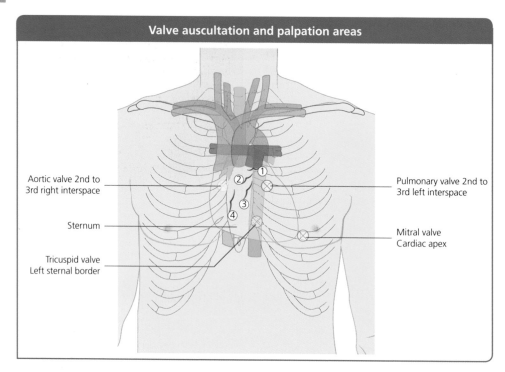

Valve auscultation and palpation areas

Aortic valve 2nd to 3rd right interspace

Sternum

Tricuspid valve Left sternal border

Pulmonary valve 2nd to 3rd left interspace

Mitral valve Cardiac apex

Figure 2.9 Location of the auscultation and palpation areas of the apex beat and heart valves. ① pulmonary valve; ② aortic valve; ③ mitral valve; ④ tricuspid valve; ⊗, aortic valve auscultation point; ⊗, pulmonary valve auscultation point; ⊗, tricuspid valve auscultation point; ⊗, mitral valve auscultation point (and apex beat).

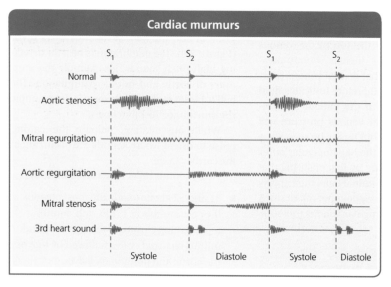

Cardiac murmurs

S_1 S_2 S_1 S_2

Normal

Aortic stenosis

Mitral regurgitation

Aortic regurgitation

Mitral stenosis

3rd heart sound

Systole Diastole Systole Diastole

Figure 2.10 Cardiac murmurs

rapid filling of a distended or poorly compliant ventricle during diastole, and is best heard with the bell of the stethoscope over the right or left ventricular apex (the left 4th or 5th intercostal space, respectively).

Lungs

Examine the chest for signs that indicate fluid within the pleural cavity or within the smaller bronchi, broncholies and alveoli.

Percuss the area overlying the lungs (**Figure 2.11**) for dullness, which may represent a pleural effusion caused by fluid overload. Normal lung is filled with air and sounds resonant when the overlying surface is tapped.

Percussion involves tapping on the surface of the body to determine what lies underneath: air, fluid or a solid organ. The non-dominant middle finger is placed on the surface (e.g. chest wall) and the distal interphalangeal joint is tapped with the tip of the dominant middle finger. The sound elicited is resonant if air lies beneath (e.g. lungs), or dull if fluid (e.g. pleural effusion) or an organ lies underneath.

Auscultate the chest with a stethoscope at the same points of percussion. Decreased air entry at one or both bases suggests pleural

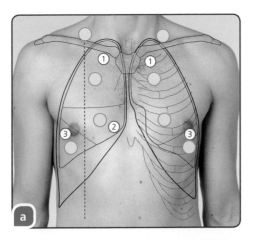

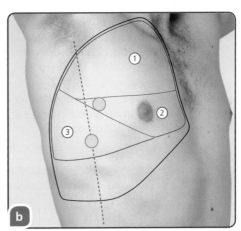

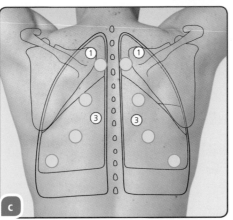

Figure 2.11 Placement of the stethoscope (blue circles) for auscultation and percussion. (a) Anterior view. (b) Axillae. (c) Posterior view. ①, upper lobes; ②, middle lobe; ③, lower lobes.

effusion. Crepitations ('crackles') at the bases may be the result of pulmonary oedema secondary to fluid overload. CKD is a cause of this, but key other causes include heart failure and liver failure. Crepitations may also indicate consolidation caused by infection.

Peripheral oedema

To complete the assessment of volume status, assess the ankles and sacrum for pitting oedema (see **Figure 2.3**). Gently press a thumb or finger against the patient's skin for a few seconds. If interstitial fluid is present, an imprint will be visible after removal of the pressure. Take care, because this can be painful for the patient.

■ Causes of pitting oedema include kidney, heart or liver failure (see **Table 2.5**)
■ Non-pitting oedema occurs when pressure on the affected area does not leave an indentation. It is caused by myxoedema, lymphoedema and lipoedema. In these conditions, the oncotic pressure within the interstitium remains high (e.g. due to blockage within the lymphatic

system in lymphoedema which results in plasma proteins that have leaked out remaining in the interstitium), preventing water from being dispersed when pressure is applied

Signs of vasculitic or connective tissue disease

Both AKI and CKD may be caused by vasculitis and connective tissue diseases. Various signs may be associated with these conditions and are sought when examining a patient presenting for the first time with renal impairment, or a patient known to have a connective tissue disease.

Rashes

Rashes are common in these disorders and represent either inflammation of small blood vessels mediated by neutrophil leukocyctes (leukocytoclastic vasculitis), and/or involvement of larger vessels with downstream ischaemia (livedo reticularis) (**Table 2.8**). Key types are:

Connective tissue diseases: rashes		
Rash	Description	Significance
Malar rash	An erythematous, butterfly-shaped rash across the nose and cheeks (see Figure 2.12)	A typical sign of SLE
Purpuric rash	Purple discoloration of the skin as a result of small bleeding vessels at the skin's surface (see Figure 2.13). Can be palpable or non-palpable (macular)	Macular purpura is typically non-inflammatory (e.g. due to trauma). Palpable purpura is a sign of blood vessel inflammation (vasculitis)
	Macular purpura is divided according to size into: ■ petechiae: small ares (<1 cm) ■ ecchymoses: larger lesions (>1cm)	A palpable purpuric rash on the buttocks is associated with Henoch–Schönlein purpura
Vasculitic rash	A palpable, non-blanching purpuric rash mainly seen in the extremities (see Figure 6.1a)	Occurs in primary vasculitides
Photosensitive rash	An erythematous eruption on sun-exposed areas	Occurs in more than 50% of patients with SLE
Livedo reticularis	A reticular, mottled discoloration of the skin, with cyanotic areas surrounding pale central areas	Seen in various vasculitides, including SLE, rheumatoid arthritis and polyarteritis nodosa, as well as in cases of cryoglobulinaemia, antiphospholipid syndrome and cholesterol emboli (see Figure 9.4)

SLE, systemic lupus erythematosus.

Table 2.8 Rashes associated with connective tissue diseases

- malar rash of SLE (**Figure 2.12**)
- vasculitic rash (see Figure 6.1a), which is characterised by purpura that is typically palpable
- purpuric rashes (**Figure 2.13**), which are characterised by purple spots on the skin that do not blanch (whiten) under pressure. It occurs due to bleeding from small blood vessels
- livedo reticularis (see Figure 9.4), which is characterised by a reticular (net-like) discolouration of the skin with red-blue cyanotic areas surrounding pale areas

A rash is best assessed by exposing the skin. This is done sequentially to maintain the patient's dignity, for example starting with the arms and face, then moving to the torso and back, and finally to the buttocks, legs and feet. The appearance and distribution of any abnormal findings should be documented in the patient's notes, ideally with a diagram. The presence of rashes prompts consideration of an autoimmune screen.

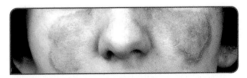

Figure 2.12 Malar rash: a rash over the cheeks and nasal bridge in patients with systemic lupus erythematosus. It is also known as a 'butterfly rash'.

Hands

Other features of vasculitis include nail fold infarcts and splinter haemorrhages. Nail fold infarcts are small brown spots around the nails and indicate small and larger vessel vasculitis. Splinter haemorrhages are thin, red-brown vertical lines underneath the nail that represent small areas of bleeding (see Figure 6.1b). These signs are detected by looking closely at the nails. They are also seen in infective endocarditis (**Figure 2.14**).

Neurological signs

Systemic lupus erythematosus (SLE) and other causes of vasculitis can affect the central and peripheral nervous systems. In SLE, this is due to autoantibody production, inflammatory and non-inflammatory SLE vasculopathies, proinflammatory cytokine production within the spinal cord and metabolic aberrations. Central nervous system manifestations of SLE are varied and include confusion, seizures and upper motor neurone signs. Up to 75% of SLE patients have neuropsychiatric manifestations of the disease.

Vasculitis also causes inflammatory occlusion of blood vessels supplying peripheral nerves, resulting in ischaemia, infarction and peripheral nerve degeneration. The clinical effects of vasculitis on the peripheral nervous system include polyneuropathy, where

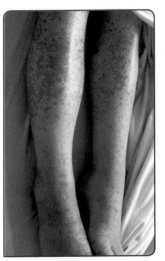

Figure 2.13 A palpable purpuric rash on the lower legs.

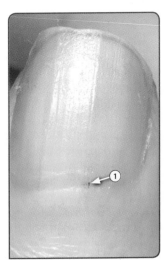

Figure 2.14 A small splinter haemorrhage ① in a woman with bacterial endocarditis.

motor and sensory peripheral nerves are affected, predominantly distally, and mononeuritis multiplex, the sequential involvement of multiple single nerves (motor and sensory components). Symptoms include sensory disturbances such as pain, numbness and paraesthesia, and focal weakness due to motor nerve involvement. The distribution is typically asymetrical. Patients often present with an acute attack and subsequently suffer relapses; however, some do experience a more indolent, progressive course.

Confusion and seizures are usually obvious on observation of the patient. However, upper and lower motor neurone signs would have to be elicited during a neurological examination.

Uraemic signs

Uraemia ('urea in the blood') is a clinical syndrome that is usually encountered in the latter stages of CKD. It also occurs in severe AKI that has developed very rapidly. The syndrome results from the constellation of fluid, electrolyte, endocrine and metabolic derangements that occur when the kidneys fail, and is responsible for many of the non-specific symptoms associated with renal disease (see page 66).

Some signs of uraemia (**Table 2.9**; see also **Figure 2.5**) may be found in a patient with AKI or CKD on general inspection. Others may be detected during examination of the cardiovascular and neurological systems.

Clinical signs of uraemia		
System	Sign	Pathophysiology
Skin	Yellow skin	Deposition of urochromes and carotene in the epidermis and subcutaneous tissue
	Scratch marks	Pruritus thought to be caused by a combination of dry skin, impaired sweating, abnormal calcium, phosphate and PTH metabolism, accumulation of uraemic toxins, systemic inflammation and common co-morbidities such as diabetes
	Uraemic frost	Deposition of crystallised urea on the skin
Cardiovascular system	Pericardial rub: a scratching noise audible on auscultation of the heart, in addition to normal heart sounds; its character changes with respiration and movement, and it is heard most clearly between the apex and the sternum	Pericarditis (inflammation of the pericardium), which has various causes The pathogenesis of uraemic pericarditis is poorly understood but it correlates with the degree of uraemia.
Respiratory system	Kussmaul's respiration, a deep, laboured pattern of breathing	Metabolic acidosis
	Pleural effusion	Inflammation of the pleura. The exact pathogenesis of uraemic pleural effusion is unclear
	Pulmonary oedema	Increased permeability of the alveolar-capillary interface
Gastrointestinal system	Nausea and vomiting	Stimulation of the vomiting centre of the brain by accumulated toxins in the blood
	Gastrointestinal bleeding	Platelet dysfunction: increased platelet turnover, impaired platelet adhesion and aggregation
Nervous system	Sensory or motor dysfunction	Distal sensorimotor neuropathy caused by uraemic toxins characterised by axonal degeneration and demyelination.
	Altered mental state: confusion, decreased consciousness, seizures and coma	Complex, multifactorial process influenced by accumulation of toxins, imbalance of neurotransmitters in the brain and hormonal disturbances (pariticularly PTH)

Table 2.9 Signs of uraemia

Signs associated with diabetes and diabetic complications

Diabetes is a leading cause of CKD, therefore its signs and complications are looked for in patients presenting with CKD. Whether or not the patient has diabetes will probably have been established from the history, so these signs do not necessarily need to be sought in non-diabetic patients. However, it is possible for patients to have diabetes without being aware of it, so a high index of suspicion is required.

Hands

On inspection of the fingertips, it may be possible to see pinpricks. This finding suggests that the patient has been monitoring their blood glucose concentration by pricking their fingertips to obtain small amounts of capillary blood for testing.

Eyes

With the patient seated, each eye is examined with an ophthalmoscope to look for signs of diabetic retinopathy, i.e. damage to the retina resulting from diabetes (**Table 2.10**). These signs indicate diabetic microvascular disease, which causes leakage of blood or blood contents from vessels, enlargement of vessels, and formation of new vessels; it also results in damage from deficiency of oxygen supply to the retina, i.e. ischaemia. The presence of these microvascular changes in the retina suggests that similar pathology is also occurring in the glomeruli, i.e. diabetic nephropathy.

Visual acuity is also checked with the use of a Snellen chart. Symptoms of diabetic retinopathy include floaters, blurred vision and progressive loss of acuity.

Diabetic retinopathy: grading		
Grade*	Sign(s)	Pathophysiology
R0: normal	None	
R1: mild non-proliferative	Microaneurysms	Small capillary dilations caused by weakening of the capillary wall
	Dot-and-blot haemorrhages	Intraretinal leakage of blood through the weakened capillary wall
	Flame haemorrhages	Superficial retinal haemorrhages that track along nerve fibres due to rupture of weakened capillaries
R2: moderate non-proliferative	Hard exudates (areas of white-yellow)	Leakage of proteins and lipoproteins from retinal blood vessels
R2: severe non-proliferative	Cotton wool spots (pale areas)	Accumulation of axonal debris at the margins of ischaemic areas, as a result of poor axonal metabolism
	Venous beading	Dilation of veins as a result of ischaemia
R3: severe proliferative	Neovascularisation	Growth of new blood vessels into hypoxic retinal tissue
	Vitreous or preretinal haemorrhage	Haemorrhage of the major retinal vessels
	Retinal detachment	Fibrovascular changes
P: treated with laser photocoagulation	Scarring	Laser treatment

*A grading of M1 requires that the signs have reached the macula. A grading of ≥ R2 indicates referral to an ophthalmologist.

Table 2.10 Grades of diabetic retinopathy according to the UK's National Health Service diabetic eye screening programme

Feet

The feet are examined for changes associated with diabetic neuropathy and arteriopathy. These include:

- deformities in shape
- reduced perfusion, as indicated by cool temperature and pale colour
- signs of sensory neuropathy, such as impaired light touch, pain, temperature, vibration and proprioception sensations in a glove-and-stocking distribution, and calluses and ulcers (**Figure 2.15**) due to abnormal weight-bearing and injury, respectively, as a part of neurological examination

Vascular examination

Diabetes is strongly associated with peripheral vascular disease, because of an increased level of atherosclerosis, i.e. fatty immune cell deposits in arterial walls. This results in decreased blood perfusion, which affects the peripheries first and is assessed clinically by checking the following.

- Colour: red and well perfused with arterial blood, or pale or blue?
- Temperature: palpate the feet and hands; cool extremeties, particularly the feet, indicate poor blood supply
- Capillary refill time: press a nail for 5 s; on letting go, the colour should return within 2 s

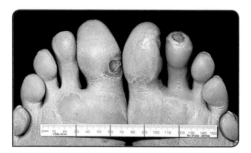

Figure 2.15 Arterial ulcers in a patient with diabetes. Arterial ulcers, in contrast to venous ulcers, are usually deep, regular in shape and painful, and have minimal exudate.

Peripheral pulses

The pulses of the lower limb (**Figure 2.16**) are palpated, or more sensitively, assessed by Doppler US, to detect their presence and determine their strength.

The ankle–brachial pressure index (ABPI) is a ratio of the blood pressure measured at the ankle and that measured at the upper arm. Peripheral vascular disease causes a decrease in ankle pressure, i.e. ABPI < 1.

Diabetic neurological examination

Diabetic peripheral neuropathy first affects the longest sensory nerve fibres, i.e. those supplying the feet and hands. This results in a 'glove and stocking' pattern of sensory neuropathy (**Figure 2.17**) and is assessed by various reproducible examination tests, such as the Ipswich touch test, which is carried out as follows.

1. Ask the patient to close their eyes and to say 'yes' when they feel a touch on their toes
2. Lightly touch one of their 1st (big) toes with a finger
3. Repeat by touching the 3rd (middle) and 5th (little) toe of the same foot, then the 1st, 3rd and 5th toes of the other foot
4. Calculate a score out of 6 for the number of times the patient correctly said 'yes' in response to a touch

A score of > 2 insensate areas indicates significant sensory neuropathy.

Signs associated with urinary tract obstruction

Obstruction of bladder outflow is a potentially reversible cause of renal failure that must not be missed. The bladder is examined by palpating the suprapubic region, i.e. above the pubic bone. If the bladder contains > 500 mL of urine, it may be palpable as a suprapubic mass that is dull to percussion over the area.

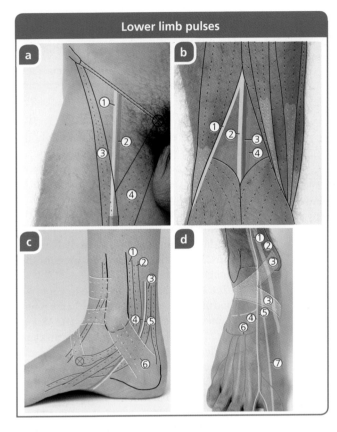

Lower limb pulses

Figure 2.16 Pulses of the lower limb: the femoral, popliteal, posterior and anterior tibial arteries. (a) ①, femoral nerve; ②, femoral artery; ③, sartorius; ④, adductor longus; ⓧ, pubic tubercle. (b) ①, common fibular nerve; ②, tibial nerve; ③, popliteal vein; ④, popliteal artery. (c) ①, tibialis posterior tendon; ②, flexor digitorum longus; ③, flexor hallucis longus; ④, posterior tibial artery; ⑤, tibial nerve; ⑥, flexor retinaculum. (d) ①, anterior tibial artery; ②, tibialis anterior tendon; ③, inferior extensor retinaculum; ④, medial branch of deep fibular nerve; ⑤, dorsalis pedis artery; ⑥, arcuate artery; ⑦, extensor hallucis longus tendon.

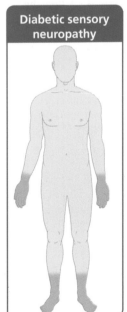

Diabetic sensory neuropathy

Figure 2.17 The 'glove and stocking' distribution of diabetic sensory neuropathy.

Bladder outflow obstruction is most commonly found in men with prostatic disease. Its presence indicates a digital rectal examination to assess prostate size.

Palpable kidneys

When examining the renal system, look for enlarged kidneys, because this finding may point towards the underlying cause of renal disease. It is rarely possible to palpate normal-sized kidneys, even in slim individuals.

Check whether the kidneys are 'ballottable', i.e. capable of being 'bounced' back and forth, during bimanual palpation (**Figure 2.18**). This is done by placing one hand posteriorly in the flank region and the other hand above it; an enlarged kidney may be balloted when palpated between the two hands.

Kidney palpation

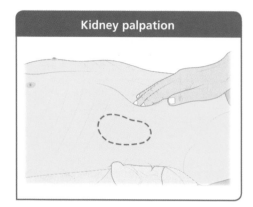

Figure 2.18 Bimanual palpation of kidney.

The most common cause of enlarged kidneys is adult polycystic kidney disease, which can be confirmed by ultrasound. Other causes include renal tumours.

A renal transplant is usually palpable beneath the scar in the left or right iliac fossa.

Renal bruits

A bruit is an abnormal harsh systolic sound audible with a stethoscope placed over an artery; it is generated by turbulent flow. Renal artery bruits are best heard by placing the stethoscope on either side of the midline above the umbilicus (**Figure 2.19**), and indicate renal artery stenosis. If a bruit is present, all peripheral pulses are examined and bruits sought elsewhere, for example the carotid artery, to look for signs of atheromatous disease.

Blood pressure

Blood pressure is an estimate of the force that blood is exerting against the walls of the arteries and represents the balance between cardiac output and vascular tone. It is an extremely useful clinical tool as it can be used to gauge disease severity in cases of volume depletion (e.g. due to blood loss), the systemic inflammatory response syndrome (e.g. due to infection), cardiac dysfunction of any cause, and to diagnose, monitor and manage hypertension.

The kidney has a central role in control of blood pressure, largely via its role in the renin–angiotensin–aldosterone system (RAAS; see page 35). Renal disease of any kind can cause hypertension. Hypertension, in turn, can cause and accelerate renal disease.

Blood pressure is measured with the use of a sphygmomanometer and a stethoscope (**Figure 2.20**) or an automated monitor. Blood pressure measurement with a sphygmomanometer and stethoscope is carried out as follows.

1. Ask the patient to remain still and rest their arm on a desk or similar

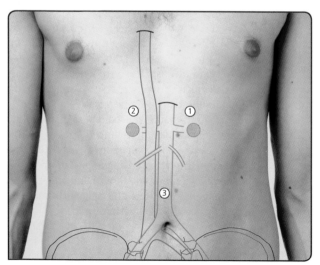

Figure 2.19 Auscultation points for renal bruit. ①, left renal artery; ②, right renal artery; ③, abdominal aorta.

Blood pressure measurement

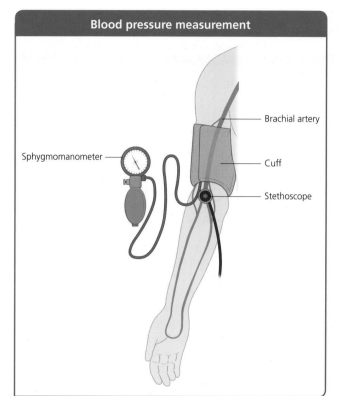

- Sphygmomanometer
- Brachial artery
- Cuff
- Stethoscope

Figure 2.20 Measurement of blood pressure using a sphygmomanometer and stethoscope.

2. Place the sphygmomanometer cuff around the patient's upper arm, at about heart height
3. Place the diaphragm over the brachial artery
4. Inflate the cuff until the radial pulse is obliterated
5. Listen as the cuff is steadily deflated
6. Record the pressure at which Korotkoff sounds of turbulent flow are heard: this is the highest, systolic, pressure

7. Record the pressure at which they disappear: this is the lowest, diastolic, pressure.

The definition of high blood pressure (hypertension) depends on a patient's characteristic but is generally considered to be >140/90 mmHg.

Investigations

Starter questions

Answers to the following questions are on page 132.

6. Why are so many tests performed on patients presenting for the first time with renal impairment?
7. Why is a blood film sometimes requested for a patient with acute kidney injury (AKI)?
8. How is renal ultrasound useful in assessing AKI?

Once a thorough history and examination have been carried out, investigations are required to:

- confirm or refute the differential diagnoses
- assess the severity of the disease
- establish a baseline for monitoring the disease

For renal patients, the key investigations are urine tests, blood tests, imaging studies, histopathology and electrocardiography (ECG).

Choosing investigations

Not all patients require all investigations; different investigations are chosen depending on the presentation and the suspected diagnosis. For example, a patient presenting with AKI requires a range of blood and urine tests, a renal US scan and a chest radiograph at a minimum, whereas a patient with urinary tract obstruction requires fewer blood tests but possibly more detailed imaging of the renal tract with a CT scan.

Unnecessary investigations can cause more harm than good. They might detect irrelevant problems, prompting investigations that unnecessarily expose patients to radiation or painful or unpleasant procedures, and that also waste resources. Always tailor investigations to each specific case.

Most patients presenting with renal impairment for the first time undergo a 'renal screen', which consists of many of the urine and blood tests detailed below, as well as an US scan of the renal tract, a chest radiograph and an electrocardiogram. The results of the screen are used to identify common causes of renal impairment, such as diabetes, as well as rarer diseases, such as SLE. More specialised imaging or renal biopsy may be required depending on what the renal screen shows. Often, more investigations are requested for new patients in renal medicine than in other specialties.

Blood urea and creatinine concentrations and estimated GFR (eGFR) give an immediate indication of the severity of renal impairment. Other blood tests, such as measurement of sodium and potassium concentrations, blood gas analysis and the bone profile provide further information on the severity of renal impairment and confirm the presence of associated complications, such as hyperkalaemia and renal bone disease. More specialised immunological tests, such as measurement of anti-glomerular basement membrane antibodies and HIV serology, are used to exclude specific disorders.

Urine tests

Urine tests are used to test for substances that suggest:

- impaired kidney function, for example protein
- renal tract infection, for example nitrites
- the presence of renal stones, for example calcium

A range of urine tests are useful in the investigation of renal disease (**Table 2.11**).

> Disorders of antidiuretic hormone, a hormone that increases water reabsorption in the renal tubules, interfere with the ability of the kidneys to concentrate urine and the concentration of serum sodium. Paired urine and serum osmolalities are a useful laboratory test to assess this ability, and are a first-line investigation for determining the cause of hyponatraemia.

Urinalysis

Urinalysis is a bedside test used as a screening tool in patients presenting with renal impairment. Urine is collected in a clear pot and initially assessed visually to determine whether it is:

- concentrated (suggests dehydration)
- dilute (suggests good hydration or polyuria)
- cloudy (suggests infection)
- discoloured (e.g. contains blood)

The dipstick examination is then performed: a stick containing pads with different chemical reagents ('reagent strips') is dipped in the urine. The pads change colour on contact with urine and are compared to a chart to determine the presence and quantity of protein (proteinuria), glucose (glucosuria), ketones (ketonuria), haemoglobin (haematuria), nitrite and leucocytes and to test pH and specific gravity. Quantitative measurements are reported in increasing amounts as: trace, 1+, 2+, 3+ and 4+. Very large amounts of protein are therefore read as '4+'.

A normal urinary pH is 5.5–6.5, but can vary between 4.5 and 8. Filtrate initially has the same pH as blood (7.35–7.45), but acidifies as it passes through the nephron. Very high urinary pH occurs in systemic alkalosis, renal tubular acidosis and with the use of certain drugs, e.g. sodium bicarbonate. Very acidic urine is found in systemic acidosis, diabetes, starvation and high-protein diets.

Urinary specific gravity is a measure of the amount of solute dissolved in urine, compared to that of water which has a specific gravity of 1. It is therefore proportional to urine osmolality. A low specific gravity (<1.005) suggests excessive hydration or a defect in the ability of the kidneys to concentrate urine. An increased specific gravity (>1.035) occurs in dehydration, glycosuria, proteinuria and the use of intravenous contrast.

The presence of leucocytes (white blood cells), detected as leucocyte esterase activity, and nitrites in urine suggest the presence

Investigation of renal disease: urine tests	
Test	Function
Urinalysis	Tests for protein, glucose, haemoglobin, nitrite, leucocytes, ketones, pH and specific gravity
Albumin:creatinine ratio (ACR) or protein:creatinine ratio (PCR)	To detect and quantify proteinuria
Osmolality	To assess the ability of the kidneys to concentrate urine
Sodium	To assess tubular reabsorptive function
Urinary chloride	To distinguish between causes of metabolic alkalosis
Tests for stone disease, including urinary calcium, oxalate, urate, citrate and cysteine	To identify renal stone disease
Myoglobin	To identify rhabdomyolysis (muscle destruction)
Bence Jones protein	To detect an immunoglobulin light chain characteristic of multiple myeloma
Microscopy	To detect characteristic findings of particular diseases

Table 2.11 Urine tests used in the investigation of renal disease

of urinary infection; urinary nitrates are converted to nitrites when Gram negative bacteria such as *Escherichia coli* are present. A positive test for glucose occurs with an elevated serum glucose concentration (e.g. in diabetes). Ketonuria (ketone bodies in the urine) occurs when ketone bodies are produced during fat metabolism. After accumulating in plasma, they are excreted in the urine. Ketonuria is associated with low-carbohydrate diets, starvation, diabetic ketoacidosis, hyperthyroidism and alcoholism.

Protein and haemoglobin in the urine suggests glomerular disease.

Renal impairment with minimal or no proteinuria suggests tubular diseases such as acute tubular necrosis and tubulointerstitial nephritis, or vascular pathology such as renovascular disease.

> **Myoglobin in the urine causes the same colour change on the reagent strip as urinary haemoglobin.** This can cause a false positive result for haematuria in patients with rhabdomyolysis (muscle breakdown).

Albumin:creatinine ratio and protein:creatinine ratio

The albumin:creatinine ratio (ACR) and protein:creatinine ratios (PCR) are used to detect and quantify proteinuria. The ACR is a measure of the albumin fraction whereas the PCR is a measure of total protein. ACR has a greater sensitivity than PCR to low-level proteinuria (microalbuminuria) not detectable on dipstick analysis; this occurs in the early stages of diabetic nephropathy. PCR is a better measure of total urinary protein concentration and is a better test for patients with non-diabetic kidney disease.

Osmolality

This assesses the ability of the kidneys to concentrate urine. It measures the number of dissolved particles per unit of water and is a more accurate measure of urinary concentration than specific gravity.

Urinary sodium

This is measured to assess tubular reabsorptive function. Low urinary sodium suggests normal reabsorptive function (sodium is being reabsorbed from filtrate), whereas increased urinary sodium indicates renal salt wasting (loss of sodium into the urine). Urinary sodium is useful for distinguishing between the causes of AKI (see page 149) or hyponatraemia (see page 224).

Urinary myoglobin

Myoglobin is a small protein found within muscle that is released into the blood when muscle is damaged, e.g. in rhabdomyolysis. Myoglobin is excreted into the urine causing an increase in urinary myoglobin.

Bence Jones protein

The Bence Jones protein is an immunoglobulin light chain found in urine that is associated with multiple myeloma. The test is carried out as part of a myeloma screen and is considered in older patients (>40 years) presenting with renal impairment.

Urine microscopy

Urine is examined under a light microscope to look for microscopic abnormalities associated with particular diseases:

■ Dysmorphic red cells and red blood cell casts indicate glomerular pathology.
■ White blood cell casts suggest the presence of pyelonephritis or inflammatory states such as tubulointerstitial nephritis and nephrotic syndrome.
■ Granular casts are formed from degenerating cellular casts and are therefore associated with glomerular pathology, infection or inflammatory states.
■ Hyaline casts are seen in proteinuric diseases such as glomerulonephritis.
■ Urinary eosinophils suggest tubulointerstitial nephritis.
■ Crystals are visible in urine samples from patients taking certain drugs (e.g. indinavir, an anti-viral medication).

Blood tests

Biochemical, haematological and immunological blood tests are used in investigating renal disease. Abnormal renal function affects various blood parameters including haemoglobin, sodium, potassium, urea, creatinine, calcium, phosphate and bicarbonate. These are measured to assess the severity of renal impairment, determine which complications have occurred and to guide treatment. Immunological tests are employed to establish the cause of renal disease.

Different tests are carried out on different components of blood: whole blood, plasma and serum.

- Whole blood includes blood cells and plasma
- Plasma is the liquid in which blood cells, clotting factors, antibodies and other proteins, electrolytes and hormones are suspended; it is obtained by centrifuging an anticoagulated blood sample to separate out the blood cells, which sink to the bottom of the tube
- Serum is the liquid that remains after a blood sample has clotted, and is similar to plasma but without the clotting factors

Reference ranges are the values for a test that the result for 95% of the population will fall between. They are used to determine whether a test result is normal (within range) or abnormal (outside the range). Reference ranges differ between laboratories; always interpret them using the values provided by the laboratory performing the test.

Biochemistry

These include the most important blood tests for the initial work-up of a patient with renal disease, for example measurement of urea, creatinine, electrolytes and pH, the results of which are used to assess the filtering and reabsorptive functions of the kidney. Measurement of glucose concentration is also essential, because patients with diabetes are at increased risk of CKD.

Renal profile ('urea and electrolytes')

The basic renal profile – a set of tests commonly done together – consists of sodium, potassium, chloride, bicarbonate, urea, creatinine and eGFR. It is commonly referred to as 'urea and electrolytes'. These tests are used routinely to screen for abnormal renal function and electrolyte abnormalities in patients presenting with symptoms that require further investigation, and to monitor renal function in patients with existing renal disease.

Urea

Blood urea concentration is increased in renal dysfunction, because of failure to excrete urea. An increased concentration is also found in dehydration, because of enhancement of the normal tubular reabsorption of urea, and after an upper gastrointestinal bleed, because digested blood is a source of protein and, therefore, urea.

Creatinine

This waste product of muscle metabolism is excreted by the kidneys into the urine. Creatinine production is relatively constant, because muscle mass remains fairly stable from day to day.

Creatinine concentration is a sensitive marker of renal function and increases non-linearly with increasing severity of renal impairment. When creatinine is normal at baseline, smaller increases indicate a more significant decrease in GFR than a larger increase when creatinine concentration is already high (**Figure 2.21**).

Serum creatinine concentration varies with a patient's muscle mass. Individuals with greater muscle bulk have a higher creatinine concentration at baseline.

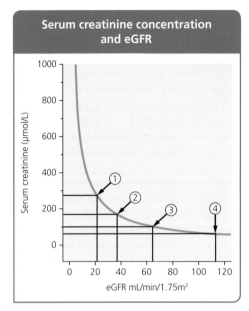

Serum creatinine concentration and eGFR

Figure 2.21 The relationship between serum creatinine concentration and glomerular filtration rate. Because the relationship is non-linear at low creatinine concentrations a small change in creatinine represents a significant change in GFR. An increase in creatinine from 75 µmol/L to 100 µmol/L (④ to ③) is associated with a decrease in GFR from around 115 mL/min/1.73 m² to 63 mL/min/1.73 m², whereas an increase in creatinine from 180 µmol/L to 280 µmol/L (② to ①) is associated with a decrease in GFR from 35 mL/min/1.73 m² to 22 mL/min/1.73 m².

> **Most filtered creatinine is excreted by the renal tubule because there is little reabsorption there.** This excretion is blocked by certain drugs, notably the antibiotic trimethoprim, which results in an increase in serum creatinine concentration unrelated to any change in GFR. A rise in creatinine should be anticipated in patients taking trimethoprim.

Glomerular filtration rate

Because GFR is difficult to measure accurately (see page 15) an estimated GFR (eGFR) is used instead. This is obtained from the Chronic Kidney Disease Epidemiology Collaboration formula, taking into account the patient's age and creatinine concentration, as well as other specific values based on age, gender and ethnicity.

Electrolytes

Commonly measured electrolyes in patients with renal disease are:

- Na^+
- K^+
- Cl^-
- HCO_3^-
- Ca^{2+}
- PO_4^{3-}

Electrolyte abnormalities are common in renal impairment, because it affects filtration of the blood and the reabsorption and excretion of various substances.

The most common electrolyte disorder in the general population are hyperkalaemia (a high serum potassium concentration) and hyponatraemia (a low serum sodium concentration). In renal patients, the most common abnormalities are hyperkalaemia, low bicarbonate, hypocalcaemia (low serum calcium concentration) and hyperphosphataemia (high serum phosphate concentration). Renal tubular pathologies also result in hypokalaemia and other electrolyte abnormalities (see page 288), due to impaired tubular reabsorption.

> **Renal impairment is commonly an incidental finding.** A patient being told a diagnosis in the absence of symptoms may find it hard to view kidney impairment as a health concern. Strike the right balance when discussing this with the patient: a mild degree of renal impairment, particularly in the elderly, is not a major clinical concern because renal function is unlikely to decline to end-stage levels over their remaining life expectancy. However, lifestyle changes, particularly the control of hypertension, are still beneficial and minimise the chances of further renal impairment.

Glucose

In diabetes, blood glucose control is abnormal because of decreased insulin production (in type 1 diabetes) and decreased insulin secretion with insulin resistance (in type 2 diabetes).

Chronic high blood glucose (hyperglycaemia) causes:

- macrovascular disease, i.e. damage to large vessels, by increasing atherogenesis
- microvascular disease, i.e. damage to small blood vessels, including those of the glomeruli and retina

Blood glucose is assessed initially by measuring a fasting blood glucose concentration (usually using capillary blood from a finger-prick test). If abnormal, an oral glucose tolerance test is performed. Here, the patient ingests an oral glucose load, after which blood glucose is recorded over time. If fasting glucose and blood glucose concentrations 2 hours after the glucose load are both elevated, the patient has impaired glucose tolerance or diabetes, depending on how high they are.

Regular monitoring of blood glucose concentrations is an essential part of managing diabetes because it enables treatment to be tailored to the individual to ensure blood glucose concentrations are kept as near to the normal range as possible. Most patients with diabetes self-monitor their blood glucose.

Haemoglobin A1c

Haemoglobin A1c is a glycated, i.e. glucose-bound, form of haemoglobin that is measured to identify average blood glucose concentrations over a period of weeks to months. Glycation bonds are permanent, so levels of haemoglobin A1c reflect average blood glucose concentrations over the lifespan of a red blood cell (110–120 days).

C-reactive protein

This acute phase protein (a protein whose plasma concentration increases in response to infection and inflammation) is produced by the liver. It has a role in the innate and adaptive immune responses. C-reactive protein binds phosphocholines on dead or damaged cells, and some microbes (e.g. the C polysaccharide of *Streptococcus pneumoniae,* hence its name) and nuclear breakdown products, and activates complement.

It acts as an opsonin by marking pathogens and damaged cells for phagocytosis by local macrophages, thereby facilitating the clearance of cellular debris and foreign molecules.

C-reactive protein is a non-specific inflammatory marker; the results of the C-reactive protein test do not indicate the site of infection or inflammation, or the underlying diagnosis. If there is no obvious cause for an increased concentration, consider an occult infection or malignancy.

Because C-reactive protein has a short half-life, a persistently increased or increasing concentration indicates an ongoing pro-inflammatory stimulus, whereas a decrease reflects resolution of an inflammatory response. In the context of renal impairment, C-reactive protein may be increased as a result of infection or an inflammatory process such as vasculitis.

> Uses of the **C-reactive protein test** include:
>
> - distinguishing viral infection from bacterial infection; the result is usually higher than normal in acute bacterial infection. In a viral infection, CRP is normal or slightly elevated
> - monitoring infections (e.g. urinary tract infection, pneumonia) or inflammatory disease (e.g. connective tissue disease)
> - assessing risk in cardiovascular disease; it is a stronger predictor of cardiovascular events than the concentration of low-density lipoprotein cholesterol

Bone profile

This is a collection of biochemical blood tests that typically include serum calcium concentration and calcium concentration corrected for albumin concentration (to account for normal binding of calcium to albumin), as well as phosphate, albumin and alkaline phosphatase concentrations. It is useful in assessment of renal disease, because abnormalities of bone metabolism are common and require treatment.

A bone profile is always requested for patients presenting with renal disease for the first time, because the results may provide evidence of renal bone disease. The bone profile should also be checked periodically in patients with CKD to monitor severity of renal bone disease and to guide treatment.

Calcium and phosphate

Renal impairment results in abnormalities of bone metabolism, so derangement of serum concentrations of calcium and phosphate are common. These include:

- hyperphosphataemia, as a consequence of decreased renal excretion of phosphate
- hypocalcaemia, resulting from decreased hydroxylation of 25-hydroxyvitamin D to active 1,25-dihydroxyvitamin D by the kidneys, and consequent poor gastrointestinal absorption of calcium

Albumin

Around 40% of serum calcium is bound to albumin and albumin concentration is required to calculate the corrected calcium concentration. Serum albumin concentration is also low (hypoalbuminaemia) in cases of malnutrition and sepsis and other inflammatory conditions (e.g. rheumatoid arthritis), but hypoalbuminaemia also makes nephrotic syndrome a possibility. In this syndrome, the integrity of the glomerular filtration membrane is compromised and albumin is lost in the urine.

Alkaline phosphatase

This is a hydrolase enzyme produced by all body tissues. Higher amounts are present in the bone, liver, and, during pregnancy, the placenta. It catalyses the removal of phosphate groups from several different types of molecule, including proteins and nucleotides.

Levels of alkaline phosphatase in the blood are increased in bone disease, liver disease and pregnancy. Alkaline phosphatase is also increased in renal disease because of secondary hyperparathyroidism and increased bone turnover.

Parathyroid hormone

This hormone is produced by the parathyroid glands and acts to increase the concentration of calcium in the blood. It also increases

renal excretion of phosphate, enhances gastrointestinal phosphate reabsorption and mobilises phosphate from bone. In renal impairment, decreased production of active vitamin D, hypocalcaemia and hyperphosphataemia all stimulate the parathyroid gland, thereby increasing the concentration of parathyroid hormone.

> **Parathyroid hormone concentrations take weeks to months to increase.** Therefore, in the context of renal impairment, an increased concentration of parathyroid hormone suggests that that this has been present for some time.

Creatine kinase

This is an enzyme found in skeletal and cardiac muscle; a small amount is also usually present in the blood. Muscle injury results in a marked increase in its serum concentration.

Rhabdomyolysis (muscle breakdown) is a cause of AKI, because of the toxic effects of the myoglobin released by damaged muscle cells on the renal tubules. In this context, creatine kinase is used to assess the extent of muscle damage and to monitor its resolution.

Blood gases

Measurements of venous or arterial blood gases are used to assess acid–base balance in renal patients. These tests usually measure pH, the partial pressures of oxygen and carbon dioxide (Po_2 and Pco_2, respectively), bicarbonate concentration and base excess, and oxygen saturation, as well as concentrations of haemoglobin, electrolytes and lactate, in venous or arterial blood. Renal impairment results in decreased acid excretion, resulting in a low pH, decreased bicarbonate and more negative base excess.

A stepwise method for interpreting a blood gas result is shown in Table 8.4.

Haematology

Full blood count

This is one of the most commonly requested blood tests. It is vital in the initial assessment of any patient, because it is used to screen for evidence of anaemia and infection. The full (or 'complete') blood count comprises several haematological variables:

- haemoglobin
- mean corpuscular volume
- total white blood cell count
- differential numbers of neutrophils, lymphocytes and eosinophils
- platelets

Haemoglobin

This is the oxygen-carrying protein tetramer of red blood cells. A low haemoglobin concentration indicates anaemia, which is a common finding in renal disease. Anaemia of renal disease is usually accompanied by normal-sized, i.e. normocytic, red blood cells and results from a lack of erythropoietin production by the diseased kidneys.

Mean corpuscular volume

Mean corpuscular volume (MCV) is a measurement of the average size of red blood cells and is routinely included in a full blood count. It is used to assess patients with anaemia and is therefore required in the work-up of patients with renal impairment. When red blood cells are smaller than normal (microcytic), the MCV is low. This occurs in iron deficiency anaemia, thalassaemia and, sometimes, anaemia of chronic disease. When red blood cells are larger than normal (macrocytic), the MCV is elevated. This occurs in B12 and folate deficiency, liver disease, hypothyroidism, reticulocytosis and myelodysplasia. Anaemia associated with CKD is usually normocytic.

White blood cell count and differential

An increased total white blood cell count is a sign of infection but can also occur in other inflammatory conditions associated with renal disease, such as vasculitis. Causes of a low white cell count include bone suppression following a viral infection, cancer, myelofibrosis, aplastic anaemia, autoimmune disorders and medications (including chemotherapeutic agents and radiotherapy). A total white cell count that is increased or decreased prompts analysis of the white blood cell differential, i.e. the different numbers of the five types of white blood cell: neutrophils, lymphocytes, basophils, monocytes and eosinophils (**Table 2.12**). This provides information on the nature of an immune response and white blood cell turnover, and is more useful when formulating possible differentials. Deranged proportions of white blood cells can occur with a normal total white cell count.

The white blood cell differential is useful in the diagnosis of the following, some of which are directly associated with renal impairment:

- infection
- inflammation
- allergies and asthma
- immunodeficiencies
- leukaemia
- bone marrow neoplasms, myelodysplasia, myeloproliferative disorders and plasma cell neoplasms
- trauma
- autoimmune diseases

Platelets

These small blood cells without a nucleus have a central role in haemostasis, the process of stopping the bleeding that occurs when blood vessels are injured. Low platelet count (thrombocytopenia) is the result of insufficient production by the bone marrow or increased consumption due to autoimmune disease, thrombosis (clot formation), infections, surgery or medications (e.g. heparin).

Thrombocytopenia is associated with conditions affecting the kidneys such as:

- microangiopathic haemolytic anaemia, which is characterised by damage to the endothelium of small blood vessel walls, resulting in platelet aggregation and fibrin deposition. This creates shearing forces which cause fragmentation of red cells
- haemolytic uraemic syndrome, a condition characterised by microangiopathic haemolytic anaemia, thrombocytopenia and progressive renal failure that is associated with certain bacterial gastrointestinal infections

Abnormalities of the differential white blood cell count

Derangement	Definition	Cause(s)
Leucocytosis	Increased total white cell count	Infection, inflammation, trauma, malignancy (e.g. leukaemias), certain medications
Leucopenia	Decreased total white cell count	Medications (e.g. chemotherapeutic agents), radiotherapy, vitamin deficiencies (B12 and folate), autoimmune diseases, sepsis, aplastic anaemia
Neutrophilia	High neutrophil count	Usually bacterial infections, but also inflammation (e.g. vasculitis, rheumatoid arthritis, IBD) or tissue death (e.g. as a consequence of trauma or surgery)
Neutropenia	Low neutrophil count	Autoimmune disorders, sepsis, chemotherapy, aplastic anaemia
Lymphocytosis	High lymphocyte count	Viral infections (e.g. viral hepatitis, cytomegalovirus, Epstein–Barr virus infection), tuberculosis, leukaemia
Lymphopenia	Low lymphocyte count	Autoimmune disorders, HIV, tuberculosis, bone marrow damage, immunodeficiency, viral infections
Monocytosis	High monocyte count	Chronic infections, bacterial endocarditis, connective tissue disease, IBD, leukaemia
Monocytopenia	Low monocyte count	Usually insignificant; sometimes bone marrow disease
Basophilia	High basophil count	Allergy, inflammation, leukaemia
Basopenia	Low basophil count	Usually insignificant
Eosinophilia	High eosinophil count	Allergy, atopy, asthma, parasitic infection, inflammation (e.g. tubulointerstitial nephritis, atheroembolic disease, eosinophilic granulomatosis with polyangiitis*, IBD, some malignancies)
Eosinopenia	Low eosinophil count	Usually insignificant

IBD, inflammatory bowel disease.

*Previously called Churg–Strauss syndrome.

Table 2.12 Abnormalities of the differential white blood cell count and their main causes

If thrombocytopenia is present, a blood film, i.e. microscopic visualisation of blood cell morphology, is requested to look for red blood cell fragments, which represent mechanical red blood cell destruction as occurs in microangiopthic haemolytic anaemia.

Increased platelet count (thrombocytosis) is caused by bone marrow disorders or infection, inflammation or malignancy. These types of increased platelet counts are classed as reactive thrombocytosis because they occur secondary to another disorder, rather than due to unregulated clonal expansion of bone marrow progenitor cells (essential thrombocythaemia).

Blood film

This is produced by spreading a drop of blood on a slide, allowing it to dry and staining it with dye. The resulting blood film is examined under the microscope to identify abnormal blood cells, which may signify the presence of certain diseases. For example, pale, round red blood cells are found in anaemia, and immature white blood cells are present in leukaemia.

In renal medicine, the blood film is used to investigate anaemias and specifically to exclude microangiopathic haemolytic anaemia, which produces red blood cell fragments.

Erythrocyte sedimentation rate

This is a non-specific test used in the diagnosis and monitoring of inflammatory conditions such as infection, malignancy and vasculitides. It is a measure of the rate at which red blood cells descend when collected in a tube of anticoagulated blood.

Normally, red blood cells descend slowly. However, in the presence of increased levels of certain proteins, such as immunoglobulins (e.g. in multiple myeloma) or fibrinogen (in inflammation), they fall more rapidly.

In renal medicine, an erythrocyte sedimentation rate is likely to be raised in patients with:

- end-stage renal disease (ESRD), because it is associated with underlying inflammation
- nephrotic syndrome, because there is often an underlying inflammatory aetiology (e.g. SLE)
- infection, due to the presence of high levels of fibrinogen which is an acute phase reactant
- malignancy, because it is associated with an inflammatory response
- vasculitis, because of increased levels of immunoglobulins

A raised erythrocyte sedimentation rate is usually a non-specific finding in renal patients because it is present in so many renal conditions. Therefore C-reactive protein is preferred as a marker of inflammation.

> **C-reactive protein is a more sensitive indicator of acute inflammation than erythrocyte sedimentation rate,** because the latter is affected by factors other than acute phase reactants, including other proteins, plasma albumin concentration and red blood cell shape, size and number.

Clotting profile

Blood coagulation is the result of a cascade of reactions in which protein clotting factors activate each other. The basic clotting profile assesses the rate at which this occurs and comprises the prothrombin time, international normalised ratio (INR) and activated partial thromboplastin time.

The clotting profile is usually requested as a part of the acute renal screen and should be checked before invasive procedures such as dialysis catheter insertion or renal biopsy are performed.

International normalised ratio

This measures the extrinsic pathway of coagulation and is a standardised ratio of the patient's prothrombin time compared to the mean prothrombin time of the healthy adult population. As it is a ratio, there are no units. It is increased by warfarin, liver dysfunction and disseminated intravascular coagulation, i.e. the systemic activation of blood coagulation caused by several conditions, including trauma and sepsis, and resulting in consumption of clotting factors. It is reduced by vitamin K supplementation and transfusion of fresh frozen plasma.

Activated partial thromboplastin time

This measures the intrinsic and final common pathway of the coagulation cascade. It is increased by the presence of heparin, and in cases of haemophilia and disseminated intravascular coagulation. It is shortened when the coagulation factor VIII is elevated, such as during an acute phase reaction, in early disseminated intravascular coagulation, and due to artefact (when samples are activated in vitro because of problems with collection).

Immunology

Immunological tests are ordered as part of an acute renal screen for certain patients presenting with renal impairment (**Table 2.13**). The results are used to rule out or diagnose autoimmune conditions, viral infections and multiple myeloma, which can all be associated with renal failure.

> **The presence of autoantibodies in SLE and other connective tissue diseases represents a dysregulation of the immune system.** Autoantibodies are produced by B lymphocytes and attack normal constituents of the body, such as DNA or phospholipids, to cause chronic and often progressive tissue destruction.

Imaging

The imaging modalities most commonly used for the initial assessment of renal

Immunological tests in renal disease

Test	Explanation
Cytoplasmic antineutrophil antibody (c-ANCA)	Autoantibody produced against protein targets (antigens) in the neutrophil cytoplasm
	The commonest antigen target is proteinase 3
	Antibodies show granular cytoplasmic staining pattern
	Proteinase 3 is targeted by ANCA in granulomatosis with polyangiitis*
	Requested in cases of suspected systemic vasculitis or as part of an acute renal screen
Perinuclear antineutrophil cytoplasmic antibody (p-ANCA)	Autoantibody produced against targets in the neutrophil cytoplasm
	Antibodies show a perinuclear staining pattern
	The commonest target is myeloperoxidase
	Associated with eosinophilic granulomatosis with polyangiitis,[†] microscopic polyangiitis, rheumatoid arthritis and ulcerative colitis
Anti-GBM antibody	Autoantibody directed against the $\alpha3$ chain of type IV collagen in the GBM
	Associated with anti-GBM disease‡ (see page 202)
Antinuclear antibody	Non-specific test to detect autoantibodies that target proteins in the cell nucleus
	Associated with various autoimmune conditions, including SLE, Sjögren's syndrome, scleroderma and mixed connective tissue disease
	Can be present in healthy individuals
Anti-double-stranded DNA	Specific autoantibody test used to support a diagnosis of SLE
	Typically carried out after a positive ANA test
	Can be used to monitor disease activity in SLE
Complement (C3 and C4)	Used in the diagnosis of SLE, and as a marker of disease activity
	Complement is consumed in the clearance of immune complexes from the blood, so low levels suggest certain autoimmune diseases or chronic infection
Cryoglobulins	Test to detect immunoglobulins that precipitate (form clumps) when cooled and dissolve when warmed
	Present in various conditions associated with renal impairment, including SLE, multiple myeloma, HIV and hepatitis C
Viral serology (hepatitis B and C, and HIV)	Tests for the presence of protein antigens specific to each virus
Serum electrophoresis	Used to detect excess production of single immunoglobulins (monoclonal antibodies) associated with multiple myeloma

ANA, antinuclear antibody; ANCA, antineutrophil antibody; GBM, glomerular basement membrane; SLE; systemic lupus erythematosus.
*Previously known as Wegener's granulomatosis.
†Previously known as Churg–Strauss syndrome.
‡Previously known as Goodpasture's disease.

Table 2.13 Immunological tests used in the investigation of renal disease

impairment are plain film radiography and ultrasound (US). These are used to exclude systemic consequences of renal failure, including fluid overload (with chest radiography) and structural renal tract abnormalities (with renal US).

More specialised tests may also be required, depending on the presentation and differential diagnoses. For example:

■ Computerised tomography of the kidneys, ureters and bladder to assess for renal stones

- Renal angiography for the detection of renovascular disease
- Nuclear medicine scans to assess renal perfusion and function

Ionising radiation

X-rays are high-energy photons (particles of electromagnetic radiation). As they pass through tissue, their energy is sufficient to ionise atoms by displacing electrons and disrupting molecular bonds, making them potentially harmful to tissues. Their effects are divided into those that occur by chance (stochastic effects), including genetic damage and cancer, and those that have a clear relationship with X-ray dose (deterministic effects), which include skin erythema and burns, cataracts, radiation sickness and death at high doses (**Table 2.14**). There is no threshold for the stochastic effects: any dose has the potential to cause genetic damage. This is why it is vital to use as low a dose as reasonably practicable, especially in children.

Radiation exposure	
Source of exposure	Dose in Sieverts
Sleeping next to someone for 8 hours	0.05 µSv
Dental radiograph	0.005 mSv
Chest radiograph	0.02 mSv
Transatlantic flight	0.07 mSv
X-ray renal tract	0.7 mSv
CT scan of the head	1.4 mSv
MAG3 scan	2.2 mSv
Average annual radiation dose in the UK	2.7 mSv
IV urogram	3 mSv
CT KUB	3 mSv
Renal angiography	9 mSv
Whole body CT scan	10 mSv
Level at which changes in blood cells are clearly visible	100 mSv
Severe radiation poisoning	2 Sv

Table 2.14 Radiation doses from different sources of exposure

X-rays are differentially absorbed (attenuated) according to tissue density:

- metal and bone have greatest absorption
- soft tissue has much lower absorption
- air has the lowest absorption

These differences underlie the contrasts produced when X-rays pass through a patient and strike the X-ray film or digital detector. Plain radiographs show poor contrast between different types of soft tissue, so they have a limited direct role in renal medicine.

Plain radiography of the chest

In chest radiography, the differing absorption of radiation by different body tissues is used to visualise structures within the thorax, predominantly the heart and major vessels, lungs and bones. In a renal patient, a chest radiograph may be requested to look for:

- fluid overload (**Figure 2.22**), which may be a result of renal failure
- enlarged lymph nodes, which are associated with infection, autoimmune conditions and underlying malignancies
- tumours

> **A chest radiograph with signs of fluid overload does not necessarily indicate renal failure.** Fluid overload also occurs in cases of heart failure and overzealous use of intravenous fluids.

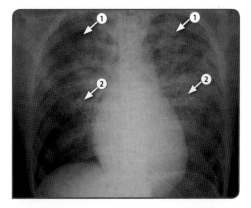

Figure 2.22 A chest radiograph showing signs of fluid overload. Perihilar airspace shadowing ②. Upper lobe venous diversion ①.

Plain radiography of the kidneys, ureters and bladder

A plain radiograph of the kidneys, ureters and bladder is not routinely requested to investigate renal disease. However, one may be used to detect renal stones in a patient with symptoms suggesting this: the radiograph will show calcium-containing stones (roughly 80% of stones; see **Table 12.2**), which are radiopaque, but it will miss smaller stones and those that are radiolucent.

Intravenous urography

An intravenous urogram is a radiographic study of the renal tract that visualises the pelvicalyceal system, the ureters and the bladder. It is used to visualise the anatomy of the renal tract, to look for obstruction (**Figure 2.23**) and to check renal function.

Intravenous contrast is injected into a vein and travels via the circulation to the kidneys. It is concentrated in the kidneys before passing into the urine via the collecting system, ureters, bladder and urethra. Because the dye is radiopaque, the kidneys, ureters and bladder appear white on radiography. A series of radiographs are taken as the dye concentrates in the kidneys and is excreted.

Intravenous urography is now used infrequently, because it has been superseded by the CT urogram which gives better visualisation of all intra-abdominal anatomy in a single study, even if radiation doses are slightly higher.

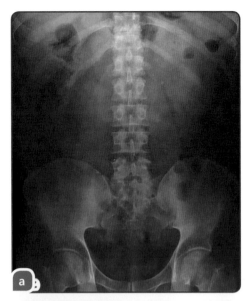
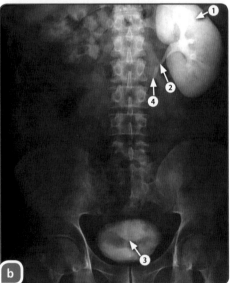

Figure 2.23 Abdominal radiographs of an intravenous urogram. (a) Before dye is injected. (b) After injection of dye; the flow of dye is impeded in the left kidney ① and proximal ureter ②. The right kidney is not visualised, because the dye has left this kidney and reached the bladder ③. This patient had a left ureteric stone causing obstruction at point ④.

Micturating cystourethrography

A micturating cystourethrogram is an X-ray examination used to evaluate bladder function. It is most commonly performed on children with recurrent urinary tract infections to exclude vesico-ureteric reflux.

A urinary catheter is inserted and water-soluble contrast medium injected through the catheter into the bladder. The patient then urinates while radiographs are obtained. If vesicoureteric reflux is present, contrast is seen moving upwards from the bladder into the ureters during micturition.

Renal ultrasound

In ultrasonography, high-frequency sound waves (2–18 MHz) are used to provide real-time images of soft tissue. Sound waves are reflected or absorbed according to tissue type. Reflected sound waves are transformed into an image. No ionising radiation is used, but the technique is limited by considerable interobserver variability and patients' body habitus because excessive body fat makes imaging difficult.

A renal US scan is carried out for virtually all patients with renal impairment to determine renal size and to detect asymmetry, identify structural abnormalities and exclude obstructive uropathy. Pre- and post-micturition bladder volumes are measured to assess bladder emptying.

- Normal kidney size is about 10–12 cm in adults
- Small kidneys (< 10 cm) suggest CKD, especially when the cortices are thin (< 1 cm)
- Large kidneys (> 12 cm) may reflect an infiltrative process such as amyloidosis or lymphoma

Ultrasound can also be used to visualise polycystic kidneys (**Figure 2.24**).

Doppler ultrasound

Doppler US is a specialised ultrasound scan that uses high frequency sound waves to evaluate the flow of blood in arteries and veins. In a renal patient, a Doppler US may be requested to assess for renal artery stenosis, renal vein thrombosis, decreased renal perfusion and renal infarction.

Computerised tomography

Computerised tomography (CT) is a radiological investigation in which a series of X-rays is taken from different angles and processed by a computer to create cross-sectional images of areas of the body. These images are much more detailed than plain X-rays. CT of the kidneys, ureters and bladder allows more detailed evaluation of the anatomy of the renal tract than US, because a sharper resolution is obtained. It is used to establish the cause of obstruction, investigate renal masses (**Figure 2.25**) and stage renal tumours.

Radioiodine contrast is used to improve image quality; however, its potential nephrotoxicity means that it must be used with caution in patients with renal impairment. The risk of nephrotoxicity must be weighed against the benefit of obtaining clear images on an individual basis, and all efforts taken to mitigate these potential effects, for example by pre-hydrating the patient with intravenous fluids before administration of contrast. Non-contrast CT of the renal tract is the imaging modality of choice to detect renal stones, because it is more sensitive than plain radiography and therefore more likely to detect smaller stones (**Figure 2.26**). However, radiation exposure should be considered when weighing the risks and benefits of CT: a single CT scan of the abdomen and pelvis is associated with 3 years' worth of background radiation, compared with a chest radiograph's 10 days.

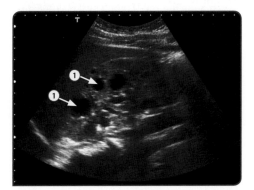

Figure 2.24 A renal US scan showing polycystic kidney disease. Renal cysts are visible within the kidney ①.

Intravenous contrast can cause renal damage, especially in patients with existing renal impairment. If contrast is required to optimise CT images, the patient should receive prehydration with intravenous fluid to minimise any adverse effects, and their renal function should be monitored closely. *N*-Acetyl cysteine has been thought to have a protective effect, but there is no solid evidence to support its use.

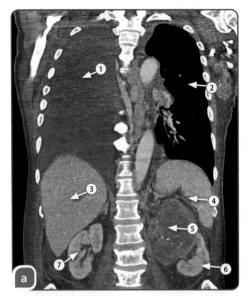

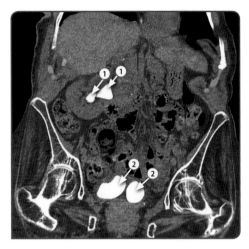

Figure 2.26 A coronal CT scan of the abdomen, showing renal calculi ① and bladder calculi ②.

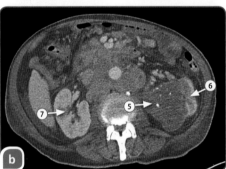

Figure 2.25 CT images of a renal mass. (a) A coronal CT scan of the kidneys, ureters and bladder. ①, large right-sided pleural effusion secondary to metastatic cancer; ②, normal left lung; ③, liver; ④, spleen; ⑤, left renal mass; ⑥, left kidney, ⑦ right kidney. (b) Transverse CT scan at level of kidneys ⑥, left kidney; ⑤, left renal mass ⑦ right kidney.

Magnetic resonance imaging

In MRI, a magnetic field at a specific resonance frequency is used to excite hydrogen atoms in the body. The resulting radiofrequency signal emitted by the atoms is detected and converted into a two-dimensional image and then a combined three-dimensional image. Soft tissues are visualised in greater detail than with CT or radiography, and although slower and more expensive, there is no radiation exposure. MRI with gadolinium contrast may be used to evaluate renovascular disease and detect renal vein thrombosis.

> **The use of the contrast gadolinium is contraindicated in patients with eGFR < 30 mL/min/1.73 m². This is because of the theoretical risk of inducing nephrogenic systemic fibrosis, a disorder resulting in fibrosis of skin, muscle and internal organs.**

Renal angiography

This uses intravenous radio-opaque contrast to visualise the renal blood vessels on X-ray. During an angiogram, procedures such as stenting narrowed vessels (angioplasty) can be performed. Newer techniques such as CT and MR angiography are also available.

Angiography of the renal vessels is the gold standard test for the detection of renovascular disease (see Figure 9.5). However, it is rarely used for this purpose, because there is little evidence that intervention (e.g. stenting of a renal artery stenosis) improves outcomes.

Nuclear medicine

Nuclear medicine uses different radioactive tracers (radioisotopes) for diagnostic and

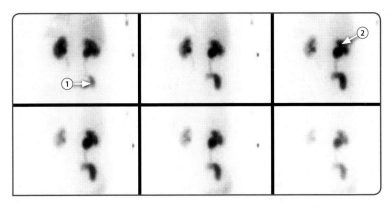

Figure 2.27 A MAG 3 dynamic nuclear medicine scan. Both ureters are connected to an ileal conduit ①. The right kidney ②; (visible on the right, because the images are posterior views) is partially obstructed, resulting in delayed excretion of isotope. Isotope is retained more on the right in the latest frame (bottom right).

therapeutic processes. During scans radioactive tracers accumulate in the area of the body being examined. They emit radioactivity which is detected by a gamma camera, enabling images to be produced. Nuclear medicine images can be integrated with CT or MRI images to produce more specialist views. They can be dynamic, i.e. enable the course of certain functional processes to be followed over time, such as the excretion of urine by the kidney, or static, where they are used to visualise the structures in which they have accumulated.

Dynamic nuclear medicine

These imaging techniques include mercaptoacetyltriglycine (MAG 3) and diethylene triamine penta-acetic acid (DTPA) scans. These use compounds labelled with technetium-99m, a gamma-emitting isotope. The radioisotope is injected into a vein and travels in the bloodstream to the kidneys, where it is taken up by the renal tubules. It is then excreted through the renal tract. A gamma camera is used to produce images as the substance is delivered to the kidney and subsequently excreted.

The images are used to identify the split function of the kidneys, i.e. the relative contribution of each kidney to total renal function, and to assess perfusion and obstruction. If perfusion is decreased, visualisation of the kidney is impaired (**Figure 2.27**). If there is a complete obstruction, the isotope does not pass beyond a certain point, and if there is a partial obstruction, its passage is delayed.

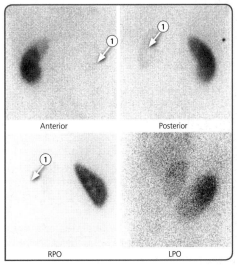

Figure 2.28 A static nuclear medicine scan using DMSA, showing marked asymmetry of renal function and little uptake of isotope by the left kidney ①. This patient had lost blood supply to the left kidney after thrombosis on the background of atheromatous renal artery stenosis. RPO, right posterior oblique; LPO, left posterior oblique

Static nuclear medicine

A radiolabelled dimercaptosuccinic acid (DMSA) scan is used to look for areas of renal scarring and to assess split renal function; the compound is not excreted, so this type of scan provides no information about obstruction. DMSA is infused into a vein, and uptake of the compound is measured after 2–4 h. Uptake is decreased in areas of scarring or ischaemia (**Figure 2.28**). This scan is useful to assess renal damage in patients with reflux disease.

Histopathology

Histopathology is the examination of tissue under a microscope to investigate disease. Tissue samples (biopsies) may be obtained from most areas of the body. Samples are then prepared and analysed using different techniques, e.g. light or electron microscopy.

Many patients with renal dysfunction present with a clinical syndrome (e.g. AKI or nephrotic syndrome) rather than a specific diagnosis (e.g. membranous glomerulonephritis). Urine tests, blood tests and imaging provide vital diagnostic information but a definitive diagnosis usually requires the examination of renal tissue obtained by percutaneous renal biopsy.

Renal biopsy

The procedure to obtain samples of renal tissue is invasive. A specialised biopsy needle is inserted into the patient's back, usually under local anaesthetic and with US guidance, to obtain renal tissue, which is then examined in the pathology laboratory using light microscopy, electron microscopy and immunohistochemical techniques.

After a renal biopsy, patients are advised that the biopsy site will be painful when the anaesthetic wears off. Following the procedure, they are required to lie in bed for 6–8 hours while their vital signs are measured and urine monitored for visible haematuria. If there are no complications after this period, the patient is discharged or, if an inpatient, allowed to end their bed rest. Patients should not be alone for 24 hours after the biopsy and should be given clear written instructions to seek medical advice if they develop increasing pain or haematuria. They are advised to avoid heavy lifting, strenuous activity or contact sports for a week after the procedure.

Indications

Renal biopsy is usually required to make a definitive diagnosis in the investigation of renal failure, especially when glomerular disease is suspected, because examination of renal tissue is required to identify the underlying pathological process. As well as being diagnostic, renal biopsies may be carried out to evaluate disease activity or stage diseases (e.g. SLE) and to provide a prognosis. The main indications are:

- AKI or CKD for which no cause can be established
- nephrotic syndrome
- a malfunctioning kidney transplant

Contraindications

Renal biopsy is contraindicated if the patient:

- has an uncorrectable bleeding diathesis
- has small kidneys
- has only a single functioning kidney
- has severe hypertension (> 170/90 mmHg)
- has an active renal infection
- is unable to follow the clinician's instructions or tolerate the procedure
- has a very large body habitus, because of technical difficulties (this is a relative contraindication)

> **The procedure to obtain samples for biopsy carries a significant risk of morbidity and a small risk of death (<0.1%), mainly as a result of bleeding complications.** Carefully consider whether the value of the information potentially provided by biopsy outweighs these risks.

Light microscopy

A light microscope uses visible light and a series of lenses to magnify small objects such as cells. Because live cells are often transparent, tissue samples are usually fixed in formalin and stained with haematoxylin and eosin (H&E) to make them more visible under the microscope (**Figure 2.29**). On a renal biopsy, additional specialised stains are also used to examine different structures and abnormalities, for example:

- Trichrome stain to assess fibrin and immune deposits
- Silver stain to assess the basement membrane, in particular to visualise spikes and double contours

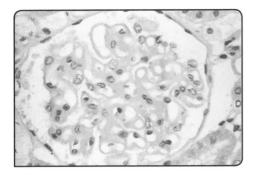

Figure 2.29 A glomerulus viewed under light microscopy, stained with haematoxylin and eosin (H&E). Nuclei are stained blue (haematoxylin), with eosin acting as a counterstain for other structures (various shades of pink).

■ Periodic acid–Schiff (PAS) stain to examine the basement membrane, mesangium and vessels

Electron microscopy

Electron microscopes use an electron beam rather than a light beam to create an image of a specimen. They are capable of much higher magnification than light microscopes, and tissues and individual cells are visualised in greater detail (**Figure 2.30**).

Tissue is fixed in glutaraldehyde and stained with toluidine blue to confirm whether any glomeruli are present, before proceeding to a detailed examination of the renal tissue ultra-structure under an electron microscope.

Immunohistochemistry

Immunohistochemical techniques are used to detect antigens, for example particular proteins, in cells of a tissue specimen by using 'tagged' antibodies that are specific for that antigen. Different techniques are used to visualise an antibody–antigen complex. Most commonly, antibodies are conjugated to an enzyme that catalyses a reaction resulting in a colour change (**Figure 2.31**). Antibodies can also be tagged with a fluorescent compound that emits light on excitation by light. Specialised light microscopes are then used to examine these samples (**Figure 2.32**).

When examining a renal biopsy, certain antigens are routinely looked for, including:

■ immunoglobulins (IgA, IgG, IgM)

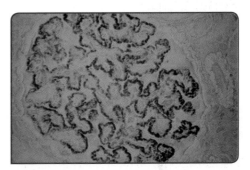

Figure 2.31 A renal biopsy specimen with immunohistochemistry showing granular deposits of immunoglobulin G in the capillary loops of a glomerulus from a case of membranous nephropathy (see Chapter 5).

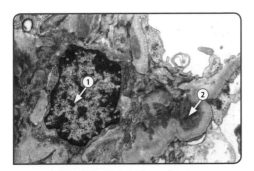

Figure 2.30 Electron micrograph of a renal biopsy specimen from a case of IgA nephropathy (see Chapter 5) showing a mesangial cell (① indicates the nucleus) with ② adjoining paramesangial immune deposits.

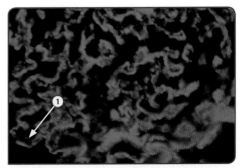

Figure 2.32 A glomerulus from a patient with membranous nephropathy (see Chapter 5) which has been stained by a fluorescein-conjugated antibody to immunoglobulin G (IgG). The resulting fluorescently stained deposits of IgG along the outside of the capillary loops have been visualised under a fluorescent microscope (one such capillary loop indicated by ①).

- components of the classical and alternative complement pathways (e.g. C1q, C4)

> **Renal biopsy provides a tissue diagnosis in about 95% of cases.** This means that for most patients undergoing a biopsy, clinically useful information will be obtained that not only confirms the diagnosis but informs prognosis and guides treatment.

Electrocardiography

An electrocardiogram (ECG) is a recording, obtained by using electrodes placed on the skin, of the heart's electrical activity. It measures the amount and direction of the heart's electrical activity. ECG is a powerful tool in the assessment of ischaemic heart disease, heart muscle disease (cardiomyopathies) and arrhythmias, as well as in the assessment of changes associated with non-cardiac disease, such as pulmonary hypertension, systemic disease and electrolyte disturbances.

Indications

For ECG, the indications include chest pain, shortness of breath, palpitations, syncope, heart murmur, hypo- or hypertension and an irregular pulse. In the context of renal medicine, it may be used to exclude electrical abnormalities of the heart associated with electrolyte derangements, particularly hyperkalaemia (see Figure 7.2). This would be particularly pertinent in a patient presenting with AKI, because severe hyperkalaemia with ECG changes is not uncommon and requires emergency management. ECG is also used to detect left ventricular hypertrophy, a common complication of hypertension.

Nerve conduction studies

Nerve conduction studies assess how well peripheral nerves conduct electrical impulses. Measurements are obtained by using recording electrodes placed on the skin. These measure electrical impulses, and a stimulating electrode is used to stimulate the nerve.

Indications

Nerve conduction studies are used in renal patients to diagnose polyneuropathies and mononeuritis multiplex in patients with connective tissue diseases, and to assess carpal tunnel syndrome caused by amyloidosis in long-term dialysis patients.

Management options

Starter questions

Answers to the following questions are on pages 132–133.

9. What types of medications are used in many patients with chronic kidney disease (CKD)?
10. What lifestyle changes might a patient with CKD need to make?
11. Which professionals are important in managing a patient with CKD?

Depending on the condition, the aims of management include some or all of the following:

- watching and waiting, i.e. monitoring of the patient for signs of disease progression
- relief of symptoms
- reversal or cure of the underlying disease
- prevention or limitation of disease progression and associated complications
- improvement of survival

Acute kidney injury may be reversible, depending on the underlying cause and severity, so the primary aim of management is usually reversal or cure of the causative disease. Conversely, there is no absolute cure for CKD, so management focuses on improvement of symptoms, reversing or limiting progression of the underlying disease, preventing complications and improving survival.

Management of renal disease may include the use of medications, surgery and renal replacement therapy, as well as psychological support, physiotherapy and occupational therapy. Most patients require a combination of these therapeutic modalities. Sometimes, management is conservative focusing on control of symptoms rather than active treatment of the disease.

The kidneys are susceptible to damage from all types of drugs, not just those prescribed for renal disease. Any possible effects should be considered before any prescriptions are made (see page 126), especially in patients who already have compromised renal function.

When treating any patient, but particularly one with a chronic disease, patient education is of great importance. Those who understand their condition are better able to cope with its effects on their life and to make the adaptations necessary to ensure optimal management.

Effective management of a disorder, especially one of a chronic nature, requires clear communication for the patient to acquire a sufficient understanding of their condition and to be involved in future decisions regarding their treatment. It is always beneficial to a patient's care to ask how they feel about their health and how much information they want from you.

The multidisciplinary team

The multidisciplinary team is a group of healthcare workers with different professional expertise who work together to deliver high-quality patient care. It typically comprises:

- doctors
- nurses
- physiotherapists
- occupational therapists
- social workers
- speech and language therapists
- dietitians
- psychologists

Not all patients require input from each professional; rather, their individual needs are assessed to allow specific services to be tailored to the patient.

Diet and lifestyle

Patients with CKD are at high risk of cardio-vascular diseases such as myocardial infarction, cerebrovascular accident and peripheral vascular disease. Cardiovascular disease is the leading cause of death worldwide, and is caused by the narrowing of arteries as a consequence of the deposition of fat-laden immune cells in arterial walls, i.e. atherosclerosis. This gradual and insidious pathology is heavily influenced by diet and lifestyle factors; it is associated with a sedentary lifestyle and a diet that is high in fat and sugar.

Atherosclerosis is increased in people with diabetes, because of the disruptive effects of a raised blood glucose concentration on the arterial wall. Diabetes is also a cause of CKD. Therefore high blood glucose is a key risk factor for both cardiovascular disease and CKD.

Modifying cardiovascular risk factors

Atherosclerosis is strongly influenced by lifestyle and dietary factors. Conservative measures aim to reduce risk factors as a means of primary prevention, and also to decrease disease progression or recurrence in established cardiovascular disease. The following are recommended:

- smoking cessation; smokers are at a fivefold increased risk of cardiovascular disease
- a healthy diet (**Table 2.15**)
- physical activity (at least 30 min, five times a week)
- weight control (body mass index < 25 kg/m^2)
- blood pressure < 140/90 mmHg
- total cholesterol concentration < 5 mmol/L
- normal glucose metabolism
- avoidance of stress
- use of antiplatelet medication, e.g. aspirin, primarily for secondary prevention of cardiovascular disease

Primary prevention consists of dietary improvement, weight loss, increased physical activity and smoking cessation, or a combination of these approaches.

Dietary guidelines for prevention of CVD	
Component of diet	Recommendation
Saturated fatty acids	< 10% of calories
Trans unsaturated fatty acids	As little as possible
Salt	< 5 g/day
Fibre	30–45 g/day
Fruit	200 g/day (two or three servings)
Vegetables	200 g/day (two or three servings)
Fish	Twice a week (at least one serving of oily fish)
Alcohol	Men: no more than two glasses (20 g)/day Women: no more than one glass (10 g)/day

Table 2.15 Dietary guidelines for the prevention of cardiovascular disease (CVD). Based on the 2012 European Society of Cardiology guidelines

Behavioural modification

There are three levels of intensity to encouraging behavioural change in patients.

1. Brief advice: opportunistic conversation to raise patient awareness and assess their desire to change
2. Brief interventions: structured advice providing more formal help, for example arranging targets and follow-up
3. Motivational interviewing: this is used to examine the patient's motivation and help them take action; it requires listening and patient-centred counselling skills that support the patient in exploring their ambivalence about changing their health-related behaviours (**Figure 2.33**)

Medication

There is no medication that provides an absolute cure for damage to the kidney; however, there are several classes of medication that are used either to minimise the complications of renal impairment or to treat the extrarenal cause of the damage. Most patients with renal disease require medication for at least one of these reasons. However

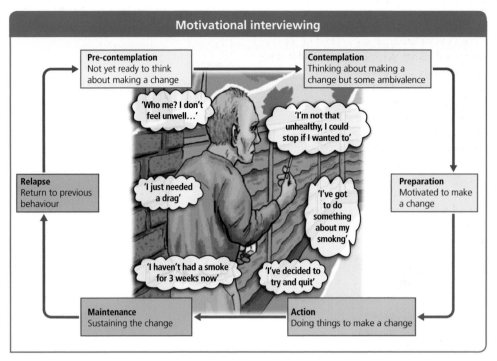

Figure 2.33 Motivational interviewing, as informed by Prochaska and DiClemente's model of behavioural change. This example concerns smoking cessation, but the theory is applicable to any behaviour.

in some patients, especially those with a very limited life expectancy, a more conservative approach is appropriate; medications are kept to a minimum and are largely restricted to palliation, for example antiemetics to control nausea and analgesics to control pain.

Special prescribing considerations in renal medicine Prescribing in renal medicine requires special care because impaired renal function alters the metabolism of many drugs. Some drugs are contraindicated in renal patients and others require dose adjustments. Accordingly, when a patient first presents with renal dysfunction, their medications are reviewed: some will need to be discontinued and others will need dose reduction. These special considerations are discussed in more detail on pages 130–131.

Blood pressure medications

Hypertension can be a cause or an effect of renal failure. Optimisation of blood pressure control limits further decline of renal function.

Antihypertensive agents are used to lower systemic blood pressure to an acceptable level. These medications are usually given in tablet form; however, intravenous preparations are used to control severely increased blood pressure in the emergency setting. There are several classes of antihypertensive drug, as listed in **Table 2.16**. Choice of drug class is made according to national and international guidelines, which are summarised in Figure 9.3.

ACE inhibitors and angiotensin II receptor blockers

These drugs are used as first-line treatment in younger, non-African-Caribbean patients with hypertension (**Table 2.16**). They are also used to treat proteinuria (particularly diabetic nephropathy) and heart failure.

Drugs in this group The most commonly prescribed ACE inhibitors are ramipril, lisinopril, elanapril and perindopril. The most commonly prescribed ARBs are losartan, valsartan, irbesartan and candesartan.

Antihypertensives: mechanisms of action and indications			
Drug class	Commonly-prescribed examples	Mechanism of action	Indication
ACE inhibitors	Ramipril Lisinopril	Block conversion of angiotensin I to angiotensin II; inhibit the RAAS	First-line agents for management of hypertension in non-African-Caribbean patients < 55 years old
Angiotensin II receptor blockers	Losartan Valsartan	Block the angiotensin II AT_1 receptor; inhibit the RAAS	Management of hypertension when ACE inhibitors are not tolerated
Calcium channel blockers	Nifedipine Amlodipine	Block L-type calcium channels to reduce calcium influx into vascular smooth muscle cells, resulting in vasodilation	First-line agents for treatment of hypertensive patients > 55 years old or African-Caribbean; second-line agents for others
Thiazide diuretics	Bendroflumethiazide	Inhibit the sodium-chloride transporter in the distal tubule Decrease systemic vascular resistance by a direct effect on blood vessels	Alternative first-line agents for patients > 55 years old or African-Caribbean in whom calcium channel blockers are unsuitable; alternative second-line agents for others. Third line agent if three drugs required.
Beta blockers	Atenolol Bisoprolol	Block β adrenergic receptors of the sympathetic nervous system	An adjunct in the management of resistant hypertension
Alpha blockers	Doxazosin	Block peripheral α_1 adrenergic receptors of the sympathetic nervous system	An adjunct in the management of resistant hypertension
Loop diuretics	Furosemide Bumetanide	Inhibit the $Na^+-K^+-2Cl^-$ cotransporter in the thick ascending limb	An adjunct in the management of resistant hypertension
Potassium-sparing diuretics	Spironolactone Amiloride	Antagonise aldosterone in the distal part of the distal tubule (spironolactone) or block epithelial sodium channels in the distal tubule and collecting duct (amiloride)	An adjunct in the management of resistant hypertension

ACE, angiotensin-converting enzyme; RAAS, renin–angiotensin–aldosterone system.

Table 2.16 Mechanisms of action and indications for blood pressure lowering medications (antihypertensive agents)

Mode of action Both ACE inhibitors and ARBs act on the RAAS (see page 35) by decreasing the activity of angiotensin II (**Figure 2.34**):

■ ACE inhibitors prevent the conversion of angiotensin I to angiotensin II
■ ARBs prevent angiotensin II from binding to angiotensin II receptors within blood vessel walls

By preventing the action of angiotensin II, these drugs promote vasodilation and inhibit aldosterone release. In this way, they reduce salt and water retention and thereby reduce blood pressure.

Angiotensin-converting enzyme inhibitors and ARBs also exert an additional protective effect on the kidneys, particularly when proteinuria is present. There is some evidence that proteinuria is toxic to the renal tubules and these agents, via their effect on intraglomerular pressure, are particularly effective at reducing the protein leak across the glomerular basement membrane.

Adverse effects These include a dry cough (ACEI only), renal impairment, hyperkalaemia, dizziness, rash and angio-oedema.

Interactions Use of ACE inhibitors and ARBs with other antihypertensives sometimes

Angiotensin-converting enzyme inhibitors

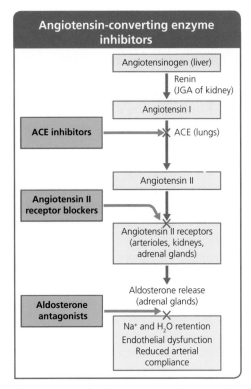

Figure 2.34 Mechanisms of action of angiotensin-converting enzyme (ACE) inhibitors and angiotensin II receptor blockers (ARBs). ACE inhibitors block ACE from converting angiotensin I to angiotensin II, leading to inhibition of the renin–angiotensin–aldosterone system (RAAS). The reduction in angiotensin II leads to peripheral vasodilation thereby reducing cardiac preload and afterload and improving impaired endothelial function, reducing sympathetic tone and reducing blood pressure. ARBs inhibit the RAAS by blocking the AT_1 receptor of angiotensin II, which leads to arteriolar and venous dilation. In this way, ARBs reduce cardiac preload and afterload, improve impaired endothelial function, and reduce sympathetic tone and blood pressure.

exacerbate this condition and in pregnancy due to the risk of teratogenicity.

> Both ACE inhibitors and ARBs are excreted by the kidneys and dosage should be carefully up- titrated (increased) in patients with renal impairment to ensure serum creatinine and potassium concentration remain within an acceptable range. They are avoided in patients with renal artery stenosis, because they interfere with renal autoregulation of blood flow to the glomerulus by relaxing the efferent arteriole (see page 19). Autoregulation in patients with renal artery stenosis is highly dependent on efferent arteriole dilation and constriction, because afferent arteriolar pressure is reduced by the narrowed renal artery. ACE inhibitors and ARBs can cause a decrease in glomerular perfusion and consequent ischaemic nephropathy.

causes hypotension. Hyperkalaemia is a result of ACE inhibitors being co-prescribed with ARBs and when either drug is taken alongside potassium-sparing diuretics, mineralocorticoid receptor antagonists, potassium supplements and NSAIDs.

Contraindications ACE inhibitors and ARBs are contraindicated in patients with previous angio-oedema and known hypersensitivity associated with these drugs. They are avoided in renal artery stenosis because they

Calcium channel blockers

These are widely used in the treatment of hypertension and are first-line agents in patients over 55 years and in African-Caribbean patients (who have lower renin levels and are therefore less responsive to ACE inhibitors and ARBs). In renal disease, calcium channel blockers are used to manage hypertension.

Drugs in this group Amlodipine, nifedepine, lercanidipine and felodipine are commonly prescribed for hypertension.

Mode of action By reducing calcium influx into vascular smooth muscle cells, they induce peripheral vasodilation, which results in decreased blood pressure.

Adverse effects These include hypotension, peripheral oedema, facial flushing, dizziness and gingival hyperplasia (swollen gums).

Interactions Hypotension occurs when calcium channel blockers are used in addition to other antihypertensives. Azole antifungals inhibit hepatic metabolism of calcium channel blockers, which increases the risk of cardiac toxicity. The antiepileptics carbamazepine and phenytoin reduce the effect of calcium channel blockers.

Contraindications Calcium channel blockers exacerbate heart failure and are avoided in such patients.

Alpha blockers

These are used as an adjunct in the treatment of resistant hypertension or in hypertension when other drugs are poorly tolerated. In renal disease, alpha blockers are commonly prescribed to bring blood pressure to within an acceptable range.

Drugs in this group Examples of alpha blockers are doxazosin, prazosin and terazosin.

Mode of action Alpha blockers act on peripheral α_1 adrenergic receptors of the sympathetic nervous system, the blockade of which results in vasodilation and a reduction in blood pressure.

Adverse effects These include hypotension, dizziness, headache, peripheral oedema and urinary incontinence.

Interactions Alpha blockers cause hypotension when co-prescribed with other antihypertensives.

Contraindications Alpha blockers are avoided in patients with existing urinary incontinence and are used with caution in patients with a history of postural hypotension and heart failure.

Beta blockers

Beta blockers are used to treat hypertension, as well as angina, arrhythmias and heart failure.

Drugs in this group Commonly used beta blockers are atenolol, bisoprolol, metoprolol, carvedilol, propranolol and labetalol.

Mode of action Beta blockers block the β adrenergic receptors of the sympathetic nervous system, thereby antagonising the effects of the catecholamines adrenaline (epinephrine) and noradrenaline (norepinephrine). There are three types of β adrenergic receptors:

- β_1 adrenergic receptors, located mainly in the heart and kidneys
- β_2 adrenergic receptors, located in the lungs, liver, gastrointestinal tract, uterus, skeletal muscle and vascular smooth muscle
- β_3 adrenergic receptors, in fat cells

Beta blockers decrease blood pressure by reducing cardiac output and by inhibiting the release of renin by juxtoglomerular cells of the kidney, an effect mediated by their action on β_1 adrenergic receptors.

Adverse effects These include fatigue, bradycardia, hypotension, cold hands and feet, nausea, vomiting, diarrhoea, bronchospasm and impaired awareness of hypoglycaemia in diabetics.

Interactions Use of beta blockers with antiarrhythmics sometimes results in bradycardia (although many patients tolerate more than one agent). Concomitant use with other antihypertensives causes hypotension in some patients.

Contraindications Beta blockers are avoided in patients with bradycardia and heart block. Non-selective beta blockers are avoided in patients with asthma and COPD due to the risk of bronchospasm.

Diuretics

These promote the urinary excretion of sodium and water by inhibiting absorption of sodium within the tubular lumen. This increases urinary osmolality and, therefore, water excretion. A diuretic is often used to treat hypertension and fluid overload at the same time, for example in heart failure. There are several classes of diuretic which each have different sites and mechanisms of action and different clinical uses (**Table 2.17** and **Figure 2.35**):

- thiazide diuretics
- loop diuretics
- potassium-sparing diuretics.

Thiazide diuretics

These diuretics are commonly used in the treatment of hypertension. They are also used to treat refractory oedema in combination with loop diuretics.

Diuretics: modes of action, adverse effects and indications					
Type	Mode of action	Location of action	Commonly prescribed examples	Common adverse effects	Indication
Loop diuretics	Block Na$^+$–K$^+$–2Cl$^-$ cotransporter	Thick ascending limb	Furosemide Bumetanide	Hyponatraemia Hypokalaemia Hyperuricaemia Renal injury	Heart failure
Thiazide diuretics	Block sodium–chloride cotransporter	Distal convoluted tubule	Bendroflumethiazide Hydrochlorothiazide Metolazone	Hypotension Dizziness Hyperglycaemia Cholestasis	Heart failure Hypertension
Potassium-sparing diuretics	Block epithelial sodium channels	Collecting duct	Amiloride Triamterene	Hyperkalaemia Dizziness Rash	Hypertension
Mineralocorticoid receptor antagonists	Block aldosterone receptors	Distal convoluted tubule	Spironolactone Eplerenone	Breast tenderness Hyperkalaemia	Heart failure Hypertension Hepatic cirrhosis

Table 2.17 Modes of action, adverse effects and indications for the different classes of diuretic agents

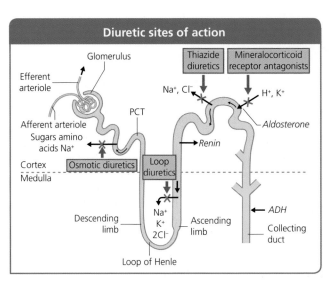

Figure 2.35 Sites of action of diuretic agents in the nephron. Osmotic diuretics (e.g. mannitol) are filtered but not reabsorbed and retain water in the renal tubule by their osmotic effect. Mannitol has a role in reducing raised intracranial pressure.

Drugs in this group Bendroflumethiazide, hydrochlorothiazide and metolozone are commonly-prescribed thiazide diuretics.

Mode of action Thiazide diuretics act on the proximal part of the distal tubule to inhibit the sodium–chloride transporter, resulting in natriuresis and diuresis.

Initially, the antihypertensive effect of thiazide diuretics is the consequence of diuresis, which decreases circulating volume. However, this effect is limited by activation of the RAAS, which increases systemic vascular resistance. The longer term antihypertensive effect of thiazides is probably the result of a direct effect on blood vessels, which causes vasodilation and a decrease in systemic vascular resistance.

In renal disease, thiazide diuretics are used in patients with eGFR > 30 mL/min/1.73 m² to lower blood pressure and reduce the risk of cardiovascular disease.

Adverse effects These include dehydration, dizziness, hypotension, hypokalaemia, hyperuricaemia, gout, hyperglycaemia and diabetes.

Interactions Use of thiazide diuretics with other antihypertensives can cause hypotension. Concomitant administration of thiazides with beta blockers increases the risk of diabetes in patients with impaired glucose tolerance, obesity and a positive family history. Hypokalaemia caused by thiazide diuretics increases the toxicity of antiarrhythmics such as digoxin.

Contraindications These include a history of gout and dyslipidaemia due to the adverse metabolic effects of thiazides. Patients with an eGFR <30 mL/min/1.73 m² should not be treated with thiazides. They are also avoided in patients with hypokalaemia and hyponatraemia because they exacerbate these disturbances, and in pregnant and breastfeeding women because they cross the placenta and are excreted in breast milk.

> **Thiazide diuretics have a synergistic effect with ACE inhibitors and ARBs.** By blocking the vasoconstrictive effect of angiotensin II, ACE inhibitors and ARBs allow thiazides to have a more powerful antihypertensive effect.

Loop diuretics

Loop diuretics are powerful diuretics that act on the loop of Henle to increase excretion of sodium and, therefore, water. They provide symptomatic relief in treatment of pulmonary oedema and peripheral oedema, and can be used in combination with thiazide diuretics.

Drugs in this group The most commonly prescribed loop diuretics are furosemide and bumetanide.

Mode of action Loop diuretics inhibit the $Na^+-K^+-2Cl^-$ cotransporter in the thick ascending limb of the loop of Henle (see page 22). This transporter reabsorbs about a quarter of filtered sodium, so its inhibition results in a substantial increase in the concentration of sodium within the distal tubule and consequently pronounced diuresis and natriuresis.

Loop diuretics have only a brief effect on blood pressure, however, because reflex stimulation of the RAAS counters any decrease in blood pressure. Therefore, although they have a stronger diuretic effect than thiazide diuretics, they are less useful in the management of hypertension because they lack a vasodilatory effect. In renal disease, loop diuretics are preferred to thiazide diuretics in patients with an eGFR < 30 mL/min/1.73 m² to treat hypertension and reduce cardiovascular risk.

Adverse effects Loop diuretics cause hyponatraemia, hypokalaemia, hypotension, hypocalcaemia, metabolic alkalosis, hyperuricaemia and ototoxicity.

Interactions Hypokalaemia potentiates the effect of antiarrhythmics such as digoxin. Concomitant use of aminoglycosides increases the risk of ototoxicity and nephrotoxicity, and NSAIDs reduce the diuretic effect of loop diuretics.

Contraindications Loop diuretics are avoided in patients with dehydration, prerenal failure, hypotension, hypokalaemia and hyponatraemia. They are also avoided in severe liver failure because hypokalaemia precipitates hepatic encephalopathy.

Potassium-sparing diuretics

In contrast to loop and thiazide diuretics, potassium-sparing diuretics induce diuresis without producing hypokalaemia. They are used in the management of resistant hypertension.

Drugs in this group These include mineralocorticoid receptor antagonists such as spironolactone and eplerenone and the epithelial sodium channel blocker, amiloride.

Mode of action Mineralocorticoid receptor antagonists, such as spironolactone, antagonise aldosterone in the distal part of the distal tubule, thereby decreasing the reabsorption of sodium and water and increasing their urinary excretion (see Figure 1.23: aldosterone release and actions). By inhibiting aldosterone-induced sodium reabsorption, fewer potassium and hydrogen ions are exchanged for sodium and lost in the urine. Amiloride blocks epithelial sodium channels in the distal tubule and collecting duct, thereby decreasing sodium and water reabsorption.

Adverse effects These include hyperkalaemia, nausea, vomiting, anorexia and diarrhoea. Spironolactone causes gynaecomastia, impotence and sexual dysfunction.

Interactions Potassium-sparing diuretics increase the risk of hyperkalaemia in patients taking ACE inhibitors or ARBs. Mineralocorticoid receptor antagonists potentiate the effects of other antihypertensives and decrease the excretion of digoxin and lithium.

Contraindications Potassium-sparing diuretics are avoided in patients with either a GFR < 30 mL/min/1.73 m² or those taking ACE inhibitors or ARBs, due to the risk of hyperkalaemia.

Diabetes medications

Diabetes is a common cause of CKD, so good glycaemic control is essential. This is achieved by a combination of structured diet and lifestyle changes as well as use of oral hypoglycaemic agents and insulin.

> All patients starting on oral hypoglycaemic agents or insulin require education about the symptoms of hypoglycaemia. These include sweating, dizziness, hunger, blurred vision, trembling and palpitations. Patients are told that if such symptoms occur, a sugary snack should be eaten immediately.

Insulin

Many diabetic patients with CKD require insulin because of inadequate glycaemic control with oral agents. Insulin is produced using recombinant DNA technology, and is administered via subcutaneous injections to replace the function of endogenous insulin. Because of its decreased renal metabolism in CKD, the starting doses of insulin for patients with CKD tend to be lower than those for people with diabetes in the general population.

Recombinant insulins vary from very short-acting to long-acting preparations. The choice of insulin regimen depends on the patient's preference; example regimens include twice-daily dosing of an intermediate-acting insulin and once-daily administration of a long-acting insulin with boluses of shorter-acting insulin with meals.

Mode of action Recombinant insulin replaces the function of endogenous insulin, therefore regulates blood glucose control.

Adverse effects Adverse effects of insulin are hypoglycaemia, weight gain, lipohypertrophy (excessive subcutaneous fat deposition) at injection sites and lipoatrophy (thinning of subcutaneous fat) at injection sites.

Interactions Concomitant use of insulin with oral hypoglycaemics increases the risk of hypoglycaemia.

Contraindications The major contraindication to insulin administration is hypoglycaemia.

> **The starting dose of insulin for a haemodialysis patient should be half that given to a patient with normal renal function.** The dose can then be increased over time, with careful monitoring of blood glucose and haemoglobin A1c concentrations.

Oral hypoglycaemics

Biguanides

Metformin is the first-line drug for treatment of type II diabetes.

Mode of action It potentiates the actions of insulin by decreasing hepatic gluconeogenesis, decreasing gastrointestinal glucose absorption and increasing peripheral glucose uptake and metabolism.

Adverse effects Gastrointestinal side effects such as bloating and diarrhoea occur in up to 50% of patients, although these are usually transient. It is associated with an increased risk of lactic acidosis in patients with renal failure, cardiac and hepatic failure.

Indications Type 2 diabetes, gestational diabetes and polycystic ovarian syndrome.

Contraindications Metformin is avoided in patients with an eGFR <30 mL/min/1.72 m^2 due to the risk of lactic acidosis.

> Metformin should be used with caution in patients with eGFR <30 mL/min/1.73 m^2 because of the risk of lactic acidosis. It is thought that this occurs because metformin impairs hepatic mitochondrial function resulting in increased anaerobic metabolism, a by-product of which is lactic acid production.

Sulfonylureas

These are often used in patients with CKD and type 2 diabetes because they are not renally-cleared and because short-acting preparations (e.g. gliclazide) are available which are less likely to cause hypoglycaemia.

Drugs in this group Examples of short-acting sulfonylureas are gliclazide and glipizide.

Mode of action Sulfonylureas increase pancreatic insulin release, which improves blood glucose control.

Adverse effects The major adverse effects are hypoglycaemia, particularly with long-acting agents, and weight gain.

Interactions Co-prescription of sulfonylureas with androgens, azole antifungals, clofibrate, H2 antagonists, salicylates or tricyclic antidepressants increases efficacy of sulfonylureas thereby increasing the risk of hypoglycaemia. Beta-blockers, calcium channel blockers and thiazide diuretics decrease the efficacy of sulfonylureas causing hyperglycaemia.

Contraindications Sulfonylureas are avoided in pregnancy and in any patient with a previous hypersensitivity reaction to this class of drug.

Metaglinides

These oral hypoglycaemics are not renally cleared and are given without increased risk of hypoglycaemia in patients with mild to moderate CKD. Other oral hypoglycaemic agents such as thiazolidinediones, dipeptidyl peptidase-4 inhibitors and alpha-glucosidase inhibitors are avoided in CKD due to limited data on their safety.

Drugs in this group Examples are repaglinide and nateglinide.

Mode of action These drugs stimulate pancreatic insulin secretion in a similar way to sulfonylureas, but have a separate binding site.

Adverse effects These are abdominal pain, diarrhoea and hypoglycaemia.

Interactions Oral contraceptives, carbamazepine, thiazides, rifampicin and corticosteroids decrease the efficacy of repaglinide.

Contraindications These are hypersensitivity to the drug, type 1 diabetes, diabetic ketoacidosis, concurrent treatment with gemfibrozil, pregnancy and lactation.

Phosphate binders

In late stage CKD, renal phosphate excretion decreases, so serum phosphate concentration increases. Chronically increased phosphate levels can result in cardiovascular damage, as well as itching, fatigue, nausea and anorexia. Phosphate binders bind to phosphate in the gut, thereby decreasing its absorption. They are started in late-stage CKD to mitigate the adverse effects of chronic hyperphosphataemia.

Drugs in this group These include simple molecules, such as calcium carbonate, and polymers, such as sevelamer.

Mode of action Phosphate binders bind to phosphate as it enters the gut to render it insoluble and therefore prevent its absorption.

Adverse effects Calcium carbonate causes hypercalcaemia and gastrointestinal side effects. Sevelamer causes varied gastrointestinal side effects comprising nausea, vomiting, diarrhoea and constipation.

Interactions Calcium carbonate decreases the therapeutic effect of various drugs including allopurinol, antipsychotics and gabapentin. Sevelamer decreases the bio-availability of ciprofloxacin.

Contraindications Sevelamer is contraindicated in cases of bowel obstruction. Calcium carbonate is avoided in patients with hypercalcaemia.

> **Phosphate binders should be taken with meals** to bind phosphate present in food as it enters the gut.

Vitamin D supplementation

Chronic kidney disease results in impaired activity of the enzyme 1-α hydroxylase, which activates vitamin D in the kidneys. Therefore patients become vitamin D-deficient, which results in hypocalcaemia and eventually secondary hyperparathyroidism, and contributes to hyperphosphataemia.

To counter this effect, vitamin D supplementation is given if the vitamin D concentration is low or the parathyroid hormone concentration increased.

Drugs in this group Ergocalciferol (vitamin D2) is used in patients with CKD stages 3 and 4 when serum 25-hydroxyvitamin D is low. Patients with CKD stage 5 require activated vitamin D in the form of alfacalcidol and calcitriol because they are less able to convert 25-hydroxyvitamin D into the active 1,25-dihydroxyvitamin D.

Mode of action Ergocalciferol undergoes 1α-hydroxylation in the kidney to become active 1,25-dihydroxyvitamin D. Alfacalcidol undergoes rapid hepatic conversion to the active 1,25-dihydroxyvitamin D and calcitriol binds directly to the vitamin D receptor.

Adverse effects Vitamin D supplementation results in hypercalcaemia.

Interactions Use of vitamin D alongside thiazide diuretics increases the risk of hypercalcaemia. Increased serum calcium concentrations associated with vitamin D supplementation potentiates the effects of digoxin.

Contraindications Vitamin D supplementation is avoided in patients with hypercalcaemia.

Calcimimetics

Calcimimetics are drugs that mimic the action of calcium on calcium-sensing receptors on the parathyroid gland. Cinacalcet is the only example in clinical use; it decreases parathyroid hormone concentrations and is used in patients with ESRD on dialysis to treat secondary hyperparathyroidism.

Drugs in this group Cinacalcet.

Mode of action Calcimimetics activate calcium-sending receptors present on parathyroid gland cells. This has a negative feedback effect and down regulates secretion of parathyroid hormone.

Adverse effects These include nausea, vomiting, hypocalcaemia and decreased bone turnover, if the concentration of parathyroid hormone becomes too low.

Interactions Cinacalcet dose may need to be decreased in patients taking CYP 450 enzyme inhibitors such as ketoconazole and itraconazole or increased in patients taking CYP 450 enzyme inducers such as rifampicin.

Contraindications Cincalcet is not given to patients with hypoalcaemia or those with CKD who are not on dialysis.

Erythropoietin and intravenous iron

Anaemia associated with renal disease (see page 53) is treated with periodic subcutaneous injections of erythropoietin and iron replacement with intravenous infusions.

Recombinant erythropoietins

Drugs in this group Examples are darbepoietin and epoetin alfa and beta.

Mode of action Recombinant erythropoietins stimulate the production of red blood cells by the bone marrow.

Adverse effects These include nausea, vomiting, diarrhoea, hypertension, headache, increased platelet count, thrombosis, influenza-like symptoms and cardiovascular events. Up to 10% of patients develop resistance to treatment and require higher doses to produce an effect.

Interactions Epoetin alfa increases the thrombogenic effects of thalidomide and lenalidomide, which are used in the treatment of multiple myeloma.

Contraindications Erythropoietins are contraindicated in uncontrolled hypertension, pure red cell aplasia associated with erythropoietin therapy and those unable to receive thromboprophylaxis.

Intravenous iron

Parenteral iron therapy is used as an adjunct to recombinant erythropoietin therapy to optimise haemoglobin concentration and minimise the dose of recombinant erythroipoietin required.

Drugs in this group These include iron sucrose, iron dextran and ferric carboxymaltose.

Mode of action Parenteral iron is processed by the reticuloendothelial system and stored as ferritin or exported out of cells and utilised in the synthesis of haemoglobin.

Adverse effects Severe hypersensitivity reactions occur in patients receiving intravenous iron, even when it has previously been tolerated. It is therefore only administered by trained staff in a setting where resuscitation equipment is available.

Interactions Dimercaprol, a chelating agent used in treatment of lead, arsenic, gold and mercury poisoning, forms toxic complexes with iron. Co-administration is therefore avoided.

Contraindications Intravenous iron is not administered to patients with allergic disorders or intercurrent infections.

Erythropoietin has been used by athletes as a performance-enhancing drug. By increasing red blood cell count, it improves oxygen delivery to tissues, resulting in enhanced aerobic respiration and improved athletic performance. The use of performance-enhancing drugs is known as doping and is banned in professional sport.

Immunosuppressants

Immunosuppressants are drugs that suppress the immune system (**Table 2.18**). They are central to the treatment of many renal conditions, including nephrotic syndrome and autoimmune diseases such as SLE and antineutrophil cytoplasmic antibody vasculitis. They are also vital for the prevention of organ rejection in renal transplant patients.

Dugs in this group Examples used in renal disease are corticosteroids, calcineurin inhibitors, alkylating agents and antiproliferative agents.

Mode of action Immunosuppressants act by various means to suppress the immune system (**Table 2.18**).

Adverse effects The most serious adverse effects are increased susceptibility to infection and malignancy, due to a weakened immune system. Other side effects vary depending on the individual drug.

Interactions These vary depending on the drug. For example, increased drug levels of tacrolimus result from co-prescription with azole antifungals and erythromycin, whereas decreased drug levels occur with carbamazepine and phenytoin. Cyclophosphamide is not coprescribed with other antiproliferative agents to avoid excessive bone marrow suppression.

Contraindications Immunosuppressats are contraindicated in patients who are already significantly immunosuppressed. Other specific contraindications depend on the individual drug.

Renal replacement therapy

Renal replacement therapy refers to the life-sustaining treatments used to replace kidney function in end-stage renal disease. These include:

- haemodialysis
- haemofiltration
- peritoneal dialysis
- renal transplantation (see pages 121–122)

Renal replacement therapy has a significant effect on patients' lives and is never

Immunosuppressive drugs: mechanisms of action and use in renal disease			
Group	Example	Mechanism of action	Use in renal disease
Corticosteroids	Prednisolone	Bind to DNA 'glucocorticoid response elements' to decrease proinflammatory gene expression and therefore T-cell activation, and increase anti-inflammatory gene expression	Immunosuppression following renal transplantation, treatment of vasculitis, certain causes of nephrotic syndrome, anti-GBM disease
Calcineurin inhibitors	Tacrolimus	Inhibit calcineurin phosphatase resulting in decreased production of IL-2 and decreased T-cell activation	Immunosuppression following renal transplantation
Alkylating agents	Cyclophosphamide	Active metabolite crosslinks DNA, adding alkyl group to guanine base of DNA. This results in inhibition of DNA replication and cell death. Immunosuppressive effect results from its action on T cells	Vasculitic renal disease, lupus nephritis, relapsing nephrotic syndrome, anti-GBM disease
Antiproliferative agents	Mycophenolate mofetil	Inhibits T and B lymphocyte proliferation resulting in suppression of cell-mediated and antibody-mediated immune responses	Immunosuppression following renal transplantation, lupus nephritis

Table 2.18 Immunosuppressive drugs used to treat renal disease and their mechanisms of action

undertaken lightly. For some patients, particularly the elderly and those with multiple comorbidities, dialysis will not improve quality or length of life and transplantation, which requires major surgery and lifelong immunosuppression, may not be appropriate. In such cases, conservative care may be chosen, which focuses on active management of symptoms and complications of renal failure, such as anaemia and bone disease.

Haemodialysis

Haemodialysis is the most commonly used form of dialysis in Europe, because it can be used in nearly all patient groups and can be performed for the patient (as opposed to peritoneal dialysis, which the patient usually manages him or herself). In 2009, 70% of UK patients starting renal replacement therapy began with haemodialysis.

In haemodialysis, a machine is used to pump blood through an artificial filter to enable the removal of waste products and fluid (**Figure 2.36**). Access to the circulation is required; this is provided via an arteriovenous

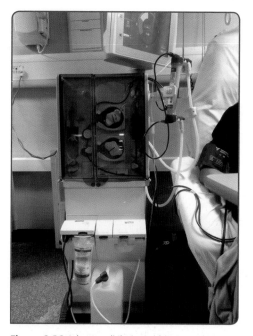

Figure 2.36 A haemodialysis machine.

fistula or graft (**Figure 2.37**) or a central venous catheter (**Figure 2.38**).

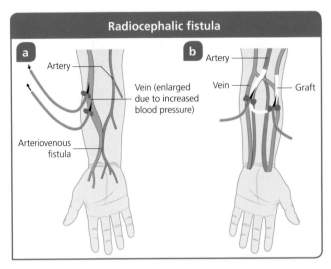

Radiocephalic fistula

a
Artery
Arteriovenous fistula

b
Artery
Vein (enlarged due to increased blood pressure)
Vein
Graft

Figure 2.37 Arteriovenous access for dialysis. (a) A radiocephalic fistula. A fistula can be made with the artery and vein end to end, side to side or end to side. The dilated vessel allows use of a larger bore catheter and enables higher flow rates. (b) The artery and vein may also be joined by a graft. This is a piece of tubing attached to an artery at one end and a vein at the other. It lies underneath the skin, and the tube is punctured during dialysis.

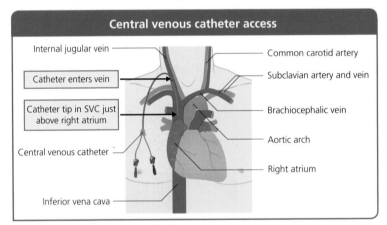

Central venous catheter access

Internal jugular vein
Catheter enters vein
Catheter tip in SVC just above right atrium
Central venous catheter
Inferior vena cava

Common carotid artery
Subclavian artery and vein
Brachiocephalic vein
Aortic arch
Right atrium

Figure 2.38 Arteriovenous access for dialysis, via a central venous catheter.

Arteriovenous fistulae

An arteriovenous fistula is a surgically constructed connection between an artery and a vein. Arterial pressure enlarges and strengthens the vein which, over time, produces a dilated blood vessel. It is used as the main point of catheter access during haemodialysis (**Figure 2.39**), because it allows large amounts of blood to flow during a dialysis treatment, provides easy access to the circulation, can withstand frequent puncture due to a thickened vessel wall and does not collapse under strong suction (unlike a normal blood vessel). An alternative form of haemodialysis access is a central venous catheter, but fistulae are preferred due to their lower risk of infection and longer lifespan.

The fistula is usually created in the upper limbs, and the blood vessel, which is dilated in consequence, may be visible. There should be a thrill, i.e. a palpable buzzing caused by turbulent blood flow, on palpation, and a bruit, i.e. a vascular sound caused by turbulent blood flow, on auscultation. Occasionally, fistulae are created in the legs.

Central venous catheters

Central venous catheters are plastic tubes inserted into large veins in the neck or thigh to allow haemodialysis. Short-term catheters are used in patients who require dialysis before insertion of a long-term central venous catheter or creation of a fistula, or those who have problems with an

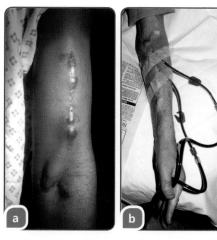

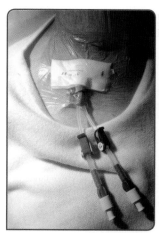

Figure 2.40
Right internal
jugular vein
vascular
catheter for
haemodialysis
access. The
point at which
the catheter
exits the skin is
hidden by the
dressing. This
catheter has a
bend and has
been inserted
low in the neck.

Figure 2.39 Upper limb arteriovenous fistulae. (a)
A brachiocephalic fistula un-needled. The shiny
areas with increased pigmentation are the sites of
repeated needling. (b) A radiocephalic fistula in use
during haemodialysis.

existing fistula (e.g. clotting preventing its
use). The most commonly used vessels are
the internal jugular and femoral veins. The
patient has a large catheter, with at least
two lumens extending from its insertion
site (**Figure 2.40**). For some patients, a fistula is not possible and long-term dialysis
access is provided by a tunnelled central
venous catheter. These long-term lines are
tunnelled into the skin, so that the exit site
of the catheter is away from its site of insertion into the blood vessel (**Figure 2.41**). This
helps to minimise the risk of line infections.

Indications

Haemodialysis may be started acutely, for
example when a patient with AKI or CKD presents with fluid overload or hyperkalaemia that
is resistant to medical management. More
often, the decision to start dialysis is planned
with the patient, taking into account their preference regarding modality (see Chapter 4).

Mechanism

Blood flows on one side of a semipermeable membrane, and dialysis fluid passes on
the other side in the opposite direction. The
dialysis fluid comprises sterile water and

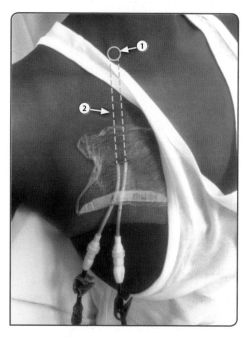

Figure 2.41 Tunnelled line in the right internal
jugular vein for haemodialysis access. ① Entry into
internal jugular vein. ② Subcutaneous track for
catheters.

solutes such as potassium, sodium, magnesium, calcium, bicarbonate and glucose.
Waste molecules, for example urea and creatinine, are transferred from the blood to the
dialysis fluid along their concentration gradients across the semipermeable membrane
(**Figures 2.42** and **2.43**).

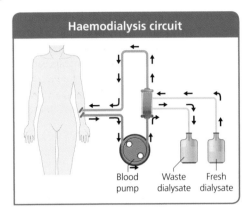

Figure 2.42 The haemodialysis circuit. Blood is removed from the patient via arteriovenous access (e.g. an arteriovenous fistula). It is then passed through the dialyser, which removes waste products. 'Clean' blood is then returned to the patient.

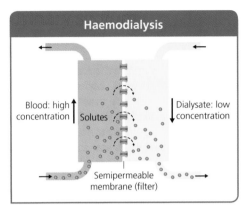

Figure 2.43 In haemodialysis, small solutes in the patient's blood diffuse across a semipermeable membrane into the dialysate fluid, which flows in the opposite direction. This countercurrent flow maintains a concentration gradient to drive solute diffusion from the blood, in which there is high concentration of the solute, and into the dialysate, in which there is a low concentration of the solute.

Dialysate contains a lower concentration of potassium and a higher concentration of bicarbonate than plasma, so potassium is lost from the blood and bicarbonate gained. Excess fluid is removed by applying a pressure gradient across the semipermeable membrane; the amount taken is altered by changing transmembrane pressure during dialysis.

> **Dialysis replaces only the filtration function of the kidneys to allow the removal of waste solutes and fluid.** It does not directly address the other effects of ESRD such as anaemia and renal bone disease. These are managed in the same way as for pre-dialysis patients.

Complications

These include hypotension, bleeding, loss of vascular access because of clotting, and bacteraemia resulting from line contamination.

Haemofiltration

Haemofiltration is another form of renal replacement therapy in which solutes move across a semipermeable membrane. Whereas in haemodialysis this occurs by diffusion, in haemofiltration solutes move by convection, across a pressure gradient. It is not used routinely for renal replacement therapy in patients with ESRD and is mostly used in the critical care setting for patients with acute kidney injury.

Indications

Haemofiltration tends to be used to treat AKI requiring renal replacement therapy in the critical care setting, where patients are more likely to be haemodynamically unstable, as it does not cause the large drops in blood pressure which may occur with haemodialysis. Haemofiltration is more effective at removing medium- and larger-sized molecules from the blood and it may remove pro-inflammatory cytokines, making it a superior option for the critically unwell. It can also be used to remove certain drugs or toxins.

Mechanism

Positive hydrostatic pressure is used to drive water and solutes across a membrane from blood into filtrate, which is then discarded (**Figure 2.44**). Because large amounts of fluid are removed from the patient, volume substitution is required. In contrast to

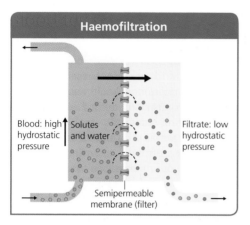

Haemofiltration

Blood: high hydrostatic pressure

Solutes and water

Filtrate: low hydrostatic pressure

Semipermeable membrane (filter)

Figure 2.44 In haemofiltration, solutes and water move across a semipermeable membrane by convection, driven by hydrostatic pressure.

haemodialysis, both small and large solutes are forced through the membrane at a similar rate, provided that the permeability of the membrane allows this.

Complications

As with haemodialysis, complications of haemofiltration include line-related sepsis, bleeding, haemodynamic instablilty (to a lesser degree), platelet consumption, and electrolyte imbalances.

> As well as being a life-saving treatment, dialysis is a life-altering treatment that results in substantial changes to patients' daily lives. Starting dialysis can be a traumatic experience for patients as they have to get used to needles, indwelling catheters and frequent visits to the hospital or dialysis unit. Many require specialist psychological support to manage this transition.

Haemodiafiltration

Haemodiafiltration combines the processes of haemodialysis and haemofiltration, resulting in solute transport by both diffusion and convection. This enables effective removal of solutes of both small and larger molecular weight, which results in better removal of waste products and may even improve

survival. Haemodiafiltration is sometimes used for maintenance renal replacement therapy in Europe but not in America; however, its use may become more widespread if a definite survival benefit can be shown.

As with haemofiltration, infusion of fluid is required to replace fluid removed from the patient's body.

Peritoneal dialysis

In Europe, about 15% of dialysis patients use peritoneal dialysis. In this mode of dialysis, the peritoneum is the semipermeable membrane used to filter the blood. Peritoneal dialysis is preferred by some patients as it allows them to carry on with their daily activities such as working and travelling, as they can perform dialysis in an ambulatory fashion, or overnight with a machine. There are also fewer restrictions on diet and fluid intake for patients using peritoneal dialysis. Some nephrologists prefer peritoneal dialysis as it avoids the fluctuations in plasma volume associated with haemodialysis, and therefore puts less strain on the heart.

Peritoneal dialysis catheters

A peritoneal dialysis catheter is a plastic tube inserted into the peritoneum for peritoneal dialysis access (**Figure 2.45**).

Indications and contraindications

Peritoneal dialysis is the preferred dialysis modality in infants and young children because it offers the least interference with

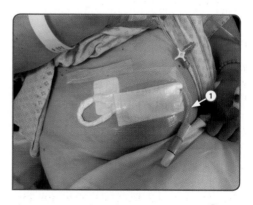

Figure 2.45 A catheter for peritoneal dialysis ①.

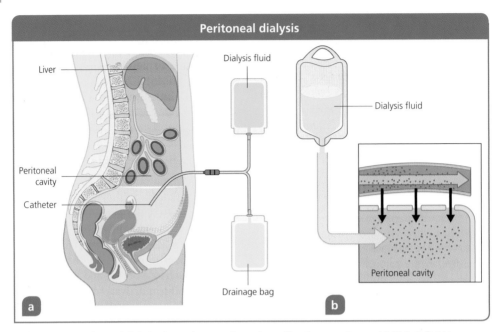

Peritoneal dialysis

Liver

Dialysis fluid

Dialysis fluid

Peritoneal cavity

Catheter

Drainage bag

Peritoneal cavity

a

b

Figure 2.46 In peritoneal dialysis, the peritoneum is used as a filtration membrane. (a) Dialysis fluid is introduced into the peritoneum and left for a few hours. Waste products move across the peritoneum into the dialysate, which is then drained from the peritoneal space into the drainage bag. (b) Waste products pass across the peritoneal membrane by diffusion and osmosis and into the dialysis fluid in the peritoneal cavity.

lifestyle and does not require the placement of intravenous catheters or needling of fistulae. It is also preferred in those with marked haemodynamic instability on haemodialysis and those with limited options for vascular access. Contraindications to peritoneal dialysis include an unsuitable peritoneum due to adhesions, fibrosis or malignancy; abdominal herniae; presence of an abdominal stoma (e.g. colostomy or ileostomy); an unsuitable home set-up (e.g. due to lack of cleanliness or space for storage of equipment); and neurological or motor problems limiting dexterity and severe psychological problems.

Mechanism

In peritoneal dialysis, fluid similar to haemodialysis fluid in composition is introduced into the peritoneum via a permanent catheter in the abdominal wall (**Figure 2.46**). The fluid is left in the peritoneum for a few hours at a time for each cycle to enable filtration to occur.

The high glucose concentration of the fluid causes water to be removed from the patient's body by osmosis. Waste products move into the dialysis fluid along their concentration gradients. The fluid is then removed and exchanged for fresh fluid.

In continuous ambulatory peritoneal dialysis, each cycle is repeated by the patient four or five times daily. In automated peritoneal dialysis, about 10 cycles, controlled by a bedside device (**Figure 2.47**), take place overnight.

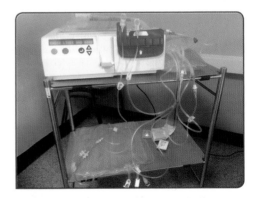

Figure 2.47 A peritoneal dialysis machine.

Complications

The major complication of peritoneal dialysis is bacterial peritonitis. Good personal hygiene and assiduous aseptic technique when changing dialysis bags helps prevent this. Because dialysis fluid has a high concentration of glucose, hyperglycaemia can occur, especially in patients with diabetes.

Surgery

Although most renal conditions are managed medically, surgery has a vital role in the management of ESRD, because surgical procedures may be required for dialysis access or renal transplantation.

Renal transplantation

Renal transplantation is the implantation of a donor kidney into a patient with ESRD, to enable them to survive without the need for dialysis. It is the gold standard management option for ESRD.

The transplanted kidney may come from a deceased donor after:

- brain death, i.e. the simultaneous and irreversible loss of the capacities for consciousness and breathing, in donation-after-brain-death ('DBD') transplants
- 'circulatory death', i.e. the irreversible loss of function of the heart and lungs in donation-after-circulatory-death ('DCD') transplants

Alternatively, the kidney is a donation from a living person, typically a family member.

Indications

Renal transplantation may be carried out pre-emptively in a patient with CKD who is not yet on dialysis, or it may be done after the patient has started dialysis.

Before transplantation, patients undergo an extensive work-up to ensure that they are fit for the procedure. Their name is then added to a waiting list for a DBD or DCD transplant. Most patients spend an average of 2–3 years on the waiting list before a transplant becomes available. Donations are allocated according to strict guidelines. If a match (according to tissue type and blood group) becomes available, children and younger adults are given priority as they are most likely to gain long-term benefit from transplantation. Older adults are allocated donations according to a scoring system based on how long that patient has been on the waiting list and how well matched the donor is. Alternatively, a live donor is found (usually a family member or friend who is an adequate match, although occasionally, people donate a kidney altruistically, and often anonymously) and an elective operation arranged.

Procedure

The procedures for live and deceased donor kidney transplants differ slightly. A live kidney donation is an elective process that is carefully planned and has the advantage of enabling a minimal amount of time to elapse between removal of the donor kidney and its implantation and perfusion in the recipient. On the other hand, a deceased donor transplant, while planned with the patient on the transplant waiting list, is performed as an emergency procedure when a suitable organ becomes available.

Most live donor nephrectomies are now performed laparoscopically rather than open, which minimises duration of hospital stay and recovery time following the procedure.

The procedure to transplant the donor kidney into the recipient is performed under general anaesthetic and begins with an incision, usually in the right iliac fossa, where the kidney will be implanted. The patient's native kidneys are left in place, unless they are causing problems such as recurrent infections or pain. The renal artery and vein from the donor kidney are attached to the recipient's external iliac artery and vein and the donor ureter is connected to the recipient's bladder (**Figure 2.48**). A stent is usually inserted into the ureter to ensure good flow of urine following the procedure. This is then removed several weeks later.

Complications

After transplantation, the patient requires lifelong immunosuppression to ensure that the organ is not rejected. Long-term

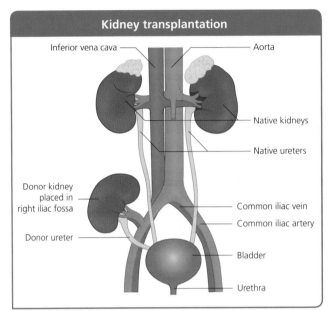

Kidney transplantation

Inferior vena cava

Aorta

Donor kidney placed in right iliac fossa

Donor ureter

Native kidneys

Native ureters

Common iliac vein

Common iliac artery

Bladder

Urethra

Figure 2.48 Implantation of a transplanted kidney. The donor renal artery and vein are anastomosed to the recipient's common (or external) iliac artery and vein and the donor ureter is attached to the bladder. The native kidneys usually remain in situ.

immunosuppression increases the risk of infection and malignancy, which are serious complications of transplantation.

A number of other complications are also associated with renal transplantation (**Table 2.19**). Not uncommonly, the donor kidney initially fails to function adequately, resulting in the need for renal replacement therapy. This is most likely with deceased donor kidneys, which have much longer ischaemia times than kidneys from a live donor. Renal artery thrombosis occurs in around 1% of renal transplants and can result in the need for a transplant nephrectomy. Transplant renal artery stenosis can also occur, usually after months or years, and causes hypertension. It can be treated percutaneously with placement of stents. Ureteric obstruction can also complicate a renal transplant, both in the short and longer term. Obstruction may result from a blood clot, stricture within the ureter, external compression, fibrosis and ureteric stones. Treatment typically involves dilatation of any stricture and stent placement. Urinary leakage can occur, usually from the anastomosis between the ureter and the bladder, and presents with urine leaking from the wound. It can be confirmed by testing any fluid leaking from the wound for creatinine and is treated with

bladder decompression if the leak is small or surgical exploration if it is large.

> Some patients who have identified a live donor find that this person is not an adequate tissue type or blood group match. Although they are unable to go ahead with donation and transplantation, the pair may be registered into a scheme to find a compatible donor with another pair. This is called a paired donation, or a pooled donation if more than two pairs are involved.

Nephrectomy

Nephrectomy is the surgical removal of a kidney. This may be required to treat cancer or to remove a diseased or injured kidney. In these cases, the nephrectomy may be complete (radical nephrectomy) or partial.

Nephrectomies are also carried on healthy individuals who wish to donate a kidney for transplantation.

Indications

These include renal cell carcinoma, chronic infection, a non-functioning kidney, a congenitally small kidney or a polycystic kidney.

Renal transplantation: complications		
Complication	Onset after transplant	Pathophysiology
Hyperacute rejection	Minutes	Pre-existing antibodies against the transplant
Transplant renal artery thrombosis	Days	Thrombosis of artery supplying donor kidney
Delayed graft function	Days to weeks	Donor kidney fails to function initially. Usually related to ischaemia time
Urine leak	Up to 1 month	Leakage of urine from anastomosis between the ureter and bladder. Presents with urine leakage from wound
Transplant artery stenosis	Weeks to months	Anastomotic stricture
Transplant ureteric obstruction	Weeks to months	Stenosis and obstruction at the ureteric anastomosis as a result of chronic fibrotic changes at the site or external compression from a haematoma, urinoma (an encapsulated collection of urine) or lymphocele (a collection of lymph)
Acute rejection	< 6 months	Anti-donor antibodies or T cells
Chronic rejection	> 1 year	Incompletely understood
Recurrence of original disease	Weeks to years	Higher risk in focal segmental glomerulosclerosis (see page 186) and immunoglobulin A nephropathy (see page 188)
Malignancies	Years	Especially of the skin and lymphoproliferative system, and caused by long-term immunosuppression from antirejection medication
Infection	Any time	Pathogens include cytomegalovirus and Pneumocystis jiroveci; this complication occurs as an adverse effect of taking immunosuppressive agents to prevent graft rejection

Table 2.19 Complications of renal transplantation

Procedure

The operation may be carried out as an open procedure through a large incision in the skin, or laparoscopically, using 'keyhole surgery'.

Complications

Complications of a nephrectomy include intra-operative injury to intra-abdominal organs or blood vessels, bleeding, post-operative ileus, atelectasis, wound infections, acute kidney injury and chronic kidney disease. Other more general complications include deep vein thrombosis, pulmonary embolism, pneumonia and myocardial infarction.

Psychological, physical and social support

Given the chronic nature of most renal disease, and the potential need for life-changing treatments such as dialysis and transplantation, many renal patients require more than just medical support; they need psychological support, physiotherapy and occupational therapy. These are a core component of management by multidisciplinary teams of health care professionals.

Psychological support

Renal units may provide access to specialised renal counsellors or psychologists, who are experts in helping renal patients come to terms with their disease and its effect on their lives, including life expectancy. Common psychosocial stressors for patients with CKD include depression, anxiety, chronic pain and lack of social support (Table 2.20).

There is some evidence that depression and a perceived lack of social support are associated with increased mortality in patients with ESRD. Outcomes are poorer in patients from

Chronic renal disease: psychological stressors		
Psychosocial stressor	Association and effects	Treatment options
Depression	Common in end-stage renal disease; may worsen health outcomes via its negative effects on nutrition, lack of concordance to treatment and possibly even changes in inflammatory response	Counselling, cognitive behavioural therapy, use of antidepressants such as selective serotonin reuptake inhibitors. Most antidepressants are hepatically metabolised and can therefore be used, with caution, in CKD. SSRIs are usually first-line treatment
Chronic pain	Common in patients with ESRD, occurring in up to 60% of dialysis patients. Associated with poor quality of life scores, insomnia and depression	Exercise programmes, counselling, judicious use of analgesia
Lack of social support	May be experienced by patients with CKD. Associated with impaired quality of life, increased risk of depression, increased morbidity and mortality	Peer support groups, psychological support (counselling), spiritual support through chaplaincy teams
Relationship difficulties with spouse, partner or family members	Chronic diseases can be associated with strain on close relationships	Counselling, peer support groups

Table 2.20 Common psychosocial stressors associated with chronic renal disease and potential treatment and intervention strategies

lower socioeconomic groups or with family or marital disturbances. Psychosocial interventions significantly improve quality of life and adherence to lifestyle recommendations and prescribed treatments.

> The multidisciplinary team plays a central role in non-medical aspects of a patient's management. This includes assessment of their physical, social and psychological needs and, where necessary, the provision of support (e.g. physiotherapy to improve strength, and occupational therapy, making adjustments to accommodation to maximise the patient's independence).

Physiotherapy

Physiotherapists assess and treat physical impairments caused by illness, disability, injury or ageing. They help patients improve and maintain mobility and strength in various ways, for example by teaching exercises, providing walking aids and organising falls prevention programmes.

Renal patients may receive support from physiotherapists, either in the community or on the dialysis unit if they are an outpatient, or on the hospital ward if they are an inpatient. Renal inpatients may require the assistance of physiotherapists to regain their strength and mobility postoperatively (e.g. transplant patients) or after an acute illness. On the haemodialysis unit, physiotherapists are involved in initiatives to encourage patients to exercise while undergoing their dialysis (e.g. using an exercise bicycle attached to their bed). This has been shown to improve outcomes. Other outpatient physiotherapy interventions include helping patients to manage their weight and maintain their strength through exercise programmes.

Occupational therapy

Occupational therapists help patients manage the effects of both physical disability and psychological difficulties, thereby enabling them to function at the highest level possible. They work closely with physiotherapists and social services to achieve this aim.

Occupational therapists carry out comprehensive assessments of individual patient's abilities to complete their activities of daily living, such as washing, dressing, preparing meals, cleaning and shopping. This usually necessitates visits to the patient's home. They then provide equipment and arrange home adaptations to optimise the patient's ability to carry out their activities, facilitate the delivery of care packages and refer patients to other agencies that may be able to offer support in the community.

> **Physiotherapists and occupational therapists play a key role in planning hospital discharges for many patients, such as the elderly or those with multiple medical conditions.** After assessing the patient's needs, they work with social services to help arrange the support a patient may need to ensure that they are able to manage at home or in the care of others after discharge from hospital.

Social support

Specialist renal social workers support patients with CKD by providing advice on practical, financial and emotional matters. They help patients to:

- access benefits (e.g. disability living allowance in the UK) or charity grants
- arrange adequate housing, particularly for patients receiving haemodialysis at home or using peritoneal dialysis, for which some homes would be unsuitable (e.g. due to lack of storage space for equipment or poor cleanliness)
- organise home care
- organise holidays

Effects of drugs on the kidney

The kidneys have a central role in the elimination of waste products such as drug metabolites. Therefore they are exposed to high concentrations of drugs and their metabolites, and are consequently vulnerable to drug-induced damage. Susceptibility to such damage results from factors that can be broadly divided into three main categories (**Table 2.21**):

- patient-specific factors, i.e. characteristics unique to that particular patient such as their age and past medical history
- kidney-specific factors, i.e. anatomical and physiological characteristics of the kidneys
- drug-specific factors, i.e. factors particular to the drug and how it is used, such as metabolites and dosage

Drug-induced renal damage: factors increasing susceptibility	
Category	Factors increasing susceptibility
Patient-specific	Older age (> 65 years)
	Acute kidney injury or chronic kidney disease
	Volume depletion
	Metabolic disorders (e.g. acidosis, hypokalaemia)
	Pharmacogenetics predisposing to drug toxicity
Kidney-specific	High rate of blood delivery (20–25% of cardiac output)
	High metabolic rate of tubular cells
	Generation of reactive oxygen species
	Uptake of toxins by tubular cells
	High concentration of toxins in renal medulla and interstitium
Drug-specific	Direct nephrotoxic effects of the drug or its metabolites
	Higher dose of the drug
	Prolonged use of the drug
	Drug combinations promoting nephrotoxicity

Table 2.21 Factors that increase susceptibility to drug-induced renal damage

When any drug is prescribed, the likelihood of renal toxicity must be considered, with a particular focus on patient- and drug-specific factors. Kidney-specific factors are 'fixed' and therefore present for each patient.

Many drugs have predictable, dose-dependent effects on the kidneys; resultant adverse effects can be anticipated and potentially prevented. Some drugs cause idiosyncratic reactions that result in renal damage; these unpredictable adverse reactions are rare and not possible to predict or prevent.

Drug-induced renal injury can occur in any area of the kidney, including the renal blood vessels, the glomerulus, the tubulointerstitium and the collecting system. The effect of drug-induced renal toxicity can be classified into two clinical syndromes:

- acute kidney injury, i.e. an abrupt decline in renal function resulting in accumulation of waste products and impaired fluid and electolyte balance
- chronic kidney disease, i.e. a chronic decline in renal function

The drugs responsible for these clinical syndromes are listed in **Table 2.22**. Commonly prescribed drugs that cause renal injury are discussed in more detail in the following sections.

> **Drug-induced renal injury** contributes to up to 25% of cases of AKI.

Non-steroidal anti-inflammatory drugs

Non-steroidal anti-inflammatory drugs (NSAIDs) are common medications used primarily in the management of pain. Examples include ibuprofen and naproxen. NSAIDs inhibit the enzymes cyclo-oxygenase 1 and cyclo-oxygenase 2, which are required for prostaglandin and thromboxane synthesis. This results in anti-inflammatory, analgesic and antipyretic effects.

Drug-induced renal toxicity: syndromes and causes

Clinical syndrome	Causative medication(s) and specific disorder(s)
Acute kidney injury	
Prerenal failure	Diuretics, particularly when used in combination
	Angiotensin-converting enzyme inhibitors
	Angiotensin II receptor blockers
	NSAIDs
	Cyclo-oxygenase 2 inhibitors
Intrinsic renal failure	Acute tubular injury
	■ Aminoglycosides
	■ Cisplatin
	■ Radiocontrast media
	■ Tenofovir
	Tubulointerstitial nephritis
	■ Antibiotics (e.g. penicillins, cephalosporins)
	■ NSAIDs
	■ Lithium
	■ Proton pump inhibitors
	■ Antiepileptics (e.g. valproate, carbamazepine)
	Vascular injury
	■ thrombotic microangiopathy (chemotherapeutic agents (e.g. cisplatin), calcineurin inhibitors (e.g. tacrolimus)
	■ occulsion of small arteries secondary to showers of arterial cholesteral plaques: anticoagulants (e.g. warfarin) and thrombolytics (e.g. tissue-plasminogen activator)
	Glomerular injury
	■ NSAIDs
	■ Gold
	■ Penicillamine
	■ Foscarnet
	■ Interferon α
Postrenal failure (renal tract obstruction)	Crystal-induced tubulointerstitial disease or obstructive uropathy
	■ Aciclovir
	■ Indinavir
	■ Methotrexate
	■ Ciprofloxacin
Chronic kidney disease	
Tubulointerstitial fibrosis	NSAIDs
	Paracetamol
	Aspirin
	Lithium
	Calcineurin inhibitors (e.g. tacrolimus)
Tubular dysfunction	
Fanconi's syndrome	Tenofovir

NSAID, non-steroidal anti-inflammatory drug.

Table 2.22 Drug-induced renal toxicity: clinical syndromes and causative medications

Effect on the kidneys

Prostaglandins have a vasodilatory effect on the renal afferent arteriole, thereby increasing GFR. In healthy individuals, the role of prostaglandins in the control of renal haemodynamics is minimal. However, in states of effective volume depletion, such as heart failure and dehydration, prostaglandin-induced vasodilation of the afferent arteriole is a vital compensatory mechanism (see pages 39–40). Under these conditions, inhibition of renal prostaglandin synthesis can result in vasoconstriction of the afferent arteriole and decreased GFR. Therefore NSAIDs are avoided in patients with renal impairment or with a decreased effective circulating volume.

ACE inhibitors and angiotensin II receptor blockers

Both ACE inhibitors and ARBs are used to treat hypertension and cardiac failure. By inhibiting the RAAS, they cause vasodilation, which results in decreased effective circulating volume, lower blood pressure and decreased cardiac oxygen demand (see **Figure 2.34**).

Effect on the kidneys

In the kidneys, angiotensin induces vasoconstriction of the efferent arteriole, thereby increasing intraglomerular perfusion pressure and GFR. When angiotensin is blocked by the actions of ACE inhibitors and ARBs, GFR is reduced (**Figure 2.49**). Particularly at risk are patients with CKD, heart failure and bilateral renal artery stenosis, in whom intrarenal perfusion pressure is already reduced.

This effect is not a contraindication to these patients starting on an ACE inhibitor or an ARB, but their renal function should be checked within 1 week of starting the drug and monitored thereafter. If creatinine increases or GFR decreases by > 30%, the drug is discontinued. In most cases, concentrations of these markers of renal function return to baseline levels once the drug is stopped.

Both ACE inhibitors and ARBs can also cause hyperkalaemia, because of their inhibitory effect on aldosterone release or action. Aldosterone acts on the renal tubules to cause retention of sodium and excretion of potassium, so inhibition of its secretion increases potassium levels. ACE inhibitors and ARBs cause a small increase in potassium levels in

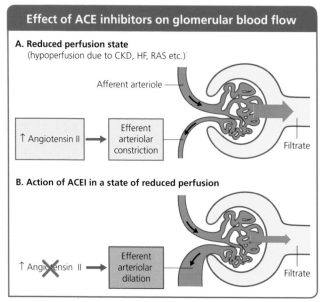

Effect of ACE inhibitors on glomerular blood flow

A. Reduced perfusion state
(hypoperfusion due to CKD, HF, RAS etc.)

Afferent arteriole

↑ Angiotensin II → Efferent arteriolar constriction

Filtrate

B. Action of ACEI in a state of reduced perfusion

↑ Angiotensin II → Efferent arteriolar dilation

Filtrate

Figure 2.49 The effect of angiotensin-converting enzyme (ACE) inhibitors on glomerular blood flow. (a) Glomerular blood flow in diseases such as chronic kidney disease (CKD), heart failure (HF) and bilateral renal artery stenosis (RAS) is already decreased (hypoperfusion), necessitating high levels of angiotensin II activity to constrict the efferent arteriole and thus maintain glomerular filtration rate (GFR). (b) ACE inhibitors block this constriction, thereby causing a significant decrease in GFR.

patients with normal renal function. However, in those with renal impairment the effect is usually more marked. In all patients, potassium concentration is monitored and the drug stopped if levels become difficult to control.

Aminoglycosides

Aminoglycosides are broad-spectrum antibiotics that are frequently used in clinical practice. They are a common cause of drug-induced nephrotoxicity and should be prescribed with caution in all patients; serum drug concentrations should be monitored closely.

Indication and mechanism of action

Aminoglycosides such as gentamicin are broad spectrum antibiotics that are effective against aerobic Gram-negative bacteria. They exert their bactericidal effect by entering the bacterial cell and binding to the 30 S ribosomal subunit. This results in misreading of the genetic code, thereby preventing normal bacterial protein synthesis.

Effect on the kidneys

Aminoglycoside antibiotics cause renal damage in 10–20% of all patients receiving them by inducing acute tubular necrosis, a disorder in which renal tubular epithelial cells die and slough into filtrate. Because new tubular cells are produced continually, the damage tends to be reversible and prognosis is usually good; however, aminoglycosides are avoided in patients at risk of AKI, such as those with volume depletion.

Aminoglycosides have a narrow therapeutic index: too much can cause toxicity, and too little is ineffective. Therefore therapeutic drug monitoring is required to ensure that the correct dose is given. A predose serum concentration is usually determined to allow the next dose to be adjusted if the level is too high.

Iodinated contrast

Iodinated contrast is a dye administered intravenously prior to certain radiographic procedures that causes renal damage in some patients.

Indication and mechanism of action

Iodinated contrast media are radiocontrast agents used during radiographic procedures to enhance the visibility of organs and blood vessels. They are commonly used for CT scans and angiograms, and are administered intravenously.

Effect on the kidneys

Iodinated contrast agents can cause AKI, usually within 12–24 h of administration. This is usually reversible; however, the use of contrast is avoided whenever possible in patients with renal impairment and those at risk of AKI. Renal injury is caused by a direct cytotoxic effect on renal tubular cells and by the induction of vasoconstriction. Different agents have different levels of toxicity. Nephrotoxicity is limited by ensuring that patients are adequately hydrated before and after contrast administration.

Prescribing in renal disease

There are special considerations when prescribing medications for renal patients. In renal disease there is a raised risk of drug-induced renal toxicity, because renal impairment alters both:

- Pharmacokinetics – the effects of the body on a drug, i.e. absorption, distribution, metabolism and excretion
- Pharmacodynamics – the effects of a drug on the body, i.e. receptor binding and post-receptor effects

The drugs that are most affected are those that are excreted via the kidneys or have active or toxic metabolites that are renally excreted.

The result is that some medications are contraindicated in patients with renal impairment, for example because they exert a toxic effect due to inadequate renal clearance (e.g. opioids) or because they damage the kidneys, risking further loss of renal function (e.g. NSAIDs and radiocontrast media). Other medications require dose alteration and close monitoring of renal function, and occasionally drug concentration, to ensure that toxicity is avoided. This is essential for renally excreted drugs with a narrow therapeutic index, i.e. those for which there is a narrow gap between therapeutic efficacy and toxicity.

> **Check prescribing guidelines** before prescribing drugs that affect renal function.

Drugs requiring dose alteration

When prescribing for patients with renal impairment, it is often necessary to alter the dose of a drug. This is because the half-life of renally excreted drugs, or their metabolites, is likely to be prolonged, resulting in accumulation of the drug and potential toxicity. Therefore doses of a given drug are reduced, or the dose frequency decreased, to prevent unwanted effects (**Table 2.23**).

Commonly used drugs that are renally excreted or have renally excreted metabolites,

Principles of prescribing for renal patients
Prescribe drugs only when there is a definite indication
Choose drugs that have minimal or no potential for nephrotoxicity
Follow guidelines for dosage regimens in renal failure
Monitor the patient for evidence of drug efficacy and toxicity
If possible, measure drug plasma concentrations to guide dose adjustments

Table 2.23 Principles of prescribing for patients with renal impairment

and that therefore require dose alteration or avoidance in renal patients, include certain antibiotics, low-molecular-weight heparins and opioid analgesics.

Monitoring

Once the drug has been given, the patient's renal function is monitored; should it deteriorate, the dose may need to be reduced further, or the drug stopped completely. Conversely, if the patient's renal function recovers, as in cases of AKI, the dose may need to be increased to ensure therapeutic efficacy.

For some drugs (e.g. aminoglycosides), it is possible to measure plasma concentrations. The results can be used to guide any further dose adjustments. If a drug has a narrow therapeutic index but it is not possible to monitor its plasma concentration, and there is potential for renal toxicity or dose-related adverse effects, an alternative should be found.

> **Extra caution should be exercised when prescribing for patients with renal impairment and hepatic dysfunction.** In these patients, pharmacokinetics and pharmacokinetics can be significantly altered, resulting in increased potential for drug toxicity.

Antibiotics

Many antibiotics are renally excreted and require dose reductions in renal patients.

These include penicillins, fluoroquinolones (e.g. ciprofloxacin and levofloxacin) and cephalosporins (e.g. cefuroxime). The dose adjustments required should be checked for individual agents, and may alter, depending on the degree of renal impairment.

Heparin

Low-molecular-weight heparins are commonly used prophylactically for patients at risk of deep vein thrombosis and for the treatment of thrombosis. They have a longer half-life in patients with renal impairment and can therefore accumulate, resulting in the potential for severe bleeding complications. Because of this, they are avoided when eGFR is < 30 mL/min/1.73 m^2; unfractionated heparin is given instead.

> **Use of unfractionated heparin at doses for treatment of thrombosis (as opposed to prophylaxis) requires monitoring of the activated partial thromboplastin time (APTT) to ensure that the correct dose is given.** If the APTT is too high, the patient is at risk of bleeding and if it becomes too low, the therapeutic effect of heparin is lost. This requires blood tests to be carried out at least every 24 hours.

Opioids

Opioids include morphine and related compounds; they are powerful analgesics. Many opioids and their metabolites are renally excreted and can therefore accumulate in patients with renal impairment to cause toxicity. Morphine and codeine have neurotoxic metabolites and are therefore avoided. Oxycodone undergoes mainly hepatic metabolism, and fentanyl is very short-acting, so the use of these agents is preferred in renal patients.

Prescribing in end-stage renal disease

As for patients with AKI and earlier stages of CKD, dose adjustments for renally excreted drugs must be made for patients with ESRD. A key consideration for dialysis patients is whether the drug is removed by dialysis; this may vary depending on whether the patient is on haemodialysis or peritoneal dialysis, as drug clearance for each modality is different. Haemodialysis is more efficient at removing renally excreted drugs than peritoneal dialysis, and drug clearance is better in automated peritoneal dialysis than in continuous ambulatory peritoneal dialysis. If a drug is removed by dialysis, administration must be at an appropriate time and dose to ensure that it has a therapeutic effect.

> **Gentamicin is removed by haemodialysis, so it is given at the end of a session.** In contrast, it is unaffected by peritoneal dialysis, so timing of administration is less important in this context.

Prescribing after renal transplantation

Dose adjustments may be required when prescribing renally excreted drugs for transplant patients, depending on the individual's renal function. Any interaction with immunosuppressive agents should also be considered. Calcineurin inhibitors such as tacrolimus are commonly used as maintenance immunosuppressants after transplantation. These are metabolised by hepatic cytochrome p450 enzymes, which can be induced or inhibited by various other drugs.

- If a cytochrome p450 enzyme–inducing drug (e.g. rifampicin) is needed, the dose of calcineurin inhibitor may need to be increased to maintain a therapeutic concentration
- If a cytochrome p450 enzyme–inhibiting drug (e.g. fluconazole) is required, the dose of calcineurin inhibitor may need to be reduced

Answers to starter questions

1. A detailed drug history is crucial when taking a renal history as many drugs have a significant effect on the kidney. These can include prescribed medications, over-the-counter medications, herbal remedies and recreational drugs. Asking about all of these will ensure a comprehensive history is taken and all causes of drug-induced renal dysfunction are addressed.

2. Tiredness may result from anaemia due to decreased renal production of erythropoietin, uraemia, acidosis, hypertension, electrolyte imbalances, drug side effects and general deconditioning due to muscle atrophy and weakness following prolonged periods of inactivity.

3. Shortness of breath may have several causes. These include pulmonary oedema secondary to fluid overload due to decreased GFR and, therefore, decreased fluid removal by the kidneys; pulmonary oedema due to congestive cardiac failure resulting from sustained hypertensive cardiac disease; anaemia due to decreased renal production of erythropoietin.

4. The renal examination may vary depending on the presenting complaint. In a patient presenting with acute kidney injury for the first time, for example, it would be important to look for both potential causes, such as volume depletion, and complications such as uraemic signs. In a stable long-term dialysis patient, however, the examination would focus more on looking for potential complications of dialysis such as an infected dialysis catheter, and fluid overload or depletion due to insufficient or excess fluid removal. Like any systems examination, a logical approach is required to ensure all aspects are covered.

5. Renal disease can affect various systems and can be caused by processes affecting different organs. When examining a renal patient, it is important to ensure all systems are examined so as to enable all relevant signs to be elicited.

6. A wide variety of diseases can cause renal impairment, many of which do not present with symptoms that are immediately diagnostic. For this reason, most patients presenting with renal impairment for the first time are screened for the common and rarer causes of renal disease. This ensures that rare but important diagnoses are not missed.

7. A blood film is a lab test in which blood cells are visualised under light microscopy. It enables the number, proportions and appearance of blood cells to be assessed and is used to detect haematological disease or blood parasites. In AKI, a blood film is requested if the patient has either anaemia or thrombocytopenia to exclude microscopic angiopathic haemolytic anaemia which is potentially life-threatening.

8. An ultrasound is performed in assessing a patient with suspected AKI to exclude structural abnormalities of the renal tract such as hydronephrosis caused by an obstructing lesion. If present, urgent intervention is necessary to prevent irreversible renal damage from occurring.

9. There are several common complications of CKD which require treatment with certain medications. These complications include hypertension, which is treated with antihypertensives; renal bone disease, which is treated with vitamin D analogues and phosphate binders; and anaemia, which is treated with intravenous iron and subcutaneous erythropoietin.

Answers *continued*

10. Patients with CKD can make certain lifestyle modifications to limit some of the associated complications. These include weight loss and exercise, to lower blood pressure and improve blood glucose control in diabetics; smoking cessation; a healthy diet high in fruit, vegetables and whole grains and low in sugar and saturated fat; dietary restriction of salt to help regulate sodium and fluid balance; dietary restriction of phosphate and potassium, to limit retention of phosphate and potassium, respectively. By empowering patients to take ownership of their condition (e.g. by encouraging diabetic patients to self-manage their insulin or hypertensive patients to monitor their blood pressure at home), doctors can further promote these behavioural and lifestyle changes.

11. A multidisciplinary team (MDT) is a group of professionals that meet regularly to discuss the assessment or management of a patient. In a patient with CKD, this includes physicians, surgeons, nurses, physiotherapists, occupational therapists, dieticians, social workers and psychologists. The MDT enables a holistic approach to the patient's care to be taken. In addition to managing the patient's medical problems, the multidisciplinary team can help optimise mobility, improve living arrangements to maximise independence, provide specialist dietary advice and provide psychological input. This support can help empower the patient to cope with their condition and, evidence suggests that it improves outcomes such as survival.

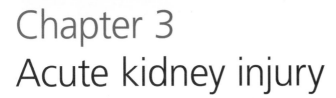

Chapter 3
Acute kidney injury

Starter questions

Answers to the following questions are on page 153.

1. What are the major causes of acute kidney injury (AKI)?
2. What tests can be used to diagnose the cause of AKI?
3. Can AKI be cured?
4. What factors increase the risk of developing AKI?
5. How can AKI be prevented?

Introduction

Acute kidney injury (AKI) is a sudden deterioration of renal function over hours or days; it is common in hospitalised adults. By comparison, chronic kidney disease (CKD) develops over a long period of time (usually years) and is usually caused by a chronic disease such as diabetes or hypertension. The two are related: AKI can result in CKD or end-stage renal disease (ESRD), and it increases the risk of developing CKD in the future, even if renal function returns to normal after an episode. Additionally, patients with CKD can develop AKI, which may resolve or cause further decline in renal function.

Because AKI is encountered so frequently across acute hospital specialties, it is often managed by non-renal doctors without the input of a nephrologist. Usually, only complex cases of AKI (e.g. if it fails to resolve with standard treatment or AKI requiring dialysis) require care by renal physicians. It is vital doctors across all specialties have a good understanding of the diagnosis, investigation and management of AKI.

Case 1 Low blood pressure and decreased urine output

Presentation

Edward Banks is a previously well 67-year-old who presented with small bowel obstruction 4 days ago. He was initially treated with intravenous fluids for hydration and a nasogastric tube to help decompress his bowel. However, his condition failed to improve and he underwent emergency surgery 3 days ago. A section of small bowel was removed.

He had been making a good recovery, but over the past 24 h his blood pressure has been low and the nurses have noticed that his urine output has reduced. He also has a postural drop in his blood pressure: a decrease in systolic blood pressure of > 20 mmHg when standing from sitting up or lying down.

Initial interpretation

Post-operative hypotension (a significant decrease in the patient's blood pressure compared with the pre-operative state) is caused by:

- dehydration
- haemorrhage
- sepsis
- autonomic dysfunction (e.g. in diabetic patients with autonomic neuropathy)

Mr Banks' hypotension could be related to any or all of these factors, although in the absence of diabetes autonomic dysfunction is unlikely. The reduced urine output indicates that his renal perfusion is being negatively affected and that his renal function is impaired.

AKI: diagnosis and explanation

Dilshad is concerned that Mr Banks is becoming very unwell. He calls Karen, the surgical trainee

After reviewing his blood results, Karen considers the differentials for his sepsis. Concerned there is an anastomotic leak, she calls the consultant Mr Ali because Mr Banks may need to go back to theatre

I feel really awful, doctor. I'm really hot, it's really hard to breathe... and my stomach hurts

He's hypotensive, oliguric, spiking temperatures and his abdomen is distended and tender. His renal function has dropped off and he's acidotic on the gas. I think he's volume depleted, septic and has gone into AKI as a result

Yes, but why?

Your blood pressure is quite low and your blood tests show that your kidneys aren't working well. This is probably because you're dehydrated, and I'm worried you might have an infection in your abdomen making this worse

Karen clearly and concisely explains the situation and current management to Mr Ali

Hi Mr Ali, I've just reviewed Mr Banks. He's hypotensive, oliguric and febrile with a distended, tender abdomen. His urea and creatinine and inflammatory markers have risen and he has a metabolic acidosis. Chest X-ray shows basal atelectasis and the abdominal CT suggests an anastomotic leak. I've started broad spectrum antibiotics and fluid resuscitation

He could be septic from his chest, but it sounds clear and the X-ray just shows atelectasis. The wound looks okay and his urine is negative. We need to rule out intra-abdominal sepsis from an anastomotic leak. Let's review him again and then call the boss…

OK. It sounds like he's dry, septic and his kidneys have taken a hit. He needs aggressive rehydration to help his kidneys and may need to go back to theatre.

What have my kidneys got to do with my belly?

Dehydration means there is less blood flowing through your kidneys. Infection is probably affecting them as well. We need to do a CT scan to see what's going on and take things from there

Taking care to avoid using medical jargon, Karen explains the diagnosis to Mr Banks

Examination

Mr Banks is tachycardic (heart rate 121 bpm) and hypotensive (blood pressure 95/50 mmHg), with decreased skin turgor and dry mucous membrane. His tongue appears to be dry and wrinkled. Two hours ago, his temperature increased suddenly to 38.7°C and has remained high. His respiratory rate is 28 breaths/min and his oxygen saturation is 94% on room air.

On auscultation of the chest, he has decreased air entry at both lung bases, and heart sounds are normal. His abdomen is tense and tender to palpation, and bowel sounds are reduced.

Interpretation of findings

Mr Banks has signs of hypovolaemia (decreased intravascular volume):

- decreased skin turgor
- dry mucous membranes
- postural drop in blood pressure

He also has signs of possible sepsis:

- low blood pressure (sepsis causes peripheral vasodilation and therefore a drop in systemic vascular resistance)
- abrupt increase in temperature

Reduced bowel sounds and a tense, tender abdomen suggest peritonitis (inflammation in the peritoneal cavity). In view of Mr Banks' recent surgery, this could be caused by leakage from the surgical connection (anastomosis) between the two parts of the bowel either side of the section removed. Another possibility would be ischaemia of the bowel due to problems with the blood supply.

On review of his fluid chart he is noted to be in a negative balance. This means he has been recorded as losing more fluid (urine and drainage from the nasogastric tube) than he has been receiving intravenously. This measured fluid deficit will be compounded by unmeasured, insensible losses (e.g. sweat, breath) and possibly by loss of circulating fluid into the peritoneal cavity and gut.

There may be two processes occurring here, hypovolaemia and sepsis, both of which impair renal function. The hypotension common to both will reduce renal perfusion and the possible circulation of endotoxins from bacteria associated with sepsis will cause a direct tubular injury. Fluid should be given, Mr Banks' volume status reassessed and further investigations carried out.

Investigations

Mr Banks' blood pressure and heart rate have responded well to boluses of intravenous fluid: his blood pressure has risen to 110/70 mmHg and his heart rate has fallen to 100 bpm. Blood tests and arterial blood gas measurements are arranged and Mr Banks is started on broad spectrum intravenous antibiotics. **Table 3.1** shows the blood test results before surgery and on the third post-operative day. The results for blood gases are shown in **Table 3.2**.

An erect chest radiograph and CT of the abdomen are also ordered. The radiograph suggests basal atelectasis (partial lung collapse usually producing linear opacities) and the CT shows free fluid in the peritoneal cavity.

Interpretation of results

The rise in serum urea and creatinine concentrations indicate that Mr Banks' renal function has deteriorated significantly. His increased C-reactive protein concentration and white cell count suggest that sepsis is possible, because the increase in both is much greater than would be expected from the normal

Case 1 *continued*

Edward Banks' blood test results			
Test	Preoperative result	Day 3 postoperative result	Normal range
Urea	5.4	18	2.5–6.7 mmol/L
Creatinine	63	238	50–110 µmol/L
Haemoglobin	136	122	135–177 g/L
White cell count	5.3	23	4–11 x10⁹/L
Neutrophils	2.2	18	2.0–7.5 x10⁹/L
C-reactive protein	< 5	207	<5 mg/L

Table 3.1 Blood test results for Edward Banks

Edward Banks' arterial blood gas results		
Test	Result	Normal range
pH	7.32	7.35–7.45
$P_a co_2$	4 kPa	4.7–6 kPa
$P_a o_2$	10 kPa	> 10 kPa
Base excess	-6.2 mmol/L	± 2 mmol/L
Bicarbonate	18 mmol/L	22–30 mmol/L
Lactate	4 mmol/L	0.7–2.1 mmol/L

$P_a co_2$, arterial partial pressure of carbon dioxide; $P_a o_2$, arterial partial pressure of oxygen.

Table 3.2 Arterial blood gas results (on room air) for Edward Banks

postoperative inflammatory response. His blood gas results show a metabolic acidosis (decrease in pH accompanied by a decrease in bicarbonate concentration) which reflects the underlying fluid depletion and sepsis. Both decrease tissue perfusion which leads to an increase in anaerobic respiration and a resulting lactic acidosis.

The clinical picture and the presence of free fluid in the peritoneal cavity on the CT strongly indicate an anastomotic leak. After review by the consultant, it is decided that Mr Banks requires investigative surgery to locate and repair any leak.

Diagnosis

An anastomotic leak is found and repaired in theatre. Mr Banks' peritoneal cavity is washed out to decrease the amount of bacteria and endotoxin, and he is continued on intravenous broad spectrum antibiotics. His fluid deficit is addressed by prescription of intravenous fluids to meet both his ongoing needs and the deficit itself.

As he recovers, his renal function slowly improves and his inflammatory markers normalise. One week after his second surgery Mr Banks' renal function is back to normal.

Acute kidney injury

Acute kidney injury is a sudden decrease in kidney function. It is characterised by rapid increases in blood urea and creatinine concentration caused by a decrease in glomerular filtration rate (GFR). These are tyically accompanied by a decrease in urine output.

AKI is usually a complication of a serious illness. It is often at least partially reversible, but the long-term consequences include chronic kidney disease, end-stage renal failure and death.

Classification

AKI is classified into stages based on serum creatinine concentration, urine output and GFR according to the international Kidney Disease: Improving Global Outcomes (KDIGO) staging classification (**Table 3.3**). Similar classification systems include the Risk, Injury, Failure, Loss of kidney function, and End-stage kidney disease (RIFLE) classification system for AKI, and the Acute Kidney Injury Network (AKIN) guidelines (**Figure 3.1**).

These classifications provide a uniform definition for comparing different patient groups and treatments. Some measures (e.g. the rise in creatinine concentration) also allow laboratories to issue automatic alerts to the clinical team when the relevant criteria are met. In the UK, the KDIGO system is used in clinical practice.

Epidemiology

Acute kidney injury is common in patients already in hospital, affecting 1–9% of inpatients, 20% of emergency admissions and 60% of patients in intensive care. Its overall incidence in the UK is about 1 in 200 (0.5%) per year. Dialysis is required in 10% of these cases.

Certain causes of AKI are particularly prevalent in certain geographical regions. For example, AKI secondary to volume depletion is more common in low- and middle-income countries, whereas AKI associated with polypharmacy or surgery is more likely to be seen in high-income countries.

Aetiology

The causes of AKI are defined according to the mechanism by which they develop (**Table 3.4** and **Figure 3.2**).

- Prerenal: any cause of decreased perfusion of the kidneys (approximately 35% of AKI cases)
- Intrarenal: any cause that lies within the kidney itself (45%)
- Postrenal: obstruction to the passage of urine from the kidney to the outside world (20%)

Categorising AKI in this manner helps select the most appropriate treatment (see page 150).

Acute tubular necrosis

Most cases of AKI in hospitalised patients are caused by a combination of prerenal and renal factors producing a pattern of injury loosely called acute tubular necrosis (the term is loosely applied because actual necrosis is unusual and a renal biopsy, which is required to demonstrate necrosis, is rarely performed).

KDIGO staging		
Stage	GFR and serum creatinine concentration	Urine output
1	Increase ≥ 26 µmol/L within 48 h or 1.5-fold increase in serum creatinine or GFR decrease > 25%	< 0.5 mL/kg/h for 6 h
2	2-fold increase in serum creatinine or GFR decrease > 50%	< 0.5 mL/kg/h for > 12 h
3	3-fold increase in serum creatinine or increase ≥ 354 µmol/L or GFR decrease > 75% or started on renal replacement therapy regardless of stage	< 0.3 mL/kg/h for 24 h or anuria for 12 h
GFR, glomerular filtration rate.		

Table 3.3 The Kidney Disease: Improving Global Outcomes (KDIGO) staging classification. This represents the current consensus classification of acute kidney injury (AKI)

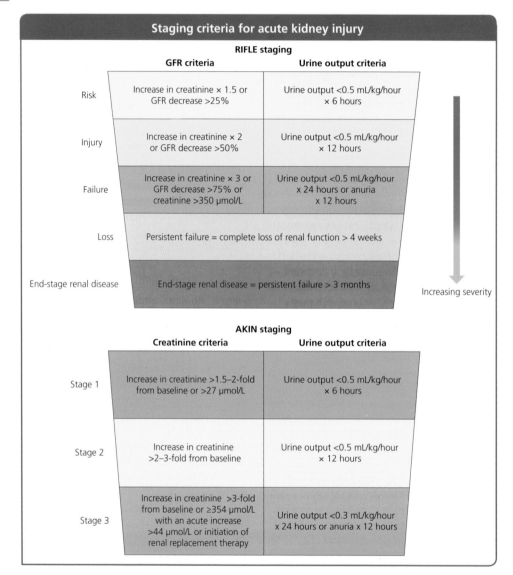

Figure 3.1 The RIFLE (Risk, Injury, Failure and Loss, and End-stage kidney disease) and AKIN (Acute Kidney Injury Network) staging criteria for acute kidney injury, based on glomerular filtration rate (GFR) and urine output variables. The KDIGO (Kidney Disease Improving Global Outcomes) classification is built on these two classification systems.

Prerenal causes of AKI

Prerenal AKI results from decreased renal perfusion causing impaired oxygenation of renal tissue. It is not associated with structural renal injury, but leads to approximately 35% of AKI cases. Specific causes of this are:

- volume depletion, e.g. as a result of haemorrhage, severe vomiting or diarrhoea, or burns
- reduced effective circulating volume (actual volume is not lost but it is inappropriately distributed or cardiac output

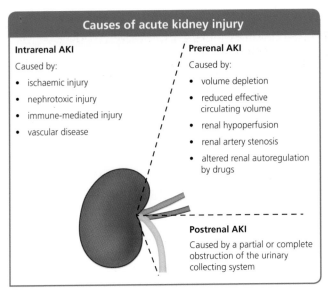

Causes of acute kidney injury

Intrarenal AKI

Caused by:
- ischaemic injury
- nephrotoxic injury
- immune-mediated injury
- vascular disease

Prerenal AKI

Caused by:
- volume depletion
- reduced effective circulating volume
- renal hypoperfusion
- renal artery stenosis
- altered renal autoregulation by drugs

Postrenal AKI

Caused by a partial or complete obstruction of the urinary collecting system

Figure 3.2 Causes of acute kidney injury (AKI) are classified into those occurring by prerenal, intrarenal and post-renal mechanisms. Prerenal causes represent decreased perfusion of the kidney, intrarenal causes are disease processes directly affecting the substance of the kidney and postrenal injury results from obstruction to the passage of urine.

Causes of postrenal AKI

Obstruction	Examples
Intrinsic upper urinary tract	Renal stones
	Blood clots
	Papillary necrosis
Extrinsic upper urinary tract	Retroperitoneal fibrosis
	Retroperitoneal or pelvic malignancy
	Retroperitoneal adenopathy
	Abdominal aortic aneurysm
Lower urinary tract	Bladder, e.g. calculus, blood clot, malignancy, neurogenic bladder
	Prostate, e.g. benign prostatic hypertrophy, malignancy
	Urethra, e.g. stricture, valves

Table 3.4 Causes of postrenal acute kidney injury (AKI)

Hepatorenal syndrome is a cause of AKI in patients with acute or chronic liver disease, when increasingly severe hepatic injury results in decreased renal perfusion. Splanchnic and peripheral vasodilation caused by increased vasodilator production leads to a decrease in effective circulating volume. This produces renal vasoconstriction and subsequently AKI.

Other forms of AKI are excluded before the diagnosis of hepatorenal syndrome is made.

Pharmacological causes

Prerenal AKI can also be caused by drugs altering renal autoregulation. Normally, prostaglandin-mediated vasodilation of afferent arterioles and angiotensin II-mediated vasoconstriction of efferent arterioles increase intraglomerular pressure and promote glomerular filtration (**Figure 3.3**).

Certain drugs produce AKI by interrupting this mechansim:

- non-steroidal anti-inflammatory drugs (NSAIDs) prevent afferent arteriolar vasodilation
- angiotensin-converting enzyme (ACE) inhibitors and angiotensin II receptor blockers prevent efferent arteriolar vasoconstriction

is decreased), e.g. in cases of sepsis, heart failure and cardiogenic shock, or cirrhosis
- renal hypoperfusion, e.g. as a result of renal artery stenosis (narrowing, e.g. as a consequence of atherosclerosis) or occlusion, abdominal aortic aneurysm (either spontaneous rupture or surgical repair), or hepatorenal syndrome

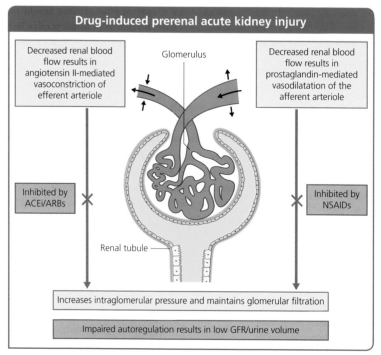

Drug-induced prerenal acute kidney injury

Decreased renal blood flow results in angiotensin II-mediated vasoconstriction of efferent arteriole

Glomerulus

Decreased renal blood flow results in prostaglandin-mediated vasodilatation of the afferent arteriole

Inhibited by ACEi/ARBs

Inhibited by NSAIDs

Renal tubule

Increases intraglomerular pressure and maintains glomerular filtration

Impaired autoregulation results in low GFR/urine volume

Figure 3.3 Pathophysiology of drug-induced prerenal acute kidney injury (AKI). The black arrows represent, on the left, the constriction of the efferent arteriole due to angiotensin II, and on the right, the dilatation of the afferent arteriole produced by prostaglandin. ACE, angiotensin-converting enzyme; ARBs, angiotensin II receptor blockers; GFR, glomerular filtration rate; NSAID, non-steroidal anti-inflammatory drug.

> **Angiotensin-converting enzyme inhibitors and angiotensin II receptor blockers can precipitate AKI** when used in patients with coincident renal artery stenosis.

Intrarenal causes of AKI

Intrarenal (intrinsic) AKI causes of 45% of cases of AKI. It results from direct damage to the renal parenchyma by:

■ ischaemic injury
■ nephrotoxic injury
■ immune-mediated injury
■ vascular disease

These factors affect the glomerulus, tubules, interstitium or a combination of the three. The tubules are generally most vulnerable to ischaemic and nephrotoxic insults, whereas immune-mediated injury tends to affect the glomerulus (causing glomerulonephritis; see Chapters 5&6) or, more rarely, the tubules and interstitium (causing tubulointerstitial nephritis; see Chapter 10). Vascular disease affects all the components of the kidney.

Ischaemic injury

Renal hypoperfusion, particularly if prolonged, results in tubular cell injury, apoptosis and acute tubular necrosis. Acute tubular necrosis is frequently multifactorial, with ischaemic and nephrotoxic injuries compounding each other.

> **The kidney is more vulnerable to ischaemia than other areas of the body;** even small decreases in oxygen can cause tubular injury and acute tubular necrosis, especially if there is already damage due to nephrotoxins. Under normal conditions the deeper areas of the medulla are already close to being hypoxic and tubular cells are so metabolically active that they are very sensitive to changes in oxygen supply.

Nephrotoxic injury

Intrarenal AKI can be caused by nephrotoxins:

- Endogenous nephrotoxins are generated during massive intravascular haemolysis, rhabdomyolysis (muscle breakdown) or breakdown of tumours with treatment (tumour lysis syndrome). They act on the renal parenchyma to cause acute tubular necrosis
- Exogenous agents with a directly toxic effect on the kidney include:
  - antibiotics (e.g. aminoglycosides)
  - chemotherapeutic agents (e.g. cisplatin)
  - radiocontrast agents
  - bacterial endotoxin

Immune-mediated injury

The kidneys can be damaged by abnormal immune responses to renal autoantigens or as a secondary effect of systemic autoimmune or inflammatory disease (**Figure 3.4**).

Antibody-associated damage typically affects the glomerulus and is characterised by decreased GFR, haematuria and proteinuria. Examples include anti-glomerular basement membrane disease (see page 202), in which

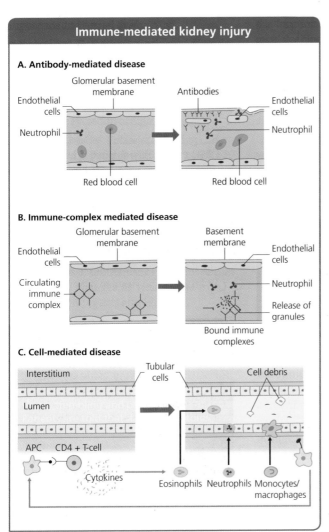

Figure 3.4 Immune-mediated causes of acute kidney injury. (a) Antibody-mediated disease: anti-glomerular basement membrane (GBM) antibodies bind directly to the GBM and then attract and activate neutrophils. (b) Immune-complex-mediated disease: immune complexes are trapped in the glomerular filter and then attract and activate neutrophils. (c) Cell-mediated immune disease in the kidney tubule: cytotoxic T cells are activated within the kidney in response to an antigen, resulting in cytokine release, recruitment of inflammatory cells to the tubulointerstitium and cell death. Chronic inflammation results when T cells continue to be activated by antigen. APC, antigen-presenting cell.

autoantibodies react with a component of collagen present in the glomerular basement membrane and antineutrophil cytoplasmic antibody (ANCA)-associated vasculitis, in which antibodies activate antigen-presenting cells expressing ANCA antigens, resulting in proinflammatory cytokine secretion.

Immune-mediated injury due to circulating antigen-antibody complexes also occurs within the glomerulus, where the filtration apparatus promotes deposition of immune complexes. Examples are:

- systemic lupus erythematosus, characterised by immune complex deposits in small blood vessels (including in the glomerulus)
- cryglobulinaemia, characterised by immunoglobulins that precipitate at low temperature within the serum

Both these conditions cause vasculitis (see page 198), thus there is a strong link between immune-mediated kidney injury and damage to the renal vasculature.

Certain drugs, such as ampicillin and rifampicin, can cause a cell-mediated hypersensitivity reaction within the tubulointerstitium (interstitial nephritis). This is characterised by the presence of lymphocytes and eosinophils (see page 290).

Vascular disease

Many of the vascular causes of intrarenal AKI are immune-mediated and are discussed above. Others are:

- thrombotic microangiopathy (e.g. haemolytic-uraemic syndrome, thrombocytopaenic purpura)
- cholesterol emboli
- accelerated hypertension
- renal infarction (e.g. bilateral renal artery stenosis and/or renal vein thrombosis)

Postrenal causes of AKI

Postrenal AKI results from an obstruction to the urinary collecting system (the renal pelvis, ureters, bladder or urethra) and accounts for 10–20% of cases of AKI. Obstruction causes irreversible damage if untreated; most patients with AKI undergo an US scan of the renal tract to rule it out.

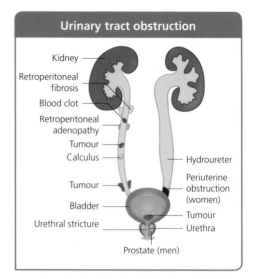

Figure 3.5 Sites and causes of urinary tract obstruction. Causes can be due to intraluminal obstruction (e.g. calculus), disease in the wall of the ureters, bladder or urethra (e.g. stricture) or compression from the outside (tumour, retroperitoneal fibrosis).

Obstruction has intrinsic and extrinsic causes (**Figure 3.5**) and is either complete or partial.

- Complete obstruction is usually associated with anuria
- Partial obstruction is either asymptomatic or presents with symptoms of voiding dysfunction such as hesitancy, poor stream and the need to strain to pass urine

Prevention

Preventing AKI is vital when managing patients in hospital, particularly the elderly and critically ill. The following are avoided:

- hypovolaemia
- nephrotoxic drugs
- contrast media

Hypovolaemia

Hypovolaemia must be anticipated and recognised promptly. If present, rapid treatment with intravenous fluids is required to maintain adequate circulating blood volume. In critically ill patients, vasopressor medications are given to induce vasoconstriction and increase mean arterial pressure. Maintaining sufficient fluid intake is also crucial in long distance runners, who are at risk of AKI.

Post-surgical hypovolaemia is a common cause of AKI. However, anticipating volume depletion can prevent its development and prompt recognition enables early treatment.

> In the intensive care setting, very close monitoring is required if vasopressors, such as noradrenaline (norepinephrine) or dobutamine are used. This is because there is a narrow margin between the dose required to maintain perfusion of vital tissues and the dose that will produce unwanted effects (excessive vasoconstriction, increased load on the heart).

Nephrotoxic drugs

Drugs that directly cause renal injury (e.g. gentamicin) or hypovolaemia (e.g. diuretics) are avoided in patients at risk of AKI. For some dugs it is possible to measure serum concentrations. Gentamicin and vancomycin are two potentially nephrotoxic drugs monitored like this.

Contrast media

Radiocontrast-induced AKI is common after cardiac catheterisation and contrast CT scans, which require infusion of radiopaque dyes. Adequate hydration before administration of contrast is key to its prevention. Also, the volume of contrast used should be minimised. In patients at increased risk of AKI, an alternative investigation that does not require the use of contrast is be considered.

To prevent contrast nephropathy in higher risk patients, for example those with diabetes or chronic kidney disease, the patient is given a 0.9% sodium chloride infusion 12 h before and 12 h after administration of contrast, and has their fluid status monitored. N-acetylcysteine is sometimes used for renal protection before contrast administration, but evidence for its use is conflicting.

Pathogenesis

AKI, whether prerenal, renal or postrenal, is characterised by a rapid decrease in GFR and a reduction in renal blood flow.

Prerenal acute kidney injury

In prerenal AKI, a reduction in renal perfusion pressure results in decreased GFR without damage to the glomerulus, renal tubules or interstitium. Under such conditions, homeostatic mechanisms ensure maximal urinary concentration and sodium reabsorption to maintain circulating blood volume and renal perfusion pressure. However, a prolonged decrease in GFR overcomes these mechanisms and results in ischaemic damage to the kidney and acute tubular necrosis (see below).

> In **prerenal AKI**, rapid restoration of renal perfusion improves renal function.

Intrarenal acute kidney injury

Intrarenal AKI results from direct damage to the kidney, which affects the:

- glomeruli
- tubules
- interstitium
- intrarenal blood vessels

Glomerular damage

AKI caused by glomerular damage is usually immune-mediated (see above) and is characteristic of acute glomerulonephritis. Acute glomerulonephritis is caused by primary renal disease or a systemic process (see Chapters 5 and 6).

Acute immune-mediated glomerular injury occurs due to either the formation or deposition of antibody–antigen complexes within the glomerulus. Small vessel vasculitis also causes glomerular injury in the absence of any immune deposits ('pauci-immune vasculitides', e.g. ANCA-associated vasculitis) (see below).

Depending upon the exact nature of the injury (see Chapters 5 and 6), there is an inflammatory response characterised by activation of the complement cascade and infiltration with inflammatory cells (predominantly neutrophils and monocytes), together with proliferation of epithelial, endothelial and mesangial cells and a consequent swelling of the glomerulus. There are also focal areas of necrosis within the glomerulus, together with proliferation of cells in Bowman's space (crescent formation).

These pathological changes compromise the glomerular barrier. They cause haematuria

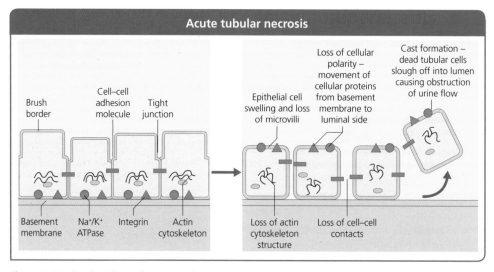

Figure 3.6 Pathophysiology of acute tubular necrosis (ATN). The left hand panel represents the normal arrangement of tubular cells on the tubular basement membrane. After injury (right hand panel) there is loss of normal cell polarity, swelling of epithelial cells and, if the injury is severe, cell death with sloughing into the lumen.

and proteinuria, and result in a reduction in GFR which causes salt and water retention and, eventually, hypertension. White cell and red cell casts are also found in the urine (urinary sediment).

Vasculitic renal disease

This is characterised by severe inflammation within small- and medium-sized blood vessels. Small vessel vasculitis is associated with necrosis and glomerular crescent formation (see Figure 6.2), whereas vasculitis affecting larger vessels causes ischaemic changes within the glomerulus due to involvement of larger upstream vessels.

In anti-glomerular basement membrane disease, the deposition of antibodies against the glomerular basement membrane provokes an inflammatory response within the glomerulus.

In antineutrophil cytoplasmic antibody (ANCA)-associated vasculitis, antibodies activate cytokine-primed neutrophils and monocytes that express the ANCA antigens, proteinase 3 and myeloperoxidase. This results in the secretion of proinflammatory cytokines and endothelial damage (see page 198).

Acute tubular necrosis

Acute tubular necrosis usually develops in the context of an acute illness, with hypotension, sepsis and the use of nephrotoxic drugs all compounding renal tubular injury. Its clinical course follows a sequence of initiation, maintenance and recovery.

Initiation:

■ Because of their high metabolic rate renal tubular cells are sensitive to insults from hypoxia and toxins. These insults decrease the production of ATP in tubular cells
■ ATP depletion damages the actin cytoskeleton within tubular cells causing changes to cell surface membrane structure and stability and damage to the adhesion molecules anchoring tubular cells to each other and to the basement membrane
■ These cause an acute but potentially reversible decrease in GFR

Maintenance:

■ In an established renal injury, cell necrosis and sloughing (shedding of dead cells) result in irreversible damage, tubular obstruction (**Figure 3.6**) and a sustained reduction in GFR. This phase can last for weeks
■ Urea and creatinine increases and urine output decreases
■ Impaired clearance of waste products results in metabolic acidosis, fluid retention and electrolyte abnormalities

Recovery:

- Recovery of renal function requires regeneration and repair of tubular epithelial cells
- The release of growth factors stimulates tubular cell proliferation
- Restoration of tubular function takes days to weeks (the more severe the initial injury the longer the recovery). It is characterised by improved urine output and a decrease in urea and creatinine concentrations
- A period of diuresis may occur during recovery, resulting in salt and water loss and therefore volume depletion

Tubulointerstitial renal disease

AKI due to tubulointerstitial renal disease is triggered by the exposure of tubular cells to exogenous antigens from drugs or pathogens, or in some cases certain endogenous antigens (page 290). Often no obvious precipitant is identified.

Whatever the precipitant, there is an inflammatory response characterised by inflammatory cell infiltrate within the intersitium (typically composed of T cells, mononuclear cells, plasma cells and eosinophils) and tubular oedema, which results in increased intrarenal pressure and impaired filtration. The inflammatory processes rapidly induce fibrogenesis, which results in tubular atrophy and a further decline in renal function unless the precipitant is removed or treatment commenced.

Vascular renal disease

Thrombotic microangiopathy AKI can result from thrombotic microangiopathy, a pathological process characterised by endothelial damage, thrombocytopenia, microangiopathic anaemia and microvascular thrombi. It typically occurs in haemolytic uraemic syndrome (HUS) and thrombotic thrombocytopenic purpura (TTP). In HUS, thrombotic microangiopathy is caused by dysregulation of the complement cascade. In TTP it is caused by deficiency of the cleaving protease for von WIllibrand Factor and the subsequent excess platelet aggregation and formation of microthrombi. In both cases formation of microvascular thrombi results

in renal ischaemia and infarction, and therefore impaired renal function.

AKI in accelerated hypertension also occurs due to thrombotic microangiopathy.

Cholesterol emboli In cases of cholesterol emboli, cholesterol crystals break away from atherosclerotic plaques and lodge in the arterioles of downstream organs. This induces an inflammatory response that promotes fibrosis and eventually obliterates the vessel lumen, resulting in ischaemia.

Renal infarction Renal infarction occurs when part or all of the renal blood supply is disrupted, resulting in ischaemia and cell death. This occurs due to renal artery stenosis (where narrowing of the renal arteries severely limits renal blood flow), or in renal arterial or venous thrombosis, which are usually due to underlying hypercoagulability.

Postrenal acute kidney injury

Postrenal causes of AKI obstruct urinary flow, causing an increase in intratubular pressure that decreases the pressure gradient between the glomerulus and Bowman's space, thereby reducing GFR. Urinary tract obstruction also impairs renal blood flow, which further decreases GFR.

Clinical features

Different causes of AKI present with different features and may include non-specific symptoms such as nausea and lethargy. There is often a history of decreased urine output. Other clinical features, including symptoms of fluid overload (oedema, orthopnoea) and electrolyte and acid-base disturbance (see Chapters 7 & 8) occur as a consequence of AKI.

> **Patients with AKI have impaired haemostasis as a result of platelet dysfunction and are therefore at high risk of gastrointestinal bleeding.** This causes significant morbidity. Prophylactic treatment with proton pump inhibitors or H_2 receptor blockers, which reduce stomach acid and the risk of bleeding, is usually initiated, and the use of aspirin is avoided.

Prerenal acute kidney injury

Prerenal AKI presents with symptoms of volume depletion (hypovolaemia) and hypotension, including thirst, dizziness and weakness. There may be a background of vomiting, diarrhoea or poor oral intake, or of major bleeding.

Hypovolaemia is not always obvious from the initial history. However, detailed fluid intake and output analysis will reveal this as a cause. Signs include (**Figure 3.7**):

- tachycardia
- low blood pressure
- postural hypotension
- loss of skin turgor
- dry mucous membranes

Intrarenal acute kidney injury

There are no specific features of intrarenal AKI. Instead, they reflect the precipitating cause and the consequences of AKI.

Drug-induced acute kidney injury

In most cases of drug-induced AKI there are no specific clinical features, although any

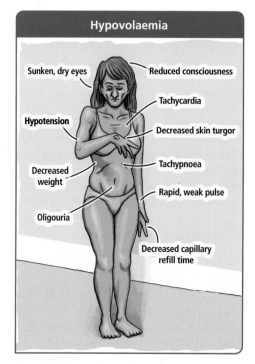

obvious side effects of drugs will provide a clue (e.g. hair loss in patients on chemotherapeutic agents). An exception is acute tubulointerstitial nephritis due to a hypersentivity reaction, which is suggested by the presence of a maculopapular rash and joint pains.

Immune-mediated acute kidney injury

Vasculitis causes:

- haematuria or smoky urine
- respiratory tract symptoms, especially haemoptysis
- palpable purpura
- joint pains or swelling

Purpura over the legs and buttocks in a young person indicates Henoch–Schlönlein purpura. Lupus nephritis presents with other signs of lupus, such as mouth ulcers, hair loss and facial rash.

Toxin-mediated acute kidney injury

A fall or crush injury in the context of dark urine suggests rhabdomyolysis (trauma to muscles that causes release of myoglobin and other intracellular components that act as nephrotoxins). Tumour lysis syndrome should be suspected if chemotherapy has just been started for large volume tumours, particularly lymphomas. Malignancy, especially myeloma, can cause hypercalcaemia that precipitates AKI.

Postrenal acute kidney injury

A history of voiding problems, such as poor urine flow and hesitancy, suggests urinary obstruction. An abdomen examination will show signs of an enlarged bladder: a mass arising from the pelvis, dull to percussion. This may be painful; however the patient may not be aware of it, especially if the obstruction is chronic.

Diagnostic approach

A fall in urine output or a change in volume status suggests AKI. A firm diagnosis relies on identifying the rise in serum creatinine and serum urea and a fall in eGFR. Subsequent investigations are used to determine the cause of AKI and include:

- urinalysis

Figure 3.7 Signs of hypovolaemia.

- specialist blood tests
- renal tract imaging
- renal biopsy

Urinalysis

Urinalysis provides information about the pathology underlying the patient's AKI (**Table 3.5**). Glomerular disease is indicated by the presence of significant proteinuria, casts and dysmorphic red cells. Urinary sodium concentration helps identify whether there is a prerenal or established renal cause of AKI. If myeloma is suspected then urine is tested for Bence Jones proteins (free immunoglobulin light chains).

> **Myoglobinuria,** the presence of myoglobin in urine found in the context of rhabdomyolysis, produces a positive reaction for haematuria without evidence of red cells on urine microscopy.

Specialist blood tests

These are tests that are done to identify specific, usually intra-renal, causes of AKI. A combination of these tests is commonly sent off as a panel (an 'acute renal screen') when an intra-renal cause is suspected on clinical grounds. They are directed at identifying toxic and immunologically-mediated injury.

Toxin-mediated injury

Calcium concentration is measured if an underlying malignancy causing hypercalcaemia is suspected. Rhabdomyolysis is characterised by:

- very high creatine kinase concentrations in the blood
- high blood phosphate
- high blood urate
- low blood calcium

The tumour lysis syndrome is associated with high blood urate concentrations; the condition is essentially an acute urate nephropathy.

Although a rare cause of AKI, massive haemolysis is associated with low haemoglobin, the presence of free haemoglobin in the serum and consumption of haptoglobin (a protein which binds free haemoglobin).

Suspected acute kidney injury: interpretation of urinalysis results	
Finding	Associated pathology
Significant proteinuria (+++ and ++++) and haematuria	Glomerular injury
Haematuria	Lower urinary tract obstruction
	Tumours
	Calculi
	Infection
	Severe renal ischaemia (e.g. arterial or venous thrombosis)
Increased white cell count (> 5 per high power field)	Acute interstitial nephritis
	Infection
	Glomerulonephritis
Eosinophiluria	Interstitial nephritis [poor positive predictive value, excellent negative predictive value (>90%)]
Low sodium concentration and high osmolality	Prerenal acute kidney injury: these results are caused by increased reabsorption of urinary sodium and water
	Sodium and osmolality results help distinguish reversible prerenal failure from established acute tubular disease; in the latter sodium concentration and osmolality approach that of plasma
Urine Bence Jones protein	Multiple myeloma
Abnormalities on microscopy	
Dysmorphic red blood cells and red cell casts	Glomerular disease
Eosinophils and white cell casts	Interstitial disease
Crystals	Toxicity from use of e.g. sulfonamides, aciclovir, indinavir
Urate crystal deposition	Tumour lysis syndrome

Table 3.5 Interpretation of urinalysis results in suspected acute kidney injury

Autoantibodies and immunological tests

Other specialist blood tests are carried out to identify specific immune causes of AKI if these are suspected on clinical grounds:

- antinuclear and related (anti-double stranded DNA, anti-extractable nuclear antigen) antibodies, which are present in lupus nephritis

- complement component (usually C3 and C4) concentrations, which are decreased in lupus nephritis and certain other immune-mediated diseases (see Chapter 6)
- antineutrophil cytoplasmic antibody, a finding in ANCA vasculitis
- anti-glomerular basement membrane antibody, which is present in anti–glomerular basement membrane disease
- serum electrophoresis, to assess for a paraprotein associated with multiple myeloma

> **Because one of the kidneys' main functions is to maintain blood volume by retaining salt and water, urinary sodium concentration is low in the initial stages of prerenal AKI.** However, prolonged insults damage the renal tubules, leaving them unable to retain salt and water; urinary sodium loss increases in consequence.

Imaging

Ultrasound is used to rule out obstructive uropathy. A postrenal (obstructive) cause is suspected if the patient is anuric, which is unusual in most causes of prerenal and intrarenal AKI. In this case it is sometimes worth repeating the ultrasound if this is normal initially because the pelvicalyceal dilatation (see Figure 12.2) characteristic of obstruction takes a while to develop.

Biopsy

Renal biopsy is indicated if glomerular disease amenable to treatment with immunosuppression is suspected. It is rarely needed if the clinical diagnosis is acute tubular necrosis, because this is usually diagnosed on clinical grounds and no specific treatment (other than supportive management) is indicated. If there is a prolonged course of renal impairment (greater then 2–3 weeks) in a suspected case of acute tubular necrosis, then a biopsy might be indicated to rule out a complicating condition (e.g. an interstitial nephritis secondary to drugs).

Management

The managment of AKI is summarised in **Figure 3.8**.

The recognition and treatment of the reversible causes of AKI prevents the development of established AKI and the resulting need for renal replacement therapy. The most important reversible causes are:

- volume depletion
- obstruction (requires a urinary catheter or radiological and/or surgical intervention)
- nephrotoxic drugs

Once AKI is diagnosed, treatment is implemented rapidly. Patients with AKI and other organ pathologies will be considered for transfer to a high-dependency or intensive therapy unit, for example if they have severe sepsis, congestive cardiac failure, encephalopathy or hypoxia.

Fluid resuscitation

Fluid replacement is the priority when hypovolaemia is contributing to a prerenal cause of AKI.

- In a hypovolaemic patient, fluid therapy using crystalloids (0.9% sodium chloride, or balanced salt solution) is started promptly
- In cases of haemorrhagic shock, colloids (blood products or plasma substitutes, such as dextran or gelatin) are considered
- If fluid balance is more complex, e.g. AKI in the context of heart failure, small boluses of crystalloid are used, for example 250 mL of 0.9% sodium chloride followed by reassessment for signs of fluid overload

> **Patients with AKI are at risk of acute hyperkalaemia, which predisposes to cardiac arrhythmias.** Therefore they require potassium restriction, typically to < 50 mmol per day. Regular electrocardiographic monitoring is warranted if potassium levels are increased. Typical changes in hyperkalaemia include flat P waves, tall tented T waves and broad QRS complexes. These electrical abnormalities can degenerate into ventricular fibrillation. Treatment of hyperkalaemia includes intravenous calcium gluconate to stabilise the myocardium and insulin–glucose infusion to drive potassium into cells.

If hypotension fails to improve despite 2 L of fluid resuscitation, senior nephrology review should be sought and treatment in a higher-dependency setting considered. Once fluid resuscitation is complete, further replacement is guided by urine output. The usual requirement is 500 mL plus the equivalent volume of daily urine output.

Close attention is paid to electrolyte balance, especially potassium levels, which can increase to dangerous levels in AKI (see page 233).

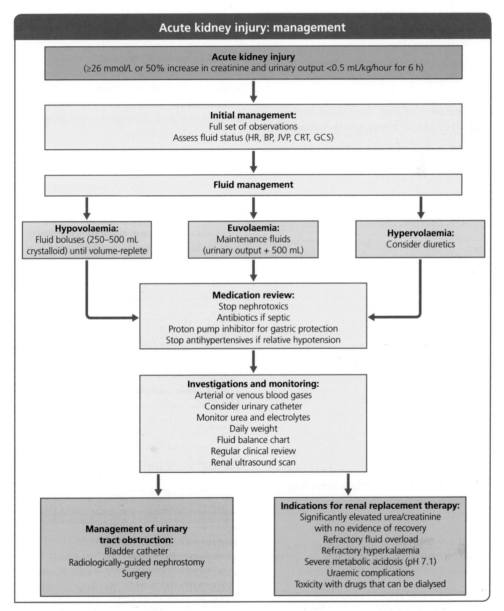

Figure 3.8 A management pathway for acute kidney injury (AKI). ABG, arterial blood gas; BP, blood pressure; CRT, capillary refill time; GCS, Glasgow coma scale score; HR, heart rate; JVP, jugular venous pulse.

Medication

Medication review

Drug charts are reviewed so that nephrotoxic agents such as ACE inhibitors, angiotensin II receptor blockers and NSAIDs are stopped. Any drug suspected of causing interstitial nephritis is also stopped. Certain other drugs require dose adjustment in the context of AKI (e.g. aminoglycoside antibiotics, digoxin).

General treatment

Once any prerenal and postrenal factors have been corrected, and relevant drugs have been stopped or had their dose altered, a number of general measures are considered:

■ Antibiotics to treat sepsis are considered in the presence of increased white cell count or C-reactive protein and with signs of infection
■ Proton pump inhibitors (e.g. omeprazole) or histamine-2 receptor antagonists (e.g. ranitidine) to reduce gastric acid production and therefore lower the risk of gastrointestinal bleeding
■ Diuretics. These agents are used to manage fluid overload once a pre-renal problem has been corrected but the urine output has not increased. There is no evidence that they significantly alter the natural history or need for haemodialysis, but they may increase urine output which can make management easier

> Patients with renal failure are particularly susceptible to infection. Therefore strict control of potential sources of sepsis is implemented and any unnecessary indwelling lines or bladder catheters removed.

Specific treatment

Specific treatments are available for certain intrarenal causes of AKI. For example:

■ immunosuppression is used for immune-mediated glomerular or tubulointerstitial disease
■ rasburicase, a recombinant form of urate oxidase is used to treat (and prevent) tumour lysis syndrome

Haemodialysis

Patients with AKI can present with life-threatening complications of renal failure that require renal replacement therapy. Indications for this include:

■ urea > 30 mmol/L and creatinine > 500–700 µmol/L, unless there is clear evidence of recovery
■ significant and intractable fluid overload
■ refractory hyperkalaemia
■ severe metabolic acidosis (pH < 7.1)
■ uraemic complications, for example pericarditis, encephalopathy, neuropathy and uraemic bleeding
■ toxicity with drugs that can be dialysed, for example barbiturates, ethylene glycol, methanol and lithium

Haemodialysis (see page 115) is the renal replacement method of choice in cases of AKI. Patients who are haemodynamically unstable require continuous renal replacement techniques, e.g. haemodiafiltration, to enable closer control of fluid balance.

> The **indications for haemodialysis** are summarised by the AEIOU mnemonic:
>
> ■ Acidaemia
> ■ Electrolytes
> ■ Ingestion/toxins
> ■ Overload (fluid)
> ■ Uraemia and uraemic complications

Prognosis

Acute kidney injury is potentially reversible, especially when it occurs in isolation in patients with few comorbidities. Mortality is associated with increasing age and burden of disease, and the presence of AKI in any inpatient increases mortality and length of hospital stay. The overall mortality is 25–40%, but this largely reflects the prognosis of the underlying condition; if this can be treated successfully then the majority of patients make a complete or near-complete recovery. However, a minority are left with chronic kidney disease and occasionally end-stage disease that requires renal replacement therapy (see Chapter 4).

Answers to starter questions

1. The major causes of AKI include prerenal, renal and postrenal causes. Prerenal AKI results from volume depletion (e.g. haemorrhage, severe vomiting or diarrhoea, burns), hypotension (due to drugs, sepsis, cardiogenic shock), renal hypoperfusion (e.g. drugs, abdominal aortic aneurysm, renal artery stenosis) or oedematous states (e.g. congestive cardiac failure, cirrhosis, nephrotic syndrome). Intrarenal AKI results from ischaemic, nephrotoxic, immune-mediated and vascular injury affecting the glomerulus, tubules, interstitium and renal blood vessels. Postrenal AKI results from obstruction within the renal tract and damage due to increased pressure.

2. AKI is investigated with tests to look for the underlying cause, including urinalysis, blood tests, renal tract imaging and renal biopsy. Urinalysis is helpful in indicating a prerenal cause (may be accompanied by a low urinary sodium concentration), or certain renal causes, e.g. casts, significant proteinuria or dysmorphic red cells suggest glomerular disease. Blood tests are helpful in diagnosing certain renal causes, primarily those due to toxins (e.g. raised creatine kinase in rhabdomyolysis) and immunologically-mediated disease (e.g. various autoantibodies). Imaging looks for evidence of a postrenal cause, i.e. obstruction. Biopsy is needed for a definitive diagnosis of certain renal causes, e.g. vasculitis.

3. AKI can sometimes be cured if the cause is rapidly reversible, for example AKI secondary to dehydration or obstruction. However, intrarenal renal injury that causes loss of renal tissue or scarring is incurable as the kidney is unable to regenerate lost tissue.

4. Risk factors for AKI include dehydration, comorbidities (e.g. diabetes), polypharmacy and the use of nephrotoxic medications. Dehydration decreases renal perfusion (i.e. prerenal AKI), whereas diabetes (and other causes of chronic kidney disease) renders the kidney more vulnerable to acute insults. Drugs that are commonly implicated include diuretics (when overused can lead to prerenal AKI), angiotensin-converting enzyme inhibitors (ACEI) and angiotensin II receptor blockers, and non-steroidal anti-inflammatory drugs (NSAIDs).

5. AKI can be prevented by maintaining adequate blood pressure and volume status in acutely unwell patients, avoiding unnecessary potentially nephrotoxic medications [especially non-steroidal anti-inflammatory drugs (NSAIDs), angiotensin-converting enzyme inhibitors (ACEIs) and angiotensin II receptor-blockers (ARBs)], and ensuring those at risk of AKI (i.e. patients with the risk factors set out in the answer to question 4 above) are prehydrated prior to procedures involving the infusion of radiological contrast.

Chapter 4
Chronic kidney disease

Starter questions

Answers to the following questions are on page 173.

1. Why are increased urinary frequency and nocturia seen in the early stages of chronic kidney disease (CKD), and not the later stages?
2. How does CKD cause acidosis?
3. How might fruit and nut chocolate be dangerous for someone with CKD?
4. Why is it necessary to be especially careful when inserting a peripheral venous line (i.e. a cannula) in someone with CKD?
5. Why might some patients with end-stage renal disease opt for conservative management?

Introduction

Chronic kidney disease (CKD) is a gradual and often progressive loss of renal function as a result of damage to the kidneys, the vessels supplying them or pathology within the lower urinary tract. Impaired functions include excretion of waste products, salt–water and acid–base homeostasis, and endocrine activity. The most common causes are diabetes and hypertension.

If CKD progresses to a stage when renal replacement therapy (dialysis or transplantation) is required for survival, the patient has developed end-stage renal disease (ESRD).

CKD develops over months to years, and its early stages are often asymptomatic. Often renal impairment is identified only when blood tests are carried out for other reasons. The kidney damage is usually irreversible, so the aim of treatment is to prevent or limit further progression. This is achieved by treating the underlying cause and managing complications due to inadequate renal function, for example hypertension, anaemia and renal bone disease.

Case 2 Nausea and swollen ankles in a patient with diabetes

Presentation

Anthony Rich, a 64-year-old African–Caribbean man, presents to his general practitioner (GP) with ankle swelling. He first noticed this a few months ago and thinks it has worsened over time. He now finds it difficult to put on certain shoes. He also reports feeling more tired recently, and complains of intermittent nausea.

Initial interpretation

The ankle swelling suggests fluid retention resulting in dependent oedema, the accumulation of fluid in the interstitial space according to gravity (**Figure 2.3**). Potential causes include right-sided heart failure or renal impairment. Men in general, and the African-Caribbean population in particular, have a higher incidence of renal failure, which increases the probability of this diagnosis in Anthony's case.

Oedema that has been present for months and is getting worse indicates a chronic disease process. Tiredness and nausea are non-specific symptoms with various causes, for example anaemia and gastrointestinal disease. In this context, they could be the result of chronic kidney disease or heart failure.

History

Five years ago Anthony was diagnosed with type 2 diabetes. He is now taking oral medications, after limited success with a trial of dietary and lifestyle modifications at diagnosis. He also takes a statin and an angiotensin-converting enzyme (ACE) inhibitor. He attends yearly retinopathy screening and sees his GP a few times a year.

Anthony's last blood test results, from over a year ago, showed a creatinine concentration of 120 µmol/L and an eGFR of 55 mL/min/1.73 m². On further questioning, he explains that he has not felt well for some months, and has noticed that his energy levels are poor. His appetite has decreased, and he has lost about 7 kg over the past 2 months as a result. He has recently had to start getting up at night to pass water and thinks that this is contributing to his tiredness.

Interpretation of history

Anthony's type 2 diabetes puts him at increased risk of renal, retinal, peripheral vascular and heart disease.

The increased creatinine concentration and eGFR of 55 mL/min/1.73 m² in his previous set of blood test results are consistent with stage 3a CKD (see Table 4.2), which means there is approximately 50% of normal renal function. The presence of nocturia may be associated with kidney disease, because failing kidneys are unable to concentrate urine. It could also signify prostatic disease causing irritative bladder symptoms, or reflect poorly controlled diabetes.

The low energy and poor appetite are non-specific symptoms found in a wide variety of acute and chronic disease. The accompanying weight loss is worrying, as it suggests significant underlying pathology.

Further history

Anthony admits that his diabetes control has been poor over recent months, because he has been under great stress from financial concerns.

Examination

Anthony looks pale. On examination, his jugular venous pressure is visible, at 4 cm, and his heart sounds are normal.

Blood pressure is 145/95 mmHg. His chest is clear to auscultation, and the abdomen is soft and non-tender, with no masses or organomegaly. He has bilateral pitting oedema, and his pedal pulses are weakly palpable. Light-touch sensation in the feet is impaired.

Interpretation of findings

Anthony's pallor could reflect an underlying anaemia, which in this case may be a consequence of his CKD.

His jugular venous pressure is slightly raised, which suggests fluid overload, which again may be a consequence of CKD, leading to failure to excrete sufficient salt and water. His bilateral pitting oedema confirms peripheral fluid retention. The impaired light-touch sensation suggests diabetic neuropathy, and the weak peripheral pulses may similarly reflect diabetic arteriopathy.

All of these findings are consistent with complications from Anthony's diabetes, and in particular with progression of his CKD. It will be important to check whether he is indeed anaemic, and whether his CKD has indeed progressed.

Investigations

Anthony's GP arranges blood tests, including urea and electrolytes to check kidney function and full blood count and haematinics (vitamin B12, folate, and ferritin as a measure of iron stores) to exclude anaemia. He also requests determination of urine albumin:creatinine ratio to assess for diabetic nephropathy. The results of these tests are shown in **Table 4.1**.

Diagnosis

The change in GFR from 55 to 25 mL/min represents a deterioration from stage 3a CKD to stage 4 CKD (see **Table 4.2**); Anthony now has severely reduced kidney function. He also has significant proteinuria, based on the albumin:creatinine ratio, which has not been noted in the past. In the light of these results, the GP refers Mr Rich to a renal physician in secondary care for further investigation and management.

This clinical picture is so typical of diabetic nephropathy that a renal biopsy is probably not necessary to confirm the diagnosis. It is worth obtaining a renal ultrasound. However, provided the result is normal, for example showing no evidence of urinary obstruction, management will consist of good control of the diabetes and blood pressure. Even with excellent control, this degree of CKD means that progression to end-stage renal failure is almost inevitable.

Anthony Rich's blood and urine test results		
Test	Result	Normal range
Serum creatinine	230 µmol/L	50–110 µmol/L
eGFR	25 mL/min/1.73 m^2	> 60 mL/min/1.73 m^2
Haemoglobin	103 g/L	120–160 g/L
Mean corpuscular volume	95 fl	78–97 fl
Haematinics (B$_{12}$, folate, ferritin)	Normal	
Urine albumin:creatinine ratio	70 mg/mmol	< 3mg/mmol

Table 4.1 Blood and urine test results for Anthony Rich

Chronic kidney disease

CKD is a sustained and irreversible deterioration in kidney function. It progresses through stages classified by the glomerular filtration rate (GFR), as described in **Table 4.2**. Clinically, CKD is defined as a reduction in GFR to < 60 mL/min for at least 3 months or persistent proteinuria or haematuria. Many systemic and intrinsic renal disease processes cause kidney injury that results in permanent damage to the kidneys.

Although diagnosis of CKD generally focusses on GFR, in CKD there is impairment of all the functions of the kidney. Clinically, it is characterised by hypertension and other cardiovascular complications, anaemia, and bone and mineral disorders.

Progression of CKD is indicated by a decline in eGFR of > 5 mL/min/1.73 m^2 within 1 year or > 10 mL/min/1.73 m^2 within 5 years. Because CKD is often asymptomatic, particularly in the early stages, certain patient groups are offered screening. In high-risk groups, strategies are implemented to prevent CKD developing (see Chapter 14).

Epidemiology

Chronic kidney disease is common; in Europe and the UK CKD stages 3–5 have a prevalence of about 6%. People with hypertension or diabetes, and the elderly, are at greater risk of developing CKD (**Figure 4.1**).

Overall prevalence is therefore likely to increase in the future. Management of CKD in the elderly is discussed in Chapter 14.

In general CKD has a higher prevalence and occurs at an earlier age in African-Caribbean or South Asian populations, probably because of the increased prevalence of hypertension in the former and type 2 diabetes in the latter.

Aetiology

CKD is caused by intrinsic renal, systemic and drug-induced diseases (**Table 4.3**). The commonest causes are diabetes, hypertension, reflux nephropathy causing chronic pyelonephritis and polycystic kidney disease.

Prevention

Prevention of CKD is based on identifying individuals at risk and modifying their risk factors, for example by controlling hypertension and diabetes. Maintenance of a healthy weight, not smoking, eating a healthy diet and exercising regularly are all beneficial in this regard.

Pathogenesis

Insults to the glomerulus, tubules, peritubular capillaries and the interstitium can all cause damage to the nephron, and all cause CKD. Once nephrons are lost (i.e. atrophy

Stages of chronic kidney disease		
Stage*	GFR (mL/min)	Description
1	> 90	Normal or increased GFR with other evidence of kidney damage
2	60–89	Slight decrease in GFR, with other evidence of kidney damage
3a	45–59	Moderate decrease in GFR, with or without other evidence of kidney damage
3b	30–44	
4	15–29	Severe decrease in GFR, with or without other evidence of kidney damage
5	< 15	End-stage renal failure

GFR, glomerular filtration rate.

*The addition of the suffix 'p' to a stage denotes the presence of proteinuria.

Table 4.2 Stages of chronic kidney disease

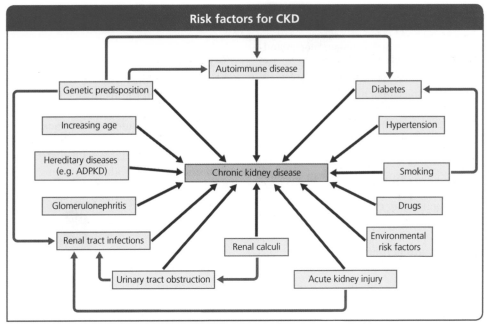

Figure 4.1 Risk factors for chronic kidney disease. ADPKD, autosomal dominant polycystic kidney disease.

Chronic kidney disease: causes	
Disease group	Disease
Intrinsic renal disease	Chronic pyelonephritis
	Polycystic kidney disease
	Glomerulonephritis
	Interstitial nephritis
	Bladder or ureteric obstruction
	Myeloma kidney disease
	Amyloidosis
Systemic disease	Diabetes mellitus
	Hypertension
	Heart failure
	Systemic lupus erythematosus
	Renovascular disease
	Vasculitides
	Gout
Drug-induced renal disease	Analgesics (especially non-steroidal anti-inflammatory drugs)
	Ciclosporin
	Lithium

Table 4.3 Causes of chronic kidney disease

and cease to function) a common pathway is established characterised by progressive interstitial fibrosis, loss of peritubular capillaries, hypoxia and tubular atrophy, resulting in loss of functioning nephrons.

Glomerular and tubulointerstitial damage

Glomerular damage occurs due to intraglomerular hypertension, immune-mediated injury, lipids, paraproteins (monoclonal proteins in the blood; see page 204) and glucose. It causes:

- alteration of all components of the filtration barrier
- altered glomerular permeability
- impaired growth factor production
- reduction in glomerular capillary surface area and blood flow.

Damage to the tubules is caused by ischaemia and the effects of toxins within the filtrate. Toxins enter the tubules via ultrafiltration or the peritubular capillaries, and include proteins, glucose, complement components, cytokines and lipids. Damage to the tubules occurs due to:

- generation of reactive oxygen species and inflammatory mediators
- altered production of growth factors
- altered extracellular matrix turnover
- tubular cell apoptosis
- tubular atrophy

Toxins, immune-mediated injury, proinflammatory mediators, ischaemia and loss of endothelial growth factors can all damage the peritubular capillaries. These insults cause endothelial cell apoptosis, capillary loss and replacement with fibrous tissue.

Damage to the tubular interstitium is caused by toxins, immune-mediated injury and ischaemia due to capillary loss. These processes generate inflammatory mediators and profibrotic cytokines, activation and proliferation of immune cells and fibroblasts, and altered extracellular matrix turnover that all result in fibrosis.

Hypertension

Common causes of CKD initiate nephron damage through different mechanisms. For example, in hypertension, damage to elastic fibres within the arterial walls results in thickening of the intimal layer and loss of autoregulatory capacity. Intraglomerular pressure rises, resulting in hyperfiltration which promotes the release of cytokines and growth factors. Hypertensive renal damage also occurs due to endothelial dysfunction, impaired vasodilatation and hypoxic injury, eventually resulting in glomerular and interstitial fibrosis and scarring.

Diabetes

In diabetes, the following glomerular changes occur:

- hyperglycaemia-induced expansion of the mesangium
- thickening of the glomerular basement membrane
- intraglomerular hypertension resulting in glomerular sclerosis

- podocyte damage resulting in a leaky filtration barrier and proteinuria

Polycystic kidney disease

In polycystic kidney disease, renal tubular cells proliferate resulting in an outpouching of the renal tubular wall. The resultant cyst fills with tubular fluid and expands, eventually separating into an isolated cyst. This cyst continues to enlarge within the tubular interstitium promoting thickening of the basement membrane, inflammatory infiltration and interstitial fibrosis. The overall result is a loss of functional tissue.

Early stages

Homeostatic mechanisms compensate for initial nephron injury by enabling the kidneys to maintain GFR despite injury and nephron loss. As a result, the early stages of renal decline are associated with an increase in serum creatinine concentration, but within the normal range. However, as more nephrons are destroyed, the adaptive capacity of nephrons is overcome, resulting in impaired clearance of waste products and a more pronounced increase in serum urea and serum creatinine concentrations (**Figure 4.2**).

Glomerular filtration rate < 50%

The serum concentration of urea and creatinine starts to increase more markedly after total GFR has decreased by 50%. Once this stage has been reached, CKD evolves the same way whatever the initial insult. This is because the mechanisms of progression (outlined below) do not depend on the initial pathology.

Hyperfiltration and hypertrophy

As result of renal injury and nephron loss the remaining nephrons filter more blood and become larger, i.e. there is hyperfiltration and hypertrophy. This contributes significantly to progressive renal dysfunction (**Figure 4.3**) because, although initially compensatory, the increased load on each functioning glomerulus activates mechanisms which lead to damage.

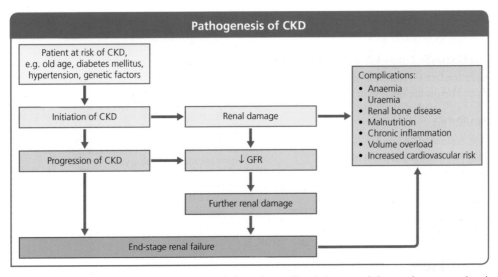

Figure 4.2 Steps in the pathogenesis of chronic kidney disease (CKD). Once renal damage has occurred and the pathogenic mechanisms underlying CKD are activated, there is further renal damage. The complications of CKD begin once this process is initiated. GFR, glomerular filtration rate.

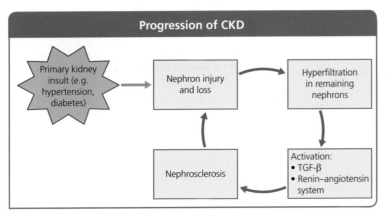

Figure 4.3
Progression of renal damage in chronic kidney disease. TGF-β, transforming growth factor-β.

RAAS activation, fibrosis and glomerulosclerosis

Hyperfiltration causes glomerular injury characterised by the proliferation of glomerular cells, infiltration of macrophages and accumulation of extracellular matrix. This is cytokine-mediated and eventually results in glomerulosclerosis (scarring of the glomerulus). Within the interstitium, there is excessive synthesis and decreased breakdown of extracellular matrix which causes interstitial fibrosis. Within both the glomeruli and the tubules, there is apoptosis of normal cells due to the presence of hypoxia and overly-abundant apoptotic cytokines. The renin–angiotensin–aldosterone system (RAAS; see page 35) is also activated because angiotensin II is produced locally within the kidneys. This causes increased glomerular capillary pressure, capillary damage and increased glomerular permeability. Angiotensin II also results in activation of profibrotic cytokines such as transforming growth factor-β.

Further nephron loss occurs as a consequence of tubulointerstitial fibrosis, driven by these profibrotic cytokines, and glomerulosclerosis occurs as increased intra-glomerular pressure damages the supporting mesangial skeleton. A vicious cycle is set up, as this progressive nephron loss increases hyperfiltration in the remaining nephrons and leads to an inexorable decline in renal function.

Anaemia

The following processes contribute to the development of anaemia in CKD:

- decreased erythropoietin production by the kidney (the principle cause)
- uraemic suppression of bone marrow
- short lifespan of erythrocytes, which is thought to be a result of the toxic effect of a uraemic environment
- a pro-inflammatory state, characteristic of CKD, resulting in altered iron homeostasis and decreased availability of iron, destruction of red cell progenitor cells and fewer erythropoietin receptors on progenitor cells
- poor dietary intake of B12, folate and iron due to anorexia and dietary restrictions associated with CKD. Deficiencies of these haematinics cause impaired erythrocyte production
- increased iron losses as a consequence of frequent blood sampling, chronic bleeding caused by uraemia-induced platelet dysfunction and blood clotting within the haemodialysis circuit.

Cardiovascular complications

In CKD, risk factors for cardiovascular disease include those that apply to the general population but there are additional risk factors: anaemia, uraemic toxins, sodium and water overload, and altered bone metabolism. The incidence of cardiac disease is increased in CKD, even in the early stages when renal function is relatively preserved. Common cardiovascular complications include coronary artery disease, myocardial infarction, congestive cardiac failure and arrhythmias such as atrial fibrillation.

The pathophysiological mechanisms underlying this are incompletely understood. However, it is likely that they are related to factors that accompany CKD, including:

- endothelial cell dysfunction
- chronic low-grade inflammation
- oxidative stress
- dyslipidaemia

In addition, pressure overload due to long-standing hypertension and vascular stiffness, volume overload and subsequent left ventricular dysfunction, and inappropriate activation of the RAAS all contribute to cardiovascular pathology.

> **Patients with CKD are more likely to die of cardiovascular disease** before they reach ESRD and require renal replacement therapy.

Bone and mineral disease

CKD alters bone and mineral metabolism; this causes metabolic bone disease, a common complication that occurs early in the course of CKD. Altered mineral metabolism affects the bone and extraskeletal sites such as the vasculature, and is characterised by:

- abnormal calcium, phosphate, parathyroid hormone (PTH) and vitamin D metabolism. In early CKD, the level of 1,25-dihydroxyvitamin D is low and the level of PTH increases. As CKD progresses, hyperphosphataemia develops as phosphate is retained by the kidneys
- abnormal bone turnover, mineralisation, strength and volume
- vascular and soft tissue calcification

Clinical features

The initial stages of CKD (stages 1–3b) are usually asymptomatic. As it progresses, patients develop non-specific symptoms such as lethargy, tiredness, loss of appetite, weight loss and nausea . These are commonly due to the abnormal retention of waste products (uraemia) and are collectively known as uraemic symptoms. Urinary frequency and nocturia are common, because the kidneys fail to concentrate urine, thereby causing production of a larger volume of more dilute urine.

Further reduction in GFR leads to salt and water retention. The clinical manifestations of water retention, impaired acid–base balance, anaemia, mineral and bone disease, and endocrine dysfunction result in other signs, symptoms and investigation findings encountered in patients with CKD (Table 4.4). Not all patients experience the same clinical manifestations of CKD, but in untreated late-stage renal disease (stages 4–5) fatigue, hypertension, hyperkalaemia, metabolic acidosis and hyperphosphataemia are seen in the majority of patients.

Cardiovascular complications

Clinical features of cardiovascular complications of CKD depend on the cardiovascular pathology:

- Coronary artery disease: either symptoms of cardiac ischaemia (e.g. chest pain, breathlessness, dizziness and nausea) or asymptomatic and presenting as sudden cardiac death
- Congestive cardiac failure: breathlessness, initially on exertion but in later stages occuring with minimal activity or at rest
- Atrial fibrillation: usually asymptomatic but occasionally causing palpitations, dizziness and chest pain

Late-stage kidney failure (stages 4–5)

In very advanced disease, symptoms and signs of uraemia worsen as the kidneys fail to sufficiently excrete urea and other nitrogenous waste compounds (Table 4.5; see also Figure 4.6):

- anorexia
- nausea and vomiting
- itching
- neuromuscular symptoms, such as restless legs

Even later stages of uraemia may be associated with platelet dysfunction, pericarditis, peripheral neuropathy and encephalopathy.

CKD: clinical manifestations and their management			
Renal abnormality	Pathophysiological effects	Clinical manifestations	Management
Abnormal excretory function	Fluid retention	Hypertension	Sodium restriction, antihypertensives
		Peripheral oedema	Sodium restriction, diuretics
		Pulmonary oedema	
	Potassium retention	Hyperkalaemia	Dietary potassium restriction, avoidance of potassium-sparing drugs
	Acid retention	Metabolic acidosis	Sodium bicarbonate
	Phosphate retention	Hyperphosphataemia	Phosphate binders
Decreased erythropoietin production	Impaired erythropoiesis and anaemia	Tiredness	Erythropoietin injections, intravenous iron
		Left ventricular hypertrophy	
Decreased production of 1,25-dihydroxyvitamin D³*	Hypocalcaemia	Bone pain	Vitamin D supplementation, phosphate binders, calcimimetics
	Increased parathyroid hormone	Hyperphosphataemia	
		Osteomalacia	
		Osteitis fibrosa	
		Fractures	

*Calcitriol, the active metabolite of vitamin D

Table 4.4 Relationships between renal abnormalities and their clinical manifestations in CKD. Management is described in more detail on pages 166–167.

Cinical effects of advanced uraemia	
Abnormality	**Clinical effects**
Uraemia-induced platelet dysfunction	Increased bleeding tendency, especially in the gastrointestinal tract
	Easy bruising
Uraemic pericarditis	Chest pain, pericardial friction rub
Uraemic neuropathy	Distal sensorimotor polyneuropathy
Uraemic encephalopathy	Headache, confusion, seizures, coma

Table 4.5 Clinical effects of advanced uraemia

These manifestations are indications for urgent renal replacement therapy if indicated, as opposed to continued conservative and palliative care.

Diagnostic approach

Early asymptomatic disease is only detected incidentally or by screening of patients who are at risk (**Table 4.6**).

In stages 4–5 disease, patients present with any of the symptoms outlined above (although some are asymptomatic, even when a diagnosis is made at stage 5). For both groups, once a diagnosis of CKD has been established investigations are carried out to determine the underlying cause of renal failure and identify its complications.

Investigations

A standard battery of urine and blood tests is carried out for all patients identified as having CKD. However, imaging and renal biopsy are reserved for specific circumstances.

Urine tests

These seek signs of non-specific renal pathology (haematuria, proteinuria) as well as more specific diagnoses (e.g. Bence Jones protein in myeloma) (**Table 4.7**).

> **The albumin:creatinine ratio** is a more sensitive test of proteinuria (protein in the urine) than the protein:creatinine ratio.

Monitoring for CKD in asymptomatic patients
Offer testing (eGFR and ACR) to patients with:
■ diabetes
■ hypertension
■ cardiovascular disease
■ structural renal tract abnormalities, renal calculi and prostatic hypertrophy
■ multisystem diseases that can have renal involvement (e.g. SLE)
■ family history of stage 5 CKD or hereditary kidney disease
■ opportunistic detection of haematuria
■ Regular use of nephrotoxic drugs (e.g. lithium, NSAIDs)
ACR, urine albumin:creatinine ration; eGFR, estimated glomerular filtration rate; SLE, systemic lupus erythematosus
*Based on the UK National Institute for Health and Care Excellence guidelines, 2014, which also recommend frequencies for re-testing (based on the eGFR and ACR results).

Table 4.6 Monitoring for CKD in asymptomatic patients

> **Proteinuria in a patient with diabetes or suspected diabetes strongly suggests diabetic nephropathy.** This is especially so in the context of other diabetic complications, such as retinopathy or neuropathy.

Blood tests

These include commonly requested tests such as full blood count and haematinics (to evaluate renal anaemia), urea, creatinine and eGFR (to stage disease), electrolytes (to look for electrolyte abnormalities), a bone profile (for metabolic bone disease), and more specialised tests if indicated (e.g. a screen for systemic lupus erythematosus might be indicated in a young woman, or a myeloma screen in a patient over 55 of either sex) (**Table 4.8**).

Imaging

Radiological investigations are carried out when an underlying renal, pulmonary or other radiologically-identifiable abnormality

Chronic kidney disease: urinary investigations

Test	Purpose
Dipstick urinalysis ('urine dip')	To identify haematuria, proteinuria or urinary infection (white blood cells and nitrites)
Protein: creatinine ratio	To detect significant proteinuria (urine protein:creatinine ratio > 100 mg/mmol); usually indicates glomerular disease or occasionally interstitial nephritis
Albumin:creatinine ratio	To detect albuminuria (> 3 mg/mmol is clinically significant)
Urine microscopy	To detect white blood cells (infection), eosinophils (interstitial nephritis), red blood cell casts and dysmorphic red blood cells (glomerulonephritis), white blood cell casts and granular casts
Urinary electrolytes (usually Ca^{2+}, Cl^-, Na^+, K^+)*	To test ability of kidneys to conserve or excrete electrolytes; also to diagnose various electrolyte disturbances
Urine protein electrophoresis	To detect multiple myeloma
Urinary Bence Jones protein	To detect multiple myeloma

*Results must be interpreted in the context of the individual patient and clinical situation.

Table 4.7 Urinary investigations in chronic kidney disease

Chronic kidney disease: blood tests

Test	Purpose
Urea, creatinine and eGFR	To enable staging of CKD
Electrolytes	To identify sodium and potassium abnormalities
Calcium	To exclude hypocalcaemia
Phosphate	To exclude hyperphosphataemia
Parathyroid hormone	To exclude secondary (or tertiary) hyperparathyroidism
Full blood count and haematinics (vitamin B_{12}, folate, ferritin)	To investigate anaemia. Further investigations if evidence of ongoing red blood cell loss (e.g. due to haemolysis or bleeding), including endoscopy to exclude bleeding and blood film, serum LDH, haptoglobin, and conjugated and unconjugated bilirubin to exclude haemolysis
Serum protein electrophoresis and immunoglobulins	To exclude multiple myeloma
Complement components and autoantibody screen	To identify immune-mediated causes of CKD, such as systemic lupus erythematosus

CKD, chronic kidney disease.

Table 4.8 Blood tests to consider when investigating chronic kidney disease

is suspected that will aid diagnosis or require specific treatment, for example:

- ultrasound of the renal tract to assess kidney size and to exclude obstruction, polycystic disease and mass lesions
- chest radiograph to look for signs of pulmonary oedema
- abdominal radiograph or CT of the renal tract to look for renal calculi

Chronic kidney disease is associated with small kidneys (except in polycystic kidney disease; see page 299). Progressive nephron loss and fibrosis both contribute to the decreased kidney volume.

Biopsy

Renal biopsy is considered if the cause of CKD is unclear after all other investigations are complete. It is usually only done if the kidneys are of normal size. If the kidneys are small biopsy is more hazardous, and the results are most unlikely to influence management because reduced size confirms irreversible damage has occurred.

Biopsy reveals:

- previously undiagnosed IgA nephropathy, focal segmental glomeruosclerosis, or other glomerular disease (see Chapters 5 and 6)
- chronic tubulointersitial inflammation and fibrosis
- less common diagnoses that are only confirmed by biopsy, for example multiple myeloma

Management

Management of CKD focuses on:

- treating the underlying cause
- preventing or delaying progression of CKD
- treating associated complications, such as anaemia, bone disease and cardiovascular disease

It also includes planning for the possibility that ESRD may develop, which requires advance discussion of renal replacement therapy (see page 169).

> Chronic kidney disease is a lifelong disease, so including the patient in their care from an early stage is vital to ensure optimal management and outcomes. This requires good, clear communication and patient education.

Medication

Drug treatment is unable to reverse CKD, but is essential to slow progression, mainly via good control of blood pressure, and to manage complications.

Because of the effect of reduced GFR on drug clearance there are special consider-ations for prescribing in renal disease, as discussed on page pages 130–131. For the newly diagnosed patient this means all medications should be reviewed. Some drugs will require dose reduction in CKD, for example digoxin.

Blood pressure control

This is essential to reduce cardiovascular complications of CKD and to slow progression of CKD, especially if the underlying cause is a glomerular disease (see Chapters 5 and 6). In CKD, target blood pressure is:

- 120–139/90 mmHg for patients without diabetes
- 120–129/80 mmHg for patients with diabetes.

Hypertension management is discussed in detail in Chapter 9. ACE inhibitors and angiotension II receptor blockers are par-ticularly effective in CKD because they target the RAAS. Most patients require two or more antihypertensives to achieve adequate con-trol of blood pressure.

Dietary salt restriction is also a crucial as-pect of blood pressure control. Patients must be advised to avoid processed foods and use of salt in cooking or at the table. A target intake of ≤ 6 g/day is suggested.

Blood glucose control

For patients with diabetes, tight control of blood glucose reduces progression of CKD. This is achieved through lifestyle and dietary modifications as well as the use of oral hypo-glycaemics and insulin therapy.

> Patients with CKD and insulin-dependent diabetes (type 1 or advanced type 2) may find that their insulin requirements decrease as CKD progresses. This is because insulin clearance, which takes place in the kidneys, slows with progressive renal dysfunction.

Fluid overload

Salt restriction can help limit fluid overload; however, a diuretic such as furosemide may also be needed.

> **The effectiveness of diuretics is reduced in renal failure, so larger doses may be required.** In particular, thiazide diuretics, or related drugs such as indapamide, are ineffective below an eGFR of about 30 mL/min/1.73 m²; loop diuretics (i.e. furosemide, bumetanide) will be needed in these circumstances.

Anaemia

This is treated by regular subcutaneous injections of erythropoietin. Before starting treatment, levels of haematinics (i.e. vitamin B_{12}, folate and ferritin) are checked; supplements are given if there is deficiency.

> **Always ensure iron stores are adequate before starting erythropoietin therapy.** Oral iron is poorly absorbed in advanced CKD, because there is an increased concentration of hepcidin, a factor produced by the liver which blocks iron absorption; therefore intravenous iron therapy is used.

Bone and mineral metabolism

Monitoring of calcium, phosphate, parathyroid hormone and vitamin D is required for all patients.

The management of renal bone disease is summarised in **Figure 4.4**. In early CKD, the level of 1,25-dihydroxyvitamin D is low and that of parathyroid hormone tends to increase. Treatment is with vitamin D supplementation.

Hyperphosphataemia requires dietary phosphate restriction and phosphate binder therapy. Once patients have started on vitamin D and phosphate binders, calcium and phosphate levels are monitored every 3–4 months to prevent hypercalcaemia and ensure that phosphate concentrations remain within the normal range.

> **Phosphate binders are medications that decrease phosphate absorption from the small intestine.** They need to be taken with food to enable them to bind phosphate in the diet.

Acidosis

Metabolic acidosis is common as CKD progresses. It is treated with oral sodium bicarbonate supplementation.

> **Multidisciplinary team management of patients with CKD is vital to ensure optimal care.** Patients benefit from support from specialist nurses, social workers and dieticians in addition to physicians.

Prognosis

With good control of risk factors such as hypertension and diabetes, progression of CKD is likely to be slow, for example a rate of loss of GFR of less than 1–2 mL/min/year. In some patients who achieve good control of complications and have no comorbidities renal function remains stable for an indefinite period. However, cardiovascular complications are common: only a small

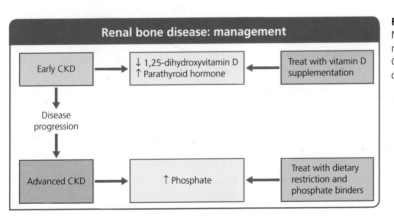

Figure 4.4
Management of renal bone disease. CKD, chronic kidney disease.

proportion of patients with CKD progress to ESRD but many experience a cardiovascular event.

Certain causes of CKD, such as diabetes and polycystic kidney disease, are associated with faster disease progression than others. Patients with more aggressive disease require early education and counselling regarding options for renal replacement therapy, preferably before ESRD develops and dialysis is required. This includes discussion of types of dialysis (haemodialysis versus peritoneal dialysis), vascular access for haemodialysis and renal transplantation (see pages 114–122).

End-stage renal disease

End-stage renal disease is irreversible chronic kidney damage that has progressed to such an extent that renal replacement therapy is required for survival. The indications for renal replacement therapy are less clearcut in ESRD than in AKI; they are listed in **Table 4.9.**

Epidemiology

The incidence of ESRD has almost doubled in the last 20–30 years in developed countries, now being approximately 110 per million per year in the UK. The rates of development of ESRD vary from country to country. Every year, for every 10,000 patients with CKD stages 3–4, between 24 and 61 patients reach end-stage. Most patients with ESRD are older; the mean age of those starting dialysis is 63 years.

Globally, the incidence of patients with ESRD starting on renal replacement therapy varies because of lack of affordability and availability. In low- and middle-income countries, very few patients are able to start on dialysis or receive a transplant. In the long term, from an economic perspective, transplantation is the most cost-effective therapy. In the UK, the number of adults on the various types of renal replacement therapy is over 750 per million of population (**Figure 4.5**).

Aetiology

The commonest causes of ESRD are the same as those of CKD (see **Table 4.3**).

Clinical features

The clinical features of ESRD are the same as those of CKD (**Figure 4.6**). A palpable renal transplant or features secondary to the

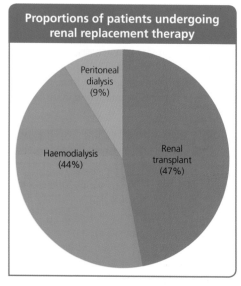

Figure 4.5 Proportions of patients undergoing different types of renal replacement therapy for end-stage renal disease (UK data).

Indications for renal replacement therapy in CKD and ESRD
■ Symptoms of uraemia
■ Fluid overload
■ Resistant hyperkalaemia
■ Resistant metabolic acidosis
■ eGFR < 10 mL/min/1.73 m^2

CKD, chronic kidney disease; ESRD, end-stage renal disease; eGFR, estimated glomerular filtration rate.

Table 4.9 Indications for renal replacement therapy as CKD progresses to ESRD

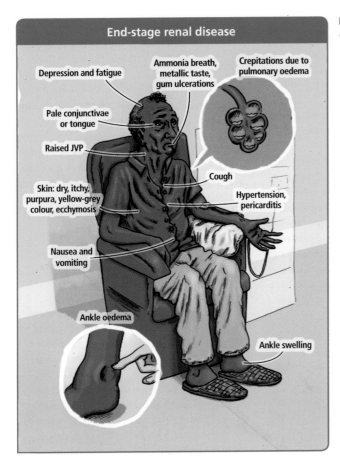

Figure 4.6 Clinical features of end-stage renal disease.

access mode used for dialysis (see Figures 2.7, 2.39–2.41, 2.45) identify a patient with established ESRD if they present in an unconscious state or are otherwise unable to communicate.

Investigations

Patients with ESRD require regular monthly monitoring of renal function, full blood count, haematinic assay, bone profile and parathyroid hormone measurement, so that complications are detected and are managed appropriately. Due to the theoretical risk of transmission of blood-borne viruses (hepatitis B and C and HIV) within haemodialysis units, patients undergoing haemodialysis have their hepatitis B, C and HIV serology monitored every 6–12 months to ensure they have not been infected with these viruses.

Patients on haemodialysis must be vaccinated against hepatitis B unless they are already immune (as demonstrated by the presence of anti-hepatitis B surface antigen antibodies (anti-HBSag) in the serum). They are at increased risk of this blood-borne virus despite improvements in infection control in haemodialysis units.

Management

Management options for ESRD include conservative management or one of the following renal replacement therapies:

- Haemodialysis: removal of excess fluid and waste products from the blood by passing it through an artificial kidney outside the body. Treatment is required three times per week

- Peritoneal dialysis: removal of waste products by using the patient's peritoneum as an exchange membrane. Treatment is continuous on a daily basis
- Renal transplantation: implantation of a healthy donor kidney to replace the function of the diseased kidney

Renal replacement therapies and their complications are described in detail in Chapter 2 (pages 114–122). Haemofiltration and haemodiafiltration are used in the management of AKI, but are not used on a routine basis in the management of end-stage renal disease.

In conservative management the focus is on preserving renal function for as long as possible, improving symptoms and maximising quality of life, without renal replacement therapy.

> Online decision tools are available to help patients explore different options for management of ESRD and decide which is best for them based on their lifestyle and values.

Patients with CKD stage 4 or 5, and those with rapidly deteriorating renal function, are referred to a nephrologist for assessment and discussion of renal replacement therapy. Ideally, this discussion takes place at least a year before the patient is expected to require renal replacement therapy, to allow time for full assessment and consideration of the patient's preferred dialysis modality as well as time for the necessary preparations (e.g. vascular access surgery).

Starting renal replacement therapy

In CKD, the point at which dialysis should be started is a matter of debate; the decision should be guided by the patient's wishes. Generally, dialysis is started when GFR reaches 10–15 mL/min, or when symptoms of uraemia and fluid overload become too difficult to manage medically (**Table 4.9**). Transplantation may take place preemptively, before the patient requires dialysis, or after they have begun dialysis,

depending on the availability of a donor kidney. Conservative care can begin at any time.

Choosing the mode of renal replacement therapy

Transplantation is the gold standard for renal replacement therapy. However, not all patients are suitable candidates, and many have to start dialysis before a kidney becomes available. Therefore most patients with ESRD are required to make a decision concerning dialysis modality. The best option depends on their personal preferences, lifestyle and capabilities, for example

- A patient with poor vision and dexterity is unsuitable for peritoneal dialysis, because they cannot set up the machine and connect themselves to it
- A patient with a busy job or living a long way from the renal unit may find having to attend three haemodialysis sessions a week too limiting and view peritoneal dialysis as a better option
- An elderly patient with multiple comorbidities and a short life expectancy may feel that the risks of dialysis outweigh the benefits, with no real effect on survival; they might opt for a conservative approach

Haemodialysis

This is the most common form of dialysis in the UK. In 2009, 70% of patients starting renal replacement therapy began with haemodialysis. It involves using a machine to pump blood through an artificial filter to enable the removal of waste products and fluid (see Figure 2.44). Access to the circulation is required and may be via an arteriovenous fistula, an arteriovenous graft or a central venous catheter (see Figures 2.39–2.41). Treatment takes place usually for 4 hours, three times per week. Most patients are treated in dialysis units in hospitals or in the community, but for motivated and able patients it is possible to set up haemodialysis in their own home.

Complications

These include hypotension, bleeding, loss of vascular access as a result of clotting and bacteraemia from line contamination.

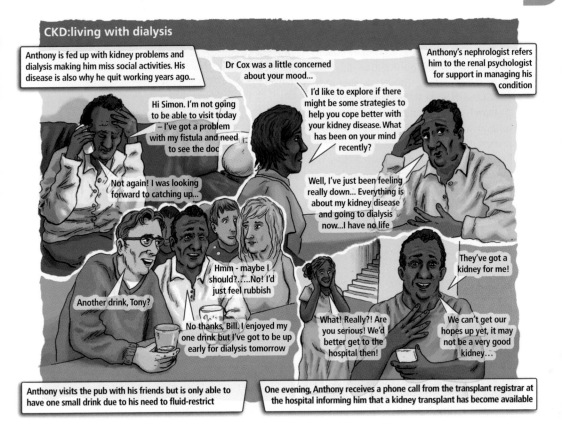

CKD: living with dialysis

Anthony is fed up with kidney problems and dialysis making him miss social activities. His disease is also why he quit working years ago...

Dr Cox was a little concerned about your mood...

Anthony's nephrologist refers him to the renal psychologist for support in managing his condition

Hi Simon. I'm not going to be able to visit today – I've got a problem with my fistula and need to see the doc

I'd like to explore if there might be some strategies to help you cope better with your kidney disease. What has been on your mind recently?

Not again! I was looking forward to catching up...

Well, I've just been feeling really down... Everything is about my kidney disease and going to dialysis now...I have no life

They've got a kidney for me!

Another drink, Tony?

Hmm - maybe I should?.....No! I'd just feel rubbish

No thanks, Bill. I enjoyed my one drink but I've got to be up early for dialysis tomorrow

What! Really?! Are you serious! We'd better get to the hospital then!

We can't get our hopes up yet, it may not be a very good kidney...

Anthony visits the pub with his friends but is only able to have one small drink due to his need to fluid-restrict

One evening, Anthony receives a phone call from the transplant registrar at the hospital informing him that a kidney transplant has become available

---

Haemodialysis involves abrupt changes in body chemistry three times a week. Patients often find this difficult to cope with, especially at first. However, if they have had significant uraemic symptoms before starting dialysis, the general improvement in chemistry may make them feel considerably better.

Peritoneal dialysis

This modality is chosen by about 15% of dialysis patients and uses the peritoneum as a semipermeable membrane. Compared with haemodialysis, peritoneal dialysis gives more independence, as the patient is not committed to attending the dialysis unit three times a week (home based haemodialysis allows similar independence).

Complications

The major complication of peritoneal dialysis is bacterial peritonitis. Good personal hygiene and assiduous aseptic technique when changing dialysis bags helps prevent this. Because dialysis fluid has a high glucose concentration, hyperglycaemia can occur, especially in patients with diabetes.

Transplantation

Renal transplantation is the gold standard for renal replacement therapy in ESRD, because compared with dialysis it improves both quality of life and long-term outcomes. However, its use is limited by the availability of organs.

Some countries, for example Wales, operate an opt-out scheme for organ donation after death, where consent to donate is presumed. There is some debate as to whether opt-out schemes increase the availability of donor organs. Other countries use an opt-in scheme, i.e. a positive decision to donate has to have been made by the donor registering their wish in advance or by the relatives making the decision after death; England is one example.

Donors may be deceased or living. With a long waiting time for kidneys from deceased donors, many patients now consider living donation, using a kidney from a close relative, partner, or friend. There is a small but increasing number of altruistic donors: people who wish to donate a kidney to someone with ESRD but not to a particular individual.

To minimise the risk of rejection, all transplant recipients require lifelong immunosuppression.

Complications

Short-term complications include hyperacute or acute rejection of the transplanted kidney (Table 2.19).

There is no treatment for hyperacute rejection; removal of the graft is necessary. However, it can be avoided by screening the recipient for graft-specific antibodies and is therefore rare.

Acute rejection is the commonest complication (10–20% of grafts) and typically occurs within 6 months of transplantation. It manifests as an acute deterioration in the function of the graft, which is usually asymptomatic but may be associated with some of the following clinical features:

■ flu-like symptoms
■ fever
■ hypertension
■ pain or tenderness around the transplanted kidney
■ sudden weight gain
■ peripheral oedema
■ a decrease in urine output

Acute rejection is confirmed by renal biopsy; characteristic pathological changes include infiltration of tubules, and sometimes vessel walls, with lymphocytes. Treatment is initially with an increased dose of corticosteroids.

It is impossible to prevent acute rejection in all cases. However, the likelihood of it occurring is reduced by the patient taking their antirejection medications as directed, ensuring that no doses are missed.

Many patients are treated for rejection based on clinical findings alone. This is because, although the diagnosis of acute rejection requires a renal transplant biopsy, the risks associated with the procedure to obtain a sample of tissue for biopsy may outweigh the benefit of a confirmed diagnosis.

Longer term complications include (Table 2.19):

■ chronic rejection, which presents with a slow decline in renal function and histological changes that involve the tubules, capillaries and interstitium of the donor kidney
■ infection with unusual organisms
■ recurrence of original disease in the transplanted kidney
■ malignancies
■ transplant ureteric obstruction
■ transplant artery stenosis

Conservative management

For some patients with advanced kidney disease, conservative management is the preferred option. This may be because of the burden of existing comorbidities, frailty or a limited life expectancy that is unlikely to improve with renal replacement therapy. These patients require ongoing care from their nephrologist, GP and palliative care team. The aim of conservative management is to enable patients to have a good quality of life by maintaining renal function at the best possible level and controlling any symptoms that occur.

The decision to opt for conservative care may be made at any time by a patient; this may be before they reach the point at which dialysis would be indicated, or after starting dialysis. Once this decision has been made, the patient may be referred to specialist advanced kidney care nurses, as well as the palliative care team, who can provide support and expert advice on symptom control.

Important aspects of conservative care are supporting families and carers, planning for the future and encouraging the patient to consider the options that are available should they become more unwell. This may include deciding where they would prefer to die, for example at home or in a hospice, or making an advance decision, a legal document that stipulates the treatments a patient would not want to undergo should they become unable to communicate their wishes. Conservative care is discussed further in Chapter 14.

Prognosis

Without renal replacement therapy, the prognosis for patients with ESRD is poor.

For those on dialysis, survival is influenced significantly by the age at which dialysis is started. Patients who start dialysis in their twenties have an average life expectancy of 20 years, whereas those over 75 years old starting dialysis have an average life expectancy of 4 years. Transplantation is associated with a reduced risk of mortality and better quality of life compared to dialysis.

As in CKD, most deaths in ESRD are caused by cardiovascular complications.

Answers to starter questions

1. Having to pass urine more frequently, and getting up at night several times to pass urine (nocturia), are seen in the early stages of CKD as the ability of the kidneys to concentrate urine is impaired. This results in larger amounts of dilute urine. As CKD progresses, however, decreasing GFR causes water retention and patients tend to pass less urine.

2. The kidneys contribute to the acid-base balance of body fluid by reabsorbing filtered bicarbonate (HCO_3^-) and excreting hydrogen (H^+) ions in the urine. Secreted H^+ combines with urinary buffers to form ammonium and hydrogen phosphate. CKD results in a decreased number of nephrons and, therefore, decreased H^+ excretion, causing an increase in plasma H^+ concentration, i.e. acidosis. Some patients also lose HCO_3^- in the urine inappropriately as a result of tubular dysfunction (see Chapter 10).

3. Fruit and nut chocolate is high in potassium. CKD patients often have impaired ability to excrete potassium, and excess dietary intake risks hyperkalaemia, which can cause cardiac arrhythmias and indeed cardiac arrest.

4. In many patients with CKD, their disease will progress to the point that they need dialysis. This often means haemodialysis, which requires high-flow blood access via a surgically-created arteriovenous fistula. If their veins have become damaged by repeated failed attempts at cannulation, this can make creating a fistula much more difficult, or even impossible. A fistula is a superior means of long term venous access as compared to a central venous line as it has far lower infection rates.

5. Conservative management is treatment that is limited to symptom control. Some patients, such as the elderly or those with multiple comorbidities and a limited life expectancy, may opt for conservative management of end-stage renal disease if they feel the burden of renal replacement therapy outweighs the benefits. Dialysis requires a huge time commitment – haemodialysis patients must attend their dialysis unit for 4 hours 3 days a week and peritoneal dialysis patients must perform exchanges several times a day or overnight. Dialysis also requires invasive procedures such as peritoneal dialysis catheter insertions, arteriovenous fistula creation or line insertion, and can have significant complications such as infections. These factors can significantly impair quality of life. In addition, dialysis may not dramatically improve life expectancy.

Chapter 5
Primary glomerular disease

Starter questions

Answers to the following questions are on page 192.

1. The glomerulus is a filter. What does a filter do and how can it go wrong?
2. Why might it be important to test the urine of a child who develops swelling (i.e. oedema) around the eyes?
3. How does loss of protein in the urine cause oedema?
4. Why might a man in his sixties diagnosed with membranous nephropathy start coughing up blood?
5. Two brothers develop a severe sore throat at the same time. One notices blood in his urine over the next day or two; the other also notices blood, but not until 2 weeks later. What underlying renal disease could they each be suffering from?

Introduction

Glomerular disease is disease affecting the glomeruli, the filtration units of the kidney:

■ in primary glomerular disease the pathology is limited to the glomeruli; this is the subject of this chapter
■ in secondary glomerular disease the kidney is only one of several organs targeted by a systemic disease process; this is covered in Chapter 6.

Understanding this distinction is essential to diagnosis and management of glomerular disease.

The pathologies underlying glomerular disease are diverse, ranging from conditions in which there are few structural changes, through those caused by deposition of various proteins, to those with aggressive inflammatory features. Of patients starting renal replacement therapy in the UK, 10–15% have a form of primary glomerulonephritis; 25% have diabetes-related secondary glomerular disease, the leading cause of end-stage renal failure in Western Europe. Other examples of secondary disease are immune complex deposition in systemic lupus erythematosus and small vessel necrosis in vasculitis.

Glomerular disease is a complex topic:

- There is often a poor correlation between the clinical presentation and the underlying cause; this is why renal biopsy is often needed. It is important to bear in mind this distinction between the clinical presentation on the one hand and the underlying cause on the other
- The histopathological nomenclature is complex
- The underlying pathogenesis for several of the diseases is unknown; furthermore

different pathogenic processes can produce the same histopathological pattern.

Regardless of the pathology, the glomerular damage equates to one, or both, of two types of filter failure: .

- the filter lets through material that it should retain, thereby causing haematuria, proteinuria or both
- the filter retains material that it should let through, thereby decreasing the glomerular filtration rate (GFR)

There are therefore a limited number of clinical presentations of glomerular disease.

> **Significant glomerular disease is unlikely in the absence of proteinuria or haematuria.** Bence Jones proteins, however, which may indicate significant disease, are not detected by the usual tests for proteinuria (see page 204).

Clinical presentations of glomerular disease

The combination of the two types of filter failure, together with the rate at which they occur, results in five different presentations of glomerular disease (**Table 5.1**). The relationship between these presentations and the primary glomerular diseases covered in this chapter is shown in **Table 5.2**.

Nephrotic syndrome

The nephrotic syndrome is defined as the triad of:

- heavy proteinuria,
- low serum albumin concentration and
- oedema

Glomerular disease: clinical presentations	
Presentation	Clinical features
Nephrotic syndrome	Heavy proteinuria (> 3–5 g/day or equivalent)
	Hypoalbuminaemia (< 30 g/L)
	Oedema
	(Depending on cause GFR is or isn't reduced)
Asymptomatic urinary abnormalities	Haematuria and/or proteinuria; GFR is normal
Nephritic syndrome	Haematuria, proteinuria and decreased GFR developing over a few days
Rapidly progressive glomerulonephritis	As for nephritic syndrome, but decreased GFR developing over weeks and months
Chronic kidney disease (see Chapter 4)	Typically small kidneys with haematuria and/or proteinuria, with decreased GFR either stable or deteriorating over years

Table 5.1 Clinical presentations of glomerular disease. GFR, glomerular filtration rate

Primary glomerular disease: clinical presentations					
Histopathology	Nephrotic syndrome	Asymptomatic urinary abnormalities	Nephritic syndrome	Rapidly progressive glomerulonephritis	Chronic kidney disease
Minimal change nephropathy	Usual	Occasional	Unknown	Unknown	Very rare or unknown
Membranous nephropathy	Usual	Occasional	Very rare	Very rare	Occasional
Focal segmental glomerulosclerosis	Usual	Occasional	Very rare	Very rare	Occasional
Immunoglobulin A nephropathy	Rare	Usual	Rare	Rare	Occasional
Post-infectious glomerulonephritis	Rare	Rare	Usual	Rare	Rare
Mesangiocapillary glomerulonephritis	Usual	Occasional	Occasional	Rare	Occasional

Table 5.2 Clinical presentations of primary glomerular disease

A number of different pathological processes (both primary and secondary) may cause the syndrome, and these may or may not be associated with a decreased GFR.

Clinically, the patient notices the development of oedema. This is usually around the feet and ankles (**Figure 5.1**), but the swelling may spread upwards; in children, there is often also swelling around the eyes (periorbital oedema). In conditions with a tendency to recur (such as minimal change nephropathy; see page 183), once the patient knows what to look for the initial sign of a relapse may be the development of frothy urine; this is a consequence of large amounts of protein in the urine acting as a detergent, lowering surface tension and producing bubbles.

In children, the nephrotic syndrome is assumed to be the result of minimal change nephropathy (see page 183) and treated as such. In adults, the underlying diseases are more diverse but, if due to primary glomerular disease, three conditions make up the majority of cases (**Table 5.3**):

- Minimal change nephropathy (20–30% of cases)
- Membranous nephropathy (30% of cases)
- Focal segmental glomerulosclerosis (20% of cases)

Diagnostic approach

For all patients there is a single initial approach to investigations and diagnosis:

- Urinalysis is required for all patients presenting with sudden onset of significant oedema; the absence of significant proteinuria excludes nephrotic syndrome as the cause
- Secondary causes of the nephrotic state (e.g. diabetes, systemic lupus erythematosus) are considered during history taking and examination, as are rare precipitants of primary causes (e.g. malignancy and use of certain drugs)

Investigations

The degree of proteinuria is quantified (see page 86) and serum albumin concentration measured. A GFR measurement is obtained (serum concentration of creatinine is usually sufficient). Serum cholesterol concentration is usually increased, occasionally to 5–6 times the upper limit of normal. This is common to all causes of nephrotic syndrome.

Investigations for secondary causes of nephrotic syndrome (see Chapter 6) are carried out as indicated by the history and examination.

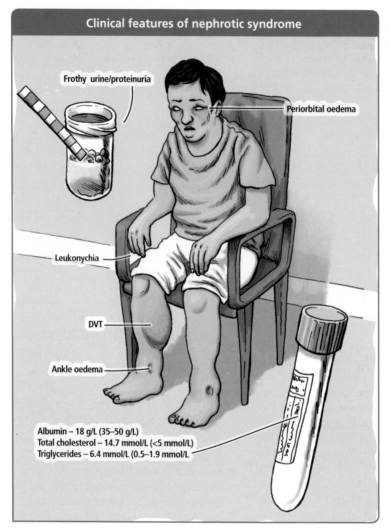

Figure 5.1 Clinical features of nephrotic syndrome.

Renal biopsy is not usually required in children because minimal change nephropathy is assumed to be the cause (see page 183 for exceptions). Biopsy is required in adults to make a definitive diagnosis.

Management

Management of the nephrotic state is common to all the causes:

- Control oedema by restricting salt intake and increasing sodium excretion, usually with loop diuretics. Intractable oedema is difficult to manage, but the synergistic use of a loop diuretic and a thiazide will help

- Treat hypertension (if present) with an angiotensin-converting enzyme (ACE) inhibitor or angiotensin II receptor blocker. These agents also reduce proteinuria
- Treat the underlying cause, if possible

Anticoagulants

The nephrotic state is associated with hypercoagulability, which occasionally results in life-threatening thromboembolic disease. Therefore anticoagulation is required if serum albumin concentration is < 20 g/L. Minimal change disease typically responds rapidly to treatment, so is an exception.

Nephrotic syndrome in adults: comparison of the commonest causes

Feature	Minimal change nephropathy	Membranous nephropathy	Focal segmental glomerulosclerosis
Pathogenesis	Unknown	High proportion of 'idiopathic' cases associated with, and possibly caused by, autoantibodies to phospholipase A2 receptor	Probably multiple different insults; unknown in most cases
Treatment (in addition to general management of nephrotic syndrome)	Corticosteroids	Immunosuppression considered for patients with deteriorating renal function	Controversial; a trial of immunosuppression may be worthwhile
Prognosis	Excellent; progresses to end-stage renal failure very rarely, if ever	One third of cases may progress to end-stage renal failure	Two thirds to three quarters of cases may progress to end-stage renal failure
Underlying conditions to consider	Rarely use of certain drugs (e.g. NSAIDs), or malignancy (Hodgkin's disease)	Underlying malignancy (10% of cases), use of certain drugs	Genetic, hyperfiltration, obesity, HIV infection

NSAID, non-steroidal anti-inflammatory drug.

Table 5.3 Comparison of the three most common primary causes of nephrotic syndrome in adults

Statins

Statins are used to treat any hypercholesterolaemia associated with the nephrotic state.

Asymptomatic urinary abnormalities

This is blood and/or protein in the urine, often detected when urinalysis is done for screening or some other indication. The diagnostic approach is the same as for IgA nephropathy (see below).

Nephritic syndrome

Nephritic syndrome involves both modes of filter failure: blood and protein in the urine with a decrease in GFR. The defining feature is that these signs develop abruptly, over a period of days. Other features are haematuria and oedema associated with salt and water retention as a consequence of the decreased GFR. Blood pressure is often raised for the same reason.

Rapidly progressive glomerulonephritis

The features are the same as for the nephritic syndrome, but the time course is longer with progression over weeks or a small number of months. The usual associated pathology is a necrotising crescentic glomerulonephritis, which can complicate some of the primary diseases in this chapter but is more commonly due to secondary conditions covered in Chapter 6 (see pages 198 and 202).

Chronic kidney disease

The presentation is with blood and/or protein in the urine (often detected incidentally), associated with a decreased GFR. Depending upon the cause, the GFR is either stable or slowly deteriorates over a number of years. A renal ultrasound will show small kidneys and if so a renal biopsy is not performed (and therefore the diagnosis of glomerular disease is presumptive rather than definitive): the risks associated with the procedure are increased with small kidneys and the results will not alter the management. If the kidneys are normal size then a biopsy is done to obtain a definitive diagnosis.

Case 3 Ankle swelling

Presentation

Mary Reynolds, a 27-year-old African–Caribbean woman, presents to her general practitioner (GP), Dr Anderson, with a 5-week history of progressive leg swelling.

Initial interpretation

Peripheral oedema – increased fluid in the interstitial tissues, particularly in dependent areas such as the feet – is common in the elderly. However, in a person of Mary's age it usually suggests significant underlying pathology, such as heart, liver or renal disease.

Further history

Mary is otherwise well, with no significant past medical history; the only medication she is taking is the combined oral contraceptive pill. Her alcohol intake is 5 units/week. She does not have orthopnoea, i.e. breathlessness on lying flat.

Examination

Dr Anderson examines Mary's feet and calves and finds pitting oedema from her ankles to her knees; pressure applied by a finger produces a visible indentation in the swelling (see Figure 2.3). She auscultates Mary's heart and lungs: there are no murmurs, and only normal breath sounds are audible. Jugular venous pressure is not raised. There are no signs of liver disease, such as jaundice or spider naevi, i.e. groups of enlarged capillaries fed by an arteriole and usually present over the upper chest.

Interpretation of findings

There is no evidence of heart or liver disease from the history or examination. Orthopnoea, had it been present, would have suggested fluid congestion in the lungs and heart failure. Raised jugular venous pressure would also have indicated possible heart failure. Together, these findings make heart or liver failure an unlikely explanation for Mary's oedema.

Testing of the urine is mandatory in such cases, to exclude nephrotic syndrome as a cause of the oedema. In nephrotic syndrome large amounts of protein are detected in urine (see **Table 5.1**).

Investigations

Dipstick urinalysis to assess for haematuria and proteinuria, and blood tests to determine the eGFR, are carried out. The results are shown in **Table 5.4**.

Mary's ethnic origin and sex prompt an autoimmune screen for systemic lupus

Mary Reynolds' blood and urine test investigation results		
Test	Result	Normal range
Dipstick urinalysis	Protein ++++	Negative
Serum creatinine	65 μmol/L	50–110 μmol/L
Serum albumin	14 g/L	35–50 g/L
Protein:creatinine ratio	369 mg/mmol	< 45 mg/mmol
eGFR	> 60 mL/min/1.73 m^2	> 60 mL/min/1.73 m^2
Autoimmune screen (complement profile and antinuclear antibody)	Negative	Negative

Table 5.4 Blood and urine test results for Mary Reynolds

erythematosus; it is more common in people of African and Caribbean origin, and far more women are affected than men (see page 200). The result is negative.

Diagnosis

Mary's serum albumin concentration of 14 g/L is low. Failure of albumin production is one possible reason for this result, but this is unlikely in the absence of significant liver disease. Another reason is excessive loss in the urine, i.e. the nephrotic syndrome.

Dr Anderson explains to Mary that the filter units in her kidney are leaking too much protein, and that there are a number of possible causes for this. Mary is obviously worried by the news, particularly when she is told that the only way to find out the exact cause is to do a kidney biopsy, i.e. obtain a sample of kidney by inserting a needle into her back under local anaesthetic to obtain a sample for examination under a microscope. Dr Anderson refers Mary to the local renal unit, where she is seen within a week as an outpatient.

The consultant explains how a renal biopsy is obtained and with Mary's consent arranges for this to be carried out the following week as a day case procedure. The biopsy report is ready the next day and shows focal segmental glomerulosclerosis (see page 186). This is managed at the renal unit, with Mary attending as an outpatient.

Case 4 Blood in the urine

Presentation

Sheila Baker, who is 23 years old and Caucasian, visits her GP, Dr Prakash, because she has noticed blood in her urine for the last 2 days (visible haematuria). Although initially alarmed, she had hoped it would go away on its own. However, she now realises she needs to see a physician.

Initial interpretation

Menstruation is a common cause of false positive haematuria, so female patients are asked about this. Urinary tract infection is a common cause of true haematuria but is nearly always accompanied by other symptoms. Haematuria can be the presenting symptom of urinary tract malignancy. Therefore, even though urinary tract malignancy is unlikely at Sheila's age, haematuria must be investigated.

Further history

Sheila is not having her period at the moment. She has had a moderately severe sore throat and has felt generally unwell for the past 3 days. She has not had any pain on passing urine (dysuria) or frequent urination. There is no significant past medical history, and she is taking no medication.

Examination

Dr Prakash notes that Sheila is a little flushed but does not appear unwell. She is apyrexial. On oral examination, he notes that her throat appears slightly red and swollen. Her blood pressure is 148/94 mmHg.

Interpretation of findings

The history suggests that the blood in Sheila's urine is not attributable to

Case 4 continued

menstruation or a urinary tract infection (there is no dysuria or urinary frequency). However, there is evidence of an upper respiratory tract infection. Sheila's blood pressure is significantly raised for a woman of her age. This finding, together with the history of visible haematuria at the same time as an upper respiratory tract infection, make this a typical presentation of immunoglobulin (Ig) A nephropathy, the commonest form of primary glomerular disease (see page 188). This type of nephropathy is more common in Caucasian and Asian people, and is most often found in patients in their twenties.

Investigations

Dipstick urinalysis to assess for haematuria and proteinuria is carried out, in addition to blood tests to estimate GFR. The results are shown in **Table 5.5**.

Diagnosis

Sheila's decreased eGFR almost certainly indicates that the haematuria has a nephrological cause, i.e. glomerular or tubulointerstitial disease, as opposed to a urological one, for example cancer or renal stones. Dr Prakash explains this to Sheila, and says that she needs to be referred to a renal physician for further tests and management.

She is seen as an outpatient at the local renal unit 2 weeks later. Blood and protein are detectable on repeat dipstick urinalysis although not visible in her urine.

The original set of blood tests is repeated. Serum creatinine concentration is now 116 µmol/L. The renal physician explains that the clinical picture strongly suggests IgA nephropathy, and gives Sheila more information about the condition. He also tells her that renal biopsy is the only way to confirm the diagnosis, and that he would recommend this because her creatinine concentration is still increased.

A renal biopsy is obtained as a day case procedure 4 weeks later. The biopsy report confirms the diagnosis of IgA nephropathy. No particular treatment or lifestyle change is indicated at the moment, but Sheila will require indefinite monitoring because 20–25% of patients with this diagnosis progress to end-stage renal disease.

Haematuria has urological and nephrological causes. The latter are indicated by decreased eGFR, significant proteinuria and dysmorphic red blood cells on urine microscopy (see page 86).

Sheila Baker's blood and urine test results		
Test	Result	Normal range
Dipstick urinalysis	Blood +++, protein ++	Negative
Serum albumin	37 g/L	35–50 g/L
Serum creatinine	124 µmol/L	50–110 µmol/L
Protein:creatinine ratio	87 mg/mmol	< 45 mg/mmol
eGFR	49 mL/min/1.73 m^2	> 60 mL/min/1.73 m^2

Table 5.5 Blood and urine test results for Sheila Baker

Minimal change nephropathy

Minimal change nephropathy is the leading cause of nephrotic syndrome in children, causing 70–80% of cases. It is the underlying cause in 20–30% of adults with primary glomerular diseases producing nephrotic syndrome. The name reflects the essentially normal results on renal biopsy using light microscopy and immunohistochemistry. In contrast, electron microscopy shows pathology in the form of fusion of podocyte foot processes.

This type of nephropathy is often viewed as a less serious condition, because it probably never leads to end-stage renal failure. However, the repeated relapses of the nephrotic state that characterise the disease, combined with the adverse effects of repeated courses of corticosteroids used to treat it, often cause great distress to patients.

Aetiology

There is no obvious precipitating cause in most patients but in a small number there is an association with an underlying malignancy, notably Hodgkin's disease, or the use of certain drugs, such as non-steroidal anti-inflammatory drugs.

The underlying pathogenesis is unknown. An abnormality of the immune system is indirectly suggested by the occasional association with other immunological disorders, for example atopy, and the response to immunosuppression.

Clinical features

Minimal change nephropathy presents clinically with the sudden development of the nephrotic syndrome (see page 176). Occasionally, lesser degrees of proteinuria are an incidental finding on urinalysis, for example in hypertensive patients.

Diagnostic approach

The approach is the same as for nephrotic syndrome (see above). The GFR is normal in minimal change nephropathy, but is increased in cases of significant hypovolaemia causing prerenal acute kidney injury.

Biopsy

Biopsy is usually unnecessary in children presenting with nephrotic syndrome, because minimal change disease is the cause in 70–80% of cases, and treatment is started on this assumption. However, renal biopsy may become necessary if the course of the child's minimal change nephropathy is not as expected, for example if the child responds poorly to corticosteroids, develops renal impairment or both.

A renal biopsy is required in adults because the underlying causes are more diverse.

For both children and adults, if a renal biopsy is indicated then a renal ultrasound is done to confirm that two normal-sized kidneys are present. Usually, in minimal change disease the only abnormality found on biopsy is fusion of podocyte foot processes (**Figure 5.2**), which is a non-specific response to heavy proteinuria of any cause.

Management

This can be divided into management of the nephrotic state, which is the same whatever the underlying cause, and specific management of minimal change nephropathy.

Management of the nephrotic state is covered on page 177.

Specific management of minimal change nephropathy

Corticosteroids are the first-line treatment. The response is typically rapid (within days) but can take several months, particularly in adults. Remission is indicated by resolution of oedema and proteinuria, and an increase in albumin to normal levels. When remission occurs, the dosage of corticosteroids is tapered over several weeks, and stopped if possible.

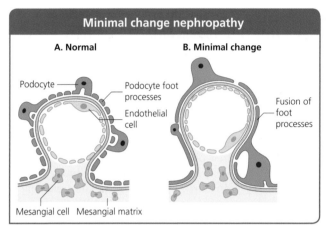

Figure 5.2 Changes in the glomerular capillary loop in minimal change nephropathy. (a) Normal glomerular capillary loop. (b) Fusion of podocyte foot processes in minimal change nephropathy.

Relapses

These are common once corticosteroids are reduced or withdrawn, and patients may require retreatment. Frequent relapses are managed with more intensive immunosuppression using cyclophosphamide or calcineurin inhibitors (e.g. ciclosporin or tacrolimus).

Prognosis for minimal change nephropathy

Prognosis is excellent in terms of preservation of renal function; the condition probably never results in progressive renal impairment. If this does occur another diagnosis, for example focal segmental glomerulosclerosis, is suspected. However, frequent relapses, which can keep happening for many years, may result in considerable morbidity secondary to corticosteroid use.

> **It is essential to clearly explain and discuss with patients the adverse effects of corticosteroids.** Over time, they usually find the mood swings, cushingoid facies ('moon face'), acne, abdominal striae, weight gain and other negative effects worse than the original swelling they presented with.

Membranous nephropathy

This is a common cause of nephrotic syndrome in adults and is the most common primary glomerular disease causing nephrotic syndrome in white adults. The name refers to the associated finding on light microscopy of thickening of the glomerular basement membrane, at least in more advanced cases.

Epidemiology

Membranous nephropathy is the underlying diagnosis in about 30% of adults presenting with nephrotic syndrome. It is the cause in about 8% of patients with end-stage renal failure resulting from primary glomerular disease.

Aetiology

Primary membranous nephropathy

About 90% of cases are idiopathic, also known as primary, membranous nephropathy. Autoantibodies to a glomerular antigen, the phospholipase A2 receptor, are found in 70% of such primary cases and probably play a role in pathogenesis.

Secondary membranous nephropathy

Up to 10% of patients have secondary disease associated with an underlying malignancy, particularly carcinoma. Certain infections (notably hepatitis B), drugs and other substances have been implicated in the pathogenesis. Most of the implicated drugs, including gold and penicillamine, are no longer used. Cosmetics containing mercury, which may also induce the disease, have been banned in many countries.

Some instances of secondary disease are probably a consequence of the deposition in the glomerulus of immune complexes containing tumour or microbial antigens, an example being HBeAg (hepatitis B e-antigen) in hepatitis B infection.

Clinical features

Presentation is usually with nephrotic syndrome (see **Figure 5.1**). Lesser degrees of proteinuria, renal impairment and hypertension may be present.

Diagnostic approach

The diagnostic approach and investigations are the same as for nephrotic syndrome (see page 177). Secondary causes are considered, particularly an underlying carcinoma (e.g. lung, colon) in more elderly patients (over 50 years of age).

Investigations

Investigations are as described for nephrotic syndrome on pages 177–178, plus any that might be appropriate for suspected secondary causes (e.g. chest X-ray for possible lung carcinoma).

Biopsy

This is required for definitive diagnosis. Histopathological analysis shows the rather uniform feature of thickening of the glomerular basement membrane, a finding that may not be visible by light microscopy in early disease. The thickening is the result of deposition of IgG-containing immune complexes, which on electron microscopy are shown to be on the outer side of the membrane and subepithelial, lying below the podocyte foot processes (**Figures 5.3** and **5.4**).

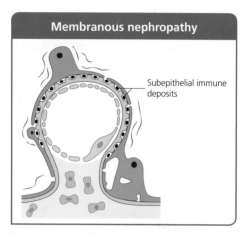

Figure 5.3 A capillary loop in membranous nephropathy, showing subepithelial (podocyte) immunoglobulin G deposits and extension of basement membrane between the deposits to produce 'spikes'.

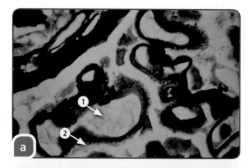

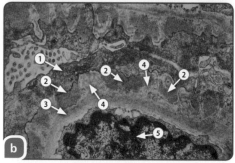

Figure 5.4 (a) Silver stain of a glomerulus from a case of membranous nephropathy, showing silver-positive spikes on the subepithelial side of the basement membrane. ①, Capillary loop; ②, spikes. (b) Electron micrograph of part of a capillary loop from a case of membranous nephropathy showing detail of immune deposits and spikes. ①, Fused podocyte foot processes; ②, electron-dense immune deposits; ③, glomerular basement membrane; ④, spikes of basement membrane material between deposits; ⑤, endothelial cell.

Systemic lupus erythematosus should be considered as a cause of apparently idiopathic membranous nephropathy if histopathology shows atypical features such as mesangial or subendothelial deposits and the presence of IgM or IgA as well as IgG (see page 200).

Management

The nephrotic state is managed as outlined above (see page 178). Any secondary causes are managed appropriately.

Disease-modifying medication

Immunosuppression with a calcineurin inhibitor (e.g. ciclosporin or tacrolimus) or the combination of corticosteroids and an alkylating agent, known as the Ponticelli regimen, may be considered. It is common practice to restrict this more intensive treatment to the subset of patients with deteriorating renal function or persisting heavy proteinuria.

Prognosis

The prognosis is in thirds:

- one third of patients will have spontaneous remission, and the long-term outlook for this group is excellent, even if they experience subsequent relapses
- one third will have persisting proteinuria but their excretory renal function is preserved
- one third will experience deteriorating renal function

Independent of underlying diagnosis, heavy proteinuria correlates with poor renal prognosis, probably because excess protein is toxic to renal tubular cells. The exception is minimal change nephropathy, in which proteinuria is usually transient because of the rapid response to treatment.

Focal segmental glomerulosclerosis

This disease causes sclerosis, mesangial matrix expansion and capillary loop collapse. As the name implies, lesions affect only some glomeruli (hence 'focal'), and only a portion of those affected (hence 'segmental'). It has the worst prognosis of the primary glomerular diseases that cause nephrotic syndrome.

Epidemiology

Focal segmental glomerulosclerosis accounts for 10–20% of cases of nephrotic syndrome in both children and adults. It is the most common primary glomerular disease causing nephrotic syndrome in African–Caribbean adults. Because the prognosis is poor, this disease is found in a high proportion of patients who present with renal impairment in addition to nephrotic syndrome.

Aetiology

In most patients the disease is idiopathic, but in a small minority it is associated with underlying conditions such as obesity, HIV infection and reduced nephron mass leading to hyperfiltration.

The histological pattern of focal segmental glomerulosclerosis probably represents a common final response to a number of different pathological processes that primarily affect the podocyte. In some patients, particularly in children, the disease is a consequence of single-gene defects. Some of the affected genes encode proteins which are part of the glomerular filtration barrier, for example nephrin, the deficiency of which underlies a congenital nephrotic syndrome known as the Finnish type.

One or more poorly characterised circulating factors are present in some patients.

These factors may be responsible for the recurrence, which can occur in days, of nephrotic syndrome in a transplanted kidney.

Clinical features

Presentation is usually with nephrotic syndrome (see **Figure 5.1**) or with lesser degrees of proteinuria. Renal impairment, hypertension or both are commonly present. A subset of patients have a rapid deterioration in renal function over a short period of time (months); this group is at particular risk of recurrence of the disease after renal transplantation.

Diagnostic approach

This is as outlined for nephrotic syndrome (see page 177). In children, it is worth screening for known single-gene defects to help inform prognosis and provide genetic counselling. However, this step is not justified in adults.

Investigations

Investigations are as given above for nephrotic syndrome, plus investigations for any suspected secondary causes (e.g. HIV).

Biopsy

A biopsy specimen is required to enable definitive diagnosis by histopathological analysis (**Figures 5.5** and **5.6**). The focal lesions affect the deep juxtamedullary glomeruli first, so they may be missed on a biopsy. Therefore some cases are initially labelled as minimal change nephropathy.

Management

The nephrotic state is managed as outlined above (see page 178). Any secondary causes are managed appropriately, for example by:

- treatment of associated HIV infection
- weight loss for obesity
- in cases of reduced nephron mass, blood pressure control with an ACE inhibitor

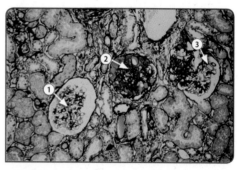

Figure 5.6 Silver stain of a renal biopsy in a case of focal segmental glomerulosclerosis showing both normal ①, globally-sclerosed ② and focally-sclerosed glomeruli in the left upper quadrant ③.

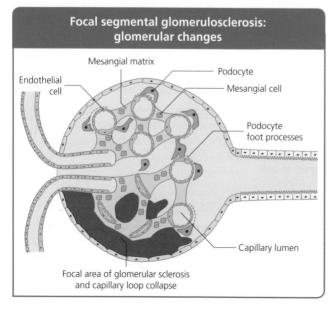

Figure 5.5 Changes to the glomerulus in focal segmental glomerulosclerosis. Part of this glomerulus is affected by a segmental lesion. Other glomeruli may be normal or globally sclerosed; the disease process is focal.

Focal segmental glomerulosclerosis: glomerular changes

Mesangial matrix
Endothelial cell
Podocyte
Mesangial cell
Podocyte foot processes
Capillary lumen
Focal area of glomerular sclerosis and capillary loop collapse

or an angiotensin II receptor blocker, which is essential to minimise glomerular hyperfiltration

Disease-modifying medication

There is no consensus as to whether more intensive treatment with immunosuppression alters the natural history of focal segmental glomerulosclerosis. In patients with persisting heavy proteinuria, deteriorating renal function or both, treatment with corticosteroids or calcineurin inhibitors is considered.

Prognosis

This cause of nephrotic syndrome is associated with the worst prognosis: up to two thirds of patients with focal segmental glomerulosclerosis experience deterioration of renal function leading to end-stage renal failure. The condition recurs in up to 50% of kidney transplant recipients and then often results in loss of the transplanted kidney.

> **Conveying a diagnosis of focal segmental glomerulosclerosis requires the skills for breaking bad news.** Most patients who receive this diagnosis will develop end-stage renal failure, and they need to be told that this is likely. The further bad news of a high rate of recurrence in transplanted kidneys is usually best left to a later session.

Immunoglobulin A nephropathy

This is the commonest primary glomerular disease worldwide. It is characterised by increased volume of mesangial matrix and number of mesangial cells in the glomerulus, associated with the deposition of IgA in the mesangium.

Epidemiology

Immunoglobulin A nephropathy is the underlying diagnosis in up to 25% of renal biopsies.

Aetiology

The vast majority of cases are idiopathic; a small number are associated with liver disease or spondyloarthropathies such as ankylosing spondylitis, but it is not clear that this is a causal association.

The cause is unknown. There is evidence of abnormal glycosylation of circulating IgA, but the connection with the pathogenesis of IgA nephropathy, if any, is unclear.

Clinical features

The most common clinical features are asymptomatic urinary abnormalities (haematuria, proteinuria), accompanied by hypertension or renal impairment, or both.

A significant proportion of patients notice visible haematuria at the same time as an upper respiratory tract infection (synpharyngitic haematuria). Rarely, patients present with other clinical patterns of glomerular disease (see **Tables 5.1** and **5.2**).

Diagnostic approach

The history of visible haematuria contemporaneous with an upper respiratory tract infection is so typical of this disease that such presentations can be managed without the necessity for renal biopsy, provided that:

- there is no significant proteinuria or renal impairment
- urological causes have been excluded

Many patients presenting with chronic kidney disease, haematuria and small kidneys, which implies long-standing disease leading to fibrosis and shrinkage, probably have underlying IgA nephropathy.

Investigations

Proteinuria is quantified and serum concentrations of albumin and creatinine are measured. Haematuria prompts consideration of investigation for urological causes, for example cystoscopy and renal imaging.

Serum concentration of IgA is increased in up to 50% of cases.

Renal biopsy is required for definitive diagnosis. It shows expansion of the mesangium, both cells and matrix, as well as mesangial deposition of IgA. On electron microscopy, the IgA deposits are typically detected in the paramesangial areas, the mesangial region immediately adjacent to a capillary loop (**Figures 5.7** and **5.8**).

Management

Because the cause, and therefore any possible specific treatment, of IgA nephropathy is unknown, management focuses on strict control of blood pressure. This includes modification of lifestyle factors (see page 278).

Hypertension is treated with an ACE inhibitor or an angiotensin II receptor blocker. Heavy proteinuria is managed as described for nephrotic syndrome (see page 178). In patients who have haematuria and renal impairment at the same time as an infection, the renal impairment usually resolves spontaneously, and no specific treatment is needed.

Medication

Immunosuppression may improve the outlook. It is considered in patients with poor prognostic features such as persisting heavy proteinuria or deteriorating renal function.

Prognosis

Up to 20% of patients with IgA nephrology eventually progress to end-stage renal failure. If these patients receive a renal transplant then recurrence of IgA deposits is seen in up to 50% of transplanted kidneys transplants, but this rarely results in graft loss.

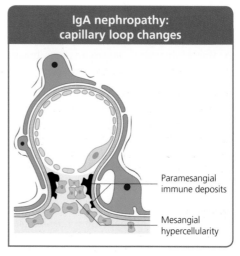

Figure 5.7 A capillary loop in immunoglobulin A nephropathy, showing expansion of mesangial matrix and cells, with paramesangial deposits of immunoglobulin A.

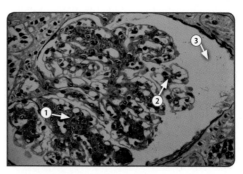

Figure 5.8 H&E stain glomerulus from a case of IgA nephropathy showing expansion of both mesangial matrix and mesangial cells. ①, mesangium showing excess matrix and cells; ②, normal mesangium; ③, Bowman's space.

Post-infectious glomerulonephritis

Post-infectious glomerulonephritis occurs after a group A streptococcal infection, i.e. invasive or non-invasive pharyngeal or skin infections by *Streptococcus pyogenes*. Despite a declining incidence of streptococcal infections, this remains a major public health problem in some populations, for example the Aboriginal people of Australia. In Western Europe, post-infectious glomerulonephritis now more commonly follows other infections.

Pathogenesis

Post-infectious glomerulonephritis is thought to develop as a result of the affinity of a bacterial antigen for the glomerular basement membrane. During an initial infection, nephritogenic strains of bacteria produce an antigen that circulates and binds to the glomerular basement membrane. This 'planted' antigen provokes an immune response resulting in fixation of complement, glomerular inflammation with proliferation of mesangial and endothelial cells, and infiltration with polymorphonuclear leucocytes.

Clinical features and investigations

The disease characteristically presents with the abrupt onset of nephritic syndrome (see page 179) 10–14 days after the initiating infection; this is the time taken for the primary immune response to develop.

Investigations show the features of the nephritic syndrome, as well as low concentrations of complement in the blood (hypocomplementaemia). This probably reflects activation of the complement system by immune complexes produced by the binding of antibodies to planted antigen. Rarely, proteinuria may be in the nephrotic range (see Table 5.1).

Typical cases of post-infectious glomerulonephritis may be managed without the need for renal biopsy. If there is doubt about the diagnosis then a biopsy is required. This shows features of glomerular inflammation (mesangial expansion, neutrophil infiltration); electron microscopy shows characteristic subepithelial hump-shaped immune deposits (Figures 5.9 and 5.10).

> A complement screen is a useful diagnostic test in the context of suspected inflammatory glomerulonephritis. Of all the primary glomerular diseases, only post-infectious and mesangiocapillary glomerulonephritis are associated with hypocomplementaemia. However, it is also seen in some glomerular diseases with secondary causes (see Chapter 6).

Management

This is largely supportive. Dialysis may be required in severe disease.

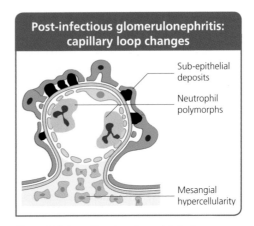

Post-infectious glomerulonephritis: capillary loop changes

Sub-epithelial deposits

Neutrophil polymorphs

Mesangial hypercellularity

Figure 5.9 A capillary loop in post-infectious glomerulonephritis, showing hump-shaped subepithelial (podocyte) immune deposits, mesangial expansion and inflammatory neutrophils.

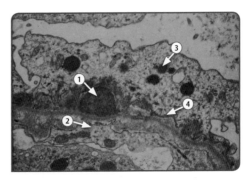

Figure 5.10 Electron micrograph of a portion of a capillary loop from a case of post-infectious glomerulonephritis, showing hump-shaped subepithelial immune deposit ①. ②, endothelium; ③, fused podocyte foot processes; ④, glomerular basement membrane.

Prognosis

There is usually spontaneous resolution of inflammation with a good long-term prognosis, particularly in children. However, post-infectious glomerulonephritis is followed by progressive renal impairment in 10–20% of adults. In some populations, such as Australian Aboriginal people, it contributes to a significant incidence of end-stage renal failure.

Mesangiocapillary glomerulonephritis

Mesangiocapillary glomerulonephritis, also known as membranoproliferative glomerulonephritis, is characterised by mesangial proliferation and thickening of capillary loops. With the exception of cases associated with hepatitis C, this is a rare condition.

Pathogenesis

Understanding of the pathogenesis of this condition is evolving, and divides cases into those with deposition of both complement component C3 and immunoglobulins (previously known as type I mesangiocapillary glomerulonephritis), and those with C3 deposition alone (previously known as type II).

C3 and immunoglobulin deposition

In a minority of patients there is no obvious cause (primary disease), but in others the disease is secondary to immune complex deposition in certain infections (notably hepatitis C and infectious endocarditis), autoimmune diseases (e.g. systemic lupus erythematosus) and monoclonal gammopathies; these are considered further in Chapter 6.

Isolated C3 deposition

Isolated C3 deposition, which includes the entities known as dense deposit disease and C3 glomerulopathy, is associated with dysregulation of the alternative pathway of complement.

In dense deposit disease, this dysregulation is caused by an autoantibody, C3 nephritic factor, which stabilises the alternative pathway C3 convertase. C3 nephritic factor may also have a role in the aetiology of the partial lipodystrophy apparent in some patients. This wasting of fat deposits, typically around the face, produces a somewhat cadaverous appearance.

Clinical features and investigations

Clinical presentation is diverse, but is often with high amounts of proteinuria, i.e. in the nephrotic range. In secondary C3 and Ig deposition, features of an underlying disease may be present (**Table 5.6**).

Blood tests show hypocomplementaemia. Renal biopsy is required for diagnosis. This shows peripheral extension of mesangial matrix and cells, and consequent thickening of capillary loops which accentuates the lobular structure of the glomerulus and produces 'double contouring' of the basement membrane of the capillary loops (**Figure 5.11**). The biopsy may suggest detailed investigation of the alternative pathway of complement if isolated C3 deposition is found.

Mesangiocapillary glomerulitis: secondary causes	
Disease	Features
Hepatitis C	Liver disease, hepatitis C serology, rheumatoid factor, type 2 cryoglobulinaemia (see page 205)
Infectious endocarditis	Pyrexia, heart murmurs, positive blood cultures
Lupus	Arthralgias, rash, lupus serology

Table 5.6 Secondary causes of mesangiocapillary glomerulonephritis and their clinical features

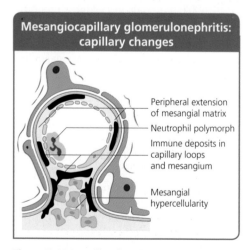

Mesangiocapillary glomerulonephritis: capillary changes

Peripheral extension of mesangial matrix

Neutrophil polymorph

Immune deposits in capillary loops and mesangium

Mesangial hypercellularity

Figure 5.11 A capillary loop in mesangiocapillary glomerulonephritis, showing peripheral extension of mesangium producing a double-contouring appearance.

Management

Nephrotic syndrome, if present, is managed as described above (see page 178). It may be possible to treat an underlying disease, if one is identified. Some cases may respond to immunosuppression.

Control of abnormal activation of complement is possible with eculizumab, a monoclonal antibody to C5. However, it is extremely expensive and of uncertain efficacy in mesangiocapillary glomerulonephritis, as opposed to its use in haemolytic uraemic syndrome (see page 209) where it is effective.

Prognosis

In the absence of a treatable underlying condition such as hepatitis C the prognosis is poor, with most cases progressing to end-stage renal failure. Recurrence in a transplanted kidney is common.

Answers to starter questions

1. Filters are designed to let some substances through, whilst selectively blocking the passage of others. Filter failure, therefore, will result in substances passing through that shouldn't, and/or in substances being retained that should pass through. Glomerular disease represents a filter failure, and therefore presents with blood and/or protein in the urine, plus or minus a decrease in glomerular filtration rate.

2. Oedema in children is often peri-orbital, in contrast to adults, where it usually occurs in gravity-dependent areas such as the ankles, or over the sacral region in bed-bound patients. An important cause of peri-orbital oedema is nephrotic syndrome, most commonly due to minimal change disease in children. If there is no proteinuria on urine dipstick testing, then this diagnosis is excluded.

3. Part of the answer is that loss of protein, primarily albumin, in the urine leads to an upset in the balance of the Starling forces in the microcirculation: the decrease in plasma oncotic pressure due to a low albumin concentration means that more fluid is retained in the interstitial compartment. However, in addition to this, the kidneys also retain more salt and water; a proportion of patients with nephrotic syndrome are in fact hypervolaemic, which cannot only be explained by changes in Starling forces.

4. There are a number of possible reasons. In 10% of patients with membranous nephropathy there is an associated underlying malignancy which, in this case, could be lung cancer. The nephrotic state (which usually accompanies membranous nephropathy) is associated with hypercoagulability; the patient could be suffering from a pulmonary embolus. Another very rare possibility is that he has anti-glomerular basement membrane (GBM) disease, which can be associated with pulmonary haemorrhage (see page 202), and can occasionally develop in the setting of membranous nephropathy.

5. This scenario emphasises the importance of an accurate history, and the different natural history of glomerular diseases that can be associated with infection. Blood in the urine at around the time of an upper respiratory tract infection (i.e. 'synpharyngitic' haematuria) is very typical of IgA nephropathy, whereas haematuria (and probably proteinuria and a reduced glomerular filtration rate) 2 weeks later would be typical timing for a post-infectious (possibly streptococcal) glomerulonephritis.

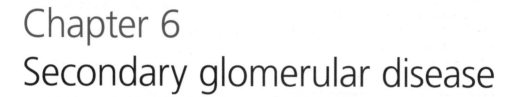

Chapter 6
Secondary glomerular disease

Starter questions

Answers to the following questions are on page 211.

1. Why is it important if a purpuric (i.e. non-blanching) rash is palpable?
2. Why might coughing up blood be a symptom of serious renal disease?
3. What connects hepatitis C infection, a skin rash, and renal disease?
4. Why might prescribing more drugs to control blood sugar and blood pressure in a diabetic patient save money in the long run?
5. Why is a recent visit to a petting zoo possibly relevant to a child presenting with acute kidney injury (AKI)?

Introduction

Secondary glomerular diseases arise when systemic disease involves the glomerular filter units. A number of renal pathological processes are responsible, including:

- direct attack by autoantibodies
- deposition of immune complexes or B-cell products
- abnormal glycosylation (in diabetes)

Secondary glomerular diseases contribute substantially to the burden of chronic kidney disease and end-stage renal failure. Diabetic nephropathy alone accounts for 25% of patients starting on renal replacement programmes in Western Europe.

Despite their diversity of pathologies, secondary glomerular diseases present with the same limited number of clinical patterns as those seen in primary glomerular diseases (see Table 5.1). However, they are by definition part of a wider disease process.

The distinction between primary and secondary disease is somewhat arbitrary. For example, anti–glomerular basement membrane (GBM) disease and vasculitis are often confined to the kidney, with no extrarenal manifestations. However, they are classified as secondary disease because of their potential for wider involvement, which must be remembered when evaluating and managing affected patients.

Generally, management of secondary glomerular diseases focuses on management of the systemic disease. Specific renal management for acute kidney injury, nephrotic syndrome, chronic kidney disease and end-stage renal failure may also be required.

Case 5 Rash, fatigue and weight loss

Presentation

Marjorie Hickson, aged 75 years, presents to her general practitioner, Dr Henderson, with a 2-week history of a rash over her lower legs. Examination confirms a palpable purpuric rash affecting both her legs and hands. Examination of Mrs Hickson's hands reveals a few splinter haemorrhages in her nails (**Figure 6.1**).

Initial interpretation

A palpable purpuric rash is a purple rash that does not blanch on pressure and is raised, allowing it to be felt above the surrounding skin. It is a useful sign, because it indicates small vessel vasculitis (inflammation of blood vessels) involving the skin. This diagnosis is supported by the presence of splinter haemorrhages. These narrow linear bleeds under the nail beds are commonly caused by minor trauma but are also signs of small vessel vasculitis.

Cutaneous vasculitis, with lesions mostly confined to the skin, usually represents milder and relatively benign vasculitic disease. However, its presence should prompt a search for evidence of systemic illness, for example fatigue, anorexia and weight loss, and involvement of other organ systems, such as the joints and kidneys.

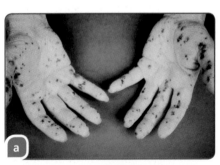

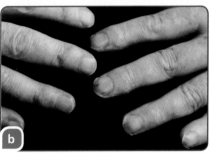

Figure 6.1 Cutaneous manifestations of vasculitis. (a) A palmar purpuric rash. (b) Splinter haemorrhages.

Further history

Further questioning reveals that Ms Hickson has been unwell for the past 2–3 months. She has been feeling tired, with progressive malaise and decreased appetite; she has lost 5–6 kg in weight. She can still do her housework and get out to the local shops, but it is now a real effort.

She initially thought that this was flu and that she would get over it. However, she is now concerned that 'it has dragged on', and that she is losing weight. She has also noted some aches and pains in her wrists and knees joints over the same time.

There is no other significant history. She is on no medication.

Examination

Further examination finds tenderness of the wrist and knee joints. Dipstick urinalysis gives the results of protein ++ and blood +++.

Interpretation of findings

Dr Henderson is concerned by the history and examination findings so far. It is common for patients to present with tiredness, but the weight loss is particularly worrying; a common broad differential diagnosis in a case like this is malignancy, chronic infection or an autoimmune process. The skin signs suggest vasculitis, an autoimmune disease. The general upset, arthralgias and the proteinuria and haematuria which indicate glomerular involvement, all point to a systemic process as the cause of Ms Hickson's symptoms.

Urgent referral to secondary care is indicated. Given Ms Hickson's main presenting features, this could be to rheumatology, dermatology or nephrology. However, because the urinary findings, together with the systemic upset and skin changes, suggest renal involvement with vasculitis, Ms Hickson needs to see a nephrologist.

Palpable purpura (indicating vasculitis), together with systemic abnormalities with or without abnormalities in the urine must be acted upon quickly. Systemic vasculitis can cause rapid damage to critical organs such as the kidney, heart and nervous system; urgent referral to a relevant specialist, determined by which particular organ is affected, is required. Immediate admission to hospital is often indicated to aid rapid diagnosis and treatment.

Investigations

Ms Hickson is seen the following week at the local renal unit as an outpatient. Dr Henderson has helpfully included in his referral letter the fact that Ms Hickson had an incidental blood test 4 months previously, which showed a normal serum creatinine concentration. The consultant goes over the history, carries out an examination, confirms the dipstick urinalysis findings of haematuria and proteinuria, and orders a number of investigations, the results of which are shown in **Table 6.1**.

In unexpected renal impairment, you must try to establish the time course of the deterioration in renal function. This is best done by obtaining previous blood results, if available. If the impairment is long-standing (over years), it probably represents chronic kidney disease. A deterioration over weeks or months suggests a more acute process requiring urgent investigation.

The test results show:

- normochromic normocyctic anaemia, i.e. low haemoglobin but with red blood cells of normal size and haemoglobin content
- significant renal impairment, indicated by increased creatinine concentration
- the presence of antineutrophil cytoplasmic antibody (ANCA) with a perinuclear staining pattern (perinuclear antineutrophil cytoplasmic antibody, p-ANCA)

Further testing shows that the p-ANCA pattern results from the presence of anti-myeloperoxidase antibodies.

Case 5 *continued*

Marjorie Hickson's blood test results		
Test	Result	Normal range
Haemoglobin	103 g/L	120–160 g/L
Mean cell volume	90 fL	80–97 fL
Mean cell haemoglobin	33.5 pg	27–34 pg
Serum creatinine	382 µmol/L	60–110 µmol/L
ANCA	Positive, p-ANCA pattern	Negative
ANCA, antineutrophil cytoplasmic antibody; p-ANCA, perinuclear antineutrophil cytoplasmic antibody.		

Table 6.1 Blood test results for Marjorie Hickson

Interpretation of findings

Ms Hickson's creatinine concentration was normal only 4 months previously. This pattern of deterioration of renal function occurring over a few weeks or months, together with blood and protein in the urine, is typical of rapidly progressive glomerulonephritis (see Table 5.1). The normochromic normocytic anaemia is consistent with the anaemia of chronic disease rather than iron deficiency (a common cause, but associated with microcytic hypochromic red cells).

In patients presenting with a clinical picture consistent with systemic vasculitis, for example rapidly progressive glomerulonephritis, the presence of a positive perinuclear (p-ANCA) pattern and anti-myeloperoxidase antibodies is a very specific finding for the diagnosis of small vessel vasculitis. The other common combination is that of a positive cytoplasmic (c-ANCA) pattern and anti-proteinase 3 antibodies, which again is very specific for the diagnosis. Histological confirmation with renal biopsy is helpful, because this is a serious diagnosis requiring intensive treatment (see page 199).

Further investigations

The consultant reviews the blood test results the next day, and given the rapidity of the decline in Mrs Hickson's renal function, arranges for her admission to hospital for renal biopsy as soon as a bed becomes available on the renal ward. The biopsy report, which is available the next day, shows a focal necrotising glomerulonephritis with crescent formation, i.e. a proliferation of cells in Bowman's space (see **Figures 6.2** and **6.3**).

> Rapidly progressive glomerulonephritis with crescentic glomerulonephritis on biopsy is usually produced by ANCA-associated small vessel vasculitis. Occasionally, it is due to anti-GBM disease or another disease that causes necrosis in the glomerular tuft (**Table 6.2**). Rarely, the same presentation of rapid deterioration of renal function with blood and protein in the urine, is caused by an acute interstitial nephritis (see page 290)

Diagnosis

The consultant explains to Ms Hickson that the renal biopsy results confirm the diagnosis of small vessel vasculitis, and gives her information about this disease. She is relieved that a diagnosis has been made but worried by the serious nature of both the disease and the treatment required. She appreciates that she has little choice but to accept the recommended treatment, and is started on high-dose corticosteroids and cyclophosphamide.

Case 5 *continued*

Crescent formation

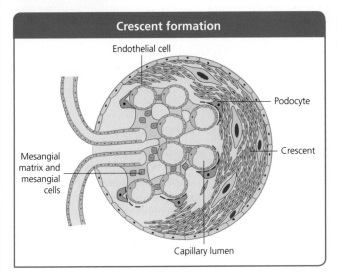

Endothelial cell

Podocyte

Crescent

Mesangial matrix and mesangial cells

Capillary lumen

Figure 6.2 Crescent formation in Bowman's space.

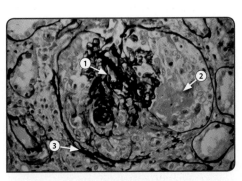

Figure 6.3 Silver stain (basement membrane stains black) of a single glomerular tuft (collapsed in this example) ① almost surrounded by a crescent (counterstained red) ②. ③, Bowman's capsule.

Crescentic nephritis: causes

Aspect	ANCA-related disease	Anti–glomerular basement membrane disease	Miscellaneous
Pathogenesis	ANCAs probably pathogenic	Autoantibodies to GBM	Immune complex disease (e.g. Henoch–Schönlein purpura, systemic lupus erythematosus), accelerated hypertension, other disorders
Immunohistochemistry	Usually negative ('pauci-immune')	Linear staining of GBM	Positive (usually mesangial) if caused by immune complex disease
Prognosis	Two thirds to three quarters recover useful renal function	Very poor for renal recovery if dependent on dialysis at presentation	Depends on underlying disease

ANCA, antineutrophil cytoplasmic antibody; GBM, glomerular basement membrane.

Table 6.2 Causes of crescentic nephritis

Vasculitis

Vasculitis is inflammation of blood vessels. It can be a primary process, with the initial pathology confined to blood vessels and other pathology caused by downstream ischaemia, or secondary to diseases such as connective tissue disorders (see page 200).

The primary vasculitides affecting the glomerulus are (**Table 6.3**):

- ANCA-associated small vessel vasculitides, the most common group of conditions that cause glomerular disease
- Henoch–Schönlein purpura, which is commoner in children but occasionally presents in adults
- Macroscopic polyarteritis nodosa, a rare disease of medium and large blood vessels with associated aneurysm formation

The latter two are far less common than ANCA-associated small vessel vasculitides, which are the subject of the rest of this section. As the name implies, these are characterised by the common features of ANCA positivity and small vessel involvement with necrosis and inflammation. The glomerulus is a modified small blood vessel, and hence subject to the same necrotising pathology; this does not occur in macroscopic polyarteritis, which is ANCA-negative and produces ischaemic glomerular changes as a result of upstream involvement of larger blood vessels.

Epidemiology

ANCA-associated vasculitis is rare; its annual incidence is 10–20 per million in the UK, for example. It predominantly affects older patients. Epidemiological studies show a weak link with exposure to silica, and some cases may be precipitated by infections or exposure to certain drugs (e.g. propylthiouracil). Most cases have no obvious causal factor.

Aetiology

The ANCAs are thought to have a direct role in the pathogenesis of this group of conditions, rather then being a mere epiphenomenon. They activate neutrophils in the vicinity of the endothelium, with resulting damage. There are some genetic associations, which are

Primary vasculitides associated with glomerular disease				
Disease	Clinical features	ANCA	Renal histopathology	Treatment
Small vessel vasculitides	Rapidly progressive glomerulonephritis; many other features possible, depending on organs involved	Positive	Glomerular necrosis, crescent formation	Immunosuppression
Henoch–Schönlein purpura	Purpuric rash, arthralgia, abdominal pain, and renal involvement (may be rapidly progressive glomerulonephritis pattern)	Negative	Similar to immunoglobulin A nephropathy (see page 188), usually with crescentic changes	Usually resolves spontaneously with supportive care; immunosuppression may be considered for progressive renal deterioration
Macroscopic polyarteritis nodosa	Systemic upset, myalgias, livedo reticularis (see Figure 9.4), variable renal involvement	Negative	Ischaemic changes: shrinking and wrinkling of the glomerular tuft	Immunosuppression

ANCA, antineutrophil cytoplasmic antibody.

Table 6.3 Clinical features, histopathology and treatment of primary vasculitides associated with glomerular disease

strongest with the type of ANCA as opposed to the particular clinical syndrome.

Clinical features

There are various patterns of presentation:

- granulomatosis with polyangiitis (previously called Wegener's granulomatosis)
- microscopic polyangiitis
- renal-limited vasculitis
- eosinophilic granulomatosis with polyangiitis (previously called Churg–Strauss syndrome)

Renal involvement usually takes the form of a rapidly progressive glomerulonephritis (Table 5.1), although fluctuating renal impairment is occasionally found. Extrarenal features may predominate initially, or occur concurrently with the renal involvement. Patients often have considerable systemic upset, with fatigue, malaise, anorexia and weight loss.

Granulomatosis with polyangiitis

This classically involves the upper and lower airways in addition to the kidney. It is usually associated with c-ANCA, representing antibodies to proteinase 3.

Microscopic polyangiitis

This can involve most organ systems, and commonly affects the kidney, lungs, nervous system and skin. It is usually associated with p-ANCA, representing antibodies to myeloperoxidase.

Renal-limited vasculitis

This represents essentially the same pathological process as the above conditions, but is limited to the kidneys; extra-renal manifestations may appear later in the course of the disease. It is usually associated with p-ANCA, representing antibodies to myeloperoxidase.

Eosinophilic granulomatosis with polyangiitis

This is characterised by vasculitis, eosinophilia and, usually, asthma or other allergic disease. ANCA positivity is not found as frequently as with the other patterns; when present, it is usually for p-ANCA representing antibodies to myeloperoxidase.

Diagnostic approach

The main challenge is for clinicians to consider the disease as a possible diagnosis, thereby enabling its recognition and early treatment. Vasculitis is not always suspected, because of the varied nature of its presentation: most organ systems may be involved, so the patient may present to many different specialties. Furthermore, the disease is occasionally confined to the kidney, in which case it may produce only non-specific systemic symptoms.

Investigations

If vasculitis is suspected, dipstick urinalysis is carried out to assess for haematuria and proteinuria. If either is present, urgent investigations are indicated, particularly estimation of glomerular filtration rate (eGFR) and testing of a blood sample for the presence of ANCA. Urine microscopy may provide additional information: dysmorphic red blood cells, and particularly red blood cell casts (proteinaceous casts of the lumen of renal tubules with red cells embedded in their matrix) indicate active glomerulonephritis with bleeding.

Biopsy

Although a positive ANCA result is highly specific for the diagnosis of small vessel vasculitis in the appropriate clinical setting, renal biopsy is usually carried out because of the serious nature of this diagnosis and the intensive treatment required.

Characteristically there is a focal necrotising glomerulonephritis with crescents (**Figure 6.2**). Staining for immune deposits is usually negative in ANCA-positive small vessel vasculitis, whereas it is positive in crescentic nephritis associated with systemic lupus erythematosus (SLE) or anti-GBM disease (see pages 200–202).

Management

Initial management is immunosuppression with corticosteroids and cyclophosphamide.

Rituximab, a monoclonal antibody targeting B cells, may be considered instead of cyclophosphamide in a woman whose fertility is at risk and in patients who do not respond to cyclophosphamide. The role of plasma exchange is unclear. Corticosteroids and azathioprine are used as maintenance therapy once the disease is in remission.

Prognosis

With treatment, most patients recover, even if they are dependent on dialysis at presentation. However, indefinite follow up is required: patients are usually left with a degree of renal impairment, and a third to a half experience a relapse of vasculitis, particularly if their disease is associated with antibodies to proteinase 3.

Systemic lupus erythematosus and other connective tissue diseases

Systemic lupus erythematosus

Systemic lupus erythematosus (SLE) is the connective tissue disease that most commonly involves the kidney. It is characterised by the production of autoantibodies to a range of self-antigens. The resulting autoantibody–antigen immune complexes deposit in many sites, including the skin, joints, nervous system, serosal surfaces and glomeruli. They therefore produce a wide range of clinical manifestations.

Because SLE is common, and renal involvement is present in the majority of cases (albeit often mildly), the disease contributes significantly to the burden of chronic kidney disease and end-stage renal failure.

Epidemiology

SLE predominantly affects woman (male:female ratio, 1:10). It is particularly common in African–Caribbean patients, with a prevalence of 1 in 250 for women in this group.

Aetiology

SLE is an autoimmune disease, i.e. a disease in which the immune system provokes and maintains a response against self-antigens. This breakdown in self-tolerance is the result of both genetic and environmental factors. For example, most connective tissue diseases, including SLE, have links to particular alleles of the major histocompatibility complex. Known environmental factors that cause SLE include exposure to sunlight and certain drugs (e.g. hydrallazine, a little used anti-hypertensive agent).

Pathogenesis

Renal SLE is caused by the deposition of immune complexes formed with various autoantigens, e.g. nuclear antigens. Depending on the properties of these complexes, a wide range of features are seen in the glomeruli, including:

- mild mesangial changes
- membranous changes
- focal necrosis with crescent formation
- ultimately, scarring with glomerular or tubular atrophy and fibrosis

Clinical features

At diagnosis, up to two thirds of patients have evidence of renal involvement, i.e. proteinuria, red blood cells or red blood cell casts in the urine, or impaired renal function. More severe forms of renal involvement are rarer but when present make a significant contribution to the morbidity and mortality of the disease.

The renal presentation of SLE reflects the diversity of the underlying renal involvement, and may include any of the patterns listed in **Table 5.1**; these may occur in combination, at the same time or at different times, in an individual patient. There is usually, but not always, evidence of the involvement of other organ systems, particularly the skin and joints.

Antiphospholipid antibodies are a particular class of autoantibody that may be found in SLE (30–40% of cases) or occur in isolation. Clinically, they are associated with recurrent miscarriage, thrombocytopenia, thrombosis and a microangiopathy that may involve the kidney (see page 209).

Diagnostic approach

Connective tissue diseases such as SLE are usually diagnosed based on their characteristic clinical pattern, together with the presence of relevant autoantibodies. SLE should be suspected in a young woman presenting with a malar rash, typical of SLE (**Figure 2.12**), or joint pains. There is occasionally an isolated renal presentation with, for example, nephrotic syndrome, and the diagnosis is made only when specific autoantibodies are detected or the results of renal biopsy show typical features: deposition of different immunoglobulin classes together with complement, or thickening of the capillary loops by immune complexes producing a 'wire loop' appearance.

Investigations

Proteinuria and GFR are quantified. The following are also measured:

- SLE-associated autoantibodies, for example anti-double-stranded DNA, anti-nuclear antibody and anti-phospholipid antibody
- complement, because decreased complement reflects consumption by immune complexes and therefore indicates active SLE

Renal biopsy is indicated if significant immunosuppressive treatment is being considered: the potential toxicity of such treatment means that the diagnosis, and the presence of salvageable renal tissue, must be confirmed.

> **Measurement of C-reactive protein is useful when investigating a febrile episode in a patient with lupus.** A lupus flare is usually not accompanied by a significant increase in concentration of C-reactive protein, whereas fever with an infective cause is.

Management

Non-steroidal anti-inflammatory drugs, hydroxychloroquine and corticosteroids are used for the general management of SLE, but are not effective for renal disease (although hydroxychloroquine has some role in reducing the chance of subsequent renal flares). The more severe forms of renal involvement are treated with corticosteroids and mycophenolate mofetil; cyclophosphamide may be considered in unresponsive cases.

> **There are many dedicated patient support groups for systemic diseases such as SLE and vasculitis.** Because systemic diseases are often chronic and progressively debilitating, patients benefit from help and information provided by these networks.

Prognosis

With modern treatment regimens, the prognosis for renal SLE has improved, but the disease may still result in end-stage renal failure. Recurrence in a renal transplant is rare.

Other connective tissue diseases

Renal involvement occurs less frequently in other connective tissue diseases. Rheumatoid arthritis, an autoimmune disease that predominantly affects synovial joints, involves the kidney via:

- amyloid deposition in glomeruli, secondary to chronic inflammation (see page 204)

- drug toxicity, particularly from the use of non-steroidal anti-inflammatory drugs
- a vasculitic flare; rarely, severe disease may extend beyond the joints, with vasculitis affecting various organs including the kidney

Systemic sclerosis, a connective tissue disease of uncertain aetiology that produces fibrotic changes affecting the skin and viscera, may be complicated by severe hypertension and rapid deterioration in renal function – a 'renal crisis'. Renal biopsy shows changes in the renal arterioles that are similar to those occurring in accelerated hypertension ('onion skinning'; see page 279).

Anti-glomerular basement membrane disease

Anti–glomerular basement membrane disease, also known as Goodpasture's disease, is caused by production of an autoantibody that reacts with the basement membrane present in the glomeruli and alveoli. Although rare, with 1 or 2 cases per million per year, it is the most severe form of glomerular inflammation, with the potential to destroy kidney function in a short period of time, i.e. days or weeks.

Goodpasture's syndrome is the combination of pulmonary haemorrhage and glomerulonephritis, a presentation more commonly seen with the small vessel vasculitides (see page 198). Goodpasture's disease refers to the rarer cases when this presentation is due to anti-glomerular basement membrane antibodies.

Aetiology

The disease is caused by circulating autoantibodies directed against the non-collagenous domain of the $\alpha 3$ chain of type IV collagen in the glomerular basement membrane (GBM).

Pathogenesis

The fenestrations in the glomerular endothelium allow the anti-GBM autoantibodies direct access to the GBM. Once bound they fix complement, attract neutrophils and set up a severe necrotising glomerulonephritis with crescent formation. The same target antigen is present in the alveolar basement membrane, but some insult (e.g. damage caused by smoking) is usually required for the autoantibody to gain access to it. Once this occurs, the same pathological process results in inflammation and bleeding into the alveoli (pulmonary haemorrhage).

Trigger

It is unclear what triggers the production of anti-GBM autoantibodies. Exposure to solvents has been implicated, but the evidence for this is weak. A genetic element is indicated by an association with a major histocompatibility allele (HLA DRB1*1501), but the vast majority of people with this allele (present in up to one third of the Caucasian population) never get the disease.

A rare situation can occur after renal transplantation in a patient with Alport's syndrome (see page 301). The disorganisation of the GBM in this condition means that some of the antigens of the GBM of the donor kidney are treated as novel by the patient's immune system, generating a response that includes formation of anti-GBM antibodies. This can occasionally cause rejection of the graft.

Clinical features

The renal presentation is with rapidly progressive glomerulonephritis (see page 179). There may also be lung haemorrhage, especially in the presence of other causes of lung injury, but this is rare in non-smokers. Smokers tend to present earlier in the natural history, because haemoptysis prompts them to seek medical attention. Some patients have the clinical features of a small vessel vasculitis (see page 198) and are positive for both ANCA and anti-GBM antibodies (so-called 'double positive' patients).

> **Absence of haemoptysis does not exclude pulmonary haemorrhage.** Substantial amounts of blood can be lost into the lungs without causing overt symptoms. This is also true for other causes of Goodpasture's syndrome, such as vasculitis.

Diagnostic approach

Anti-GBM disease is a rare disease. However, it must be considered in the appropriate clinical setting (i.e. a rapidly progressive glomerulonephritis with or without pulmonary haemorrhage), because early diagnosis is essential to avoid the development of irreversible renal damage. Relevant investigations are carried out urgently in any patient with this clinical picture.

Investigations

The key investigations are the measurement of circulating anti-GBM antibodies and renal biopsy.

Blood tests

In most patients, anti-GBM antibodies are found in the blood. Occasionally, the test is negative despite typical biopsy appearances for the disease.

Measurement of ANCA is also carried out, because the clinical presentation of small vessel vasculitis overlaps with that of anti-GBM disease, and a minority of patients may have features of both diseases.

Imaging

Pulmonary haemorrhage may produce transient consolidation (air space shadowing) on a radiograph of the chest.

Pulmonary function tests

Pulmonary haemorrhage increases the transfer factor for carbon monoxide, because there is more free haemoglobin in the lung and therefore greater uptake of carbon monoxide.

Biopsy

A necrotising crescentic glomerulonephritis is found on renal biopsy. Anti-GBM disease is distinguished from other causes of this finding by the immunohistological detection of antibody deposited linearly along the GBM (**Figure 6.4**; see also **Table 6.2**).

Management

Anti–glomerular basement membrane disease is treated with immunosuppression (using corticosteroids and cyclophosphamide), combined with plasma exchange to remove circulating anti-GBM antibodies. Plasma exchange is continued until the autoantibody is undetectable.

If the patient presents with dialysis-dependent renal impairment, the prognosis for renal recovery is poor. Under these circumstances, immunosuppression and plasma exchange may be reserved for those patients who have pulmonary haemorrhage, which can be life-threatening.

Double-positive patients, i.e. patients with both anti-GBM antibodies and ANCAs, are also treated with immunosuppression and plasma exchange, irrespective of dialysis

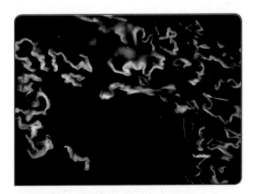

Figure 6.4 Immunofluorescence study of a renal biopsy specimen from a patient with anti-glomerular basement membrane disease. The immunofluorescence represents linear deposition of antibody along the glomerular basement membrane.

dependence. This is because of uncertainty as to the extent to which ANCA-positive disease, with its better prognosis, contributes to pathology.

Prognosis

The earlier the patient presents, the better the prognosis; if the patient is dependent on dialysis at presentation, the chance of recovery of renal function with treatment is <10%.

Once the autoantibody is removed, or if it disappears spontaneously without treatment, recurrence is rare. Transplantation is possible, but clearance of the autoantibody must be ensured first to avoid recurrent disease in the transplanted kidney.

B-cell diseases

Several glomerular diseases are caused by renal deposition of whole or parts of immunoglobulins produced by B cells and plasma cells. If these proteins are monoclonal they are collectively known as paraproteins.

In most of these conditions, the abnormal proteins deposit primarily in the glomeruli and produce one of the usual clinical patterns of glomerular disease (see Table 5.1). Myeloma is an exception because it usually affects the tubulointerstitial compartment; it is included in this chapter because glomerular involvement is also possible.

For this group of conditions, treatment and prognosis are usually determined by the underlying disease rather than the renal involvement itself.

Myeloma

Myeloma is a malignant proliferation of plasma cells. In up to 50% of patients there is renal involvement at some point during the course of the disease. Most commonly it is in the form of myeloma kidney, in which immunoglobulin light chains from the circulating paraprotein precipitate in the tubules, causing characteristic casts (**Figures 6.5**) and an associated inflammatory response. There is little detectable proteinuria, because dipstick urinalysis is not sensitive to light chains in the urine (Bence Jones proteins).

More rarely, light chains deposit in the glomerulus, in which case there is usually significant albuminuria. There are distinct patterns, including fibrillary glomerulonephritis, light chain deposition disease and, most commonly, amyloidosis (see below).

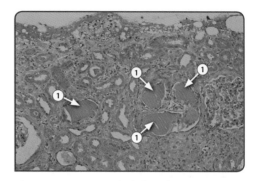

Figure 6.5 H&E stain of a kidney showing the characteristic glassy fractured casts ① within the tubular lumen of a patient with myeloma.

> **In older patients (age > 60 years) presenting with renal impairment and no detectable proteinuria, the commonest cause is probably renovascular disease (see page 281).** However, myeloma is a less common, but serious differential diagnosis.

Treatment of myeloma kidney is by treatment of the underlying malignancy, together with management of any associated hypercalcaemia (see page 240). It is unclear whether plasma exchange to remove the circulating paraprotein is helpful.

Amyloidosis

In renal amyloidosis there is renal deposition of an amyloid protein, usually in the glomerulus. This disrupts the glomerular filter and causes renal impairment and proteinuria, which may be in the nephrotic range. Other organs (e.g. heart, liver, nerves) may also be involved.

> Amyloid is an aggregate of misfolded proteins that have polymerized in stacks of beta-pleated sheets to form fibrils that are relatively resistant to proteolytic degradation. They deposit in tissues with a distinctive appearance on staining (**Figure 6.6**).

There are two main forms of amyloidosis, light chain (AL) amyloidosis and amyloid A (AA) amyloidosis, but many rarer forms are also recognised. Treatment is directed at the underlying condition.

Light chain amyloidosis

This form of amyloidosis is produced by deposition of monoclonal immunoglobulin light chains, i.e. paraproteins. In 10–15% of

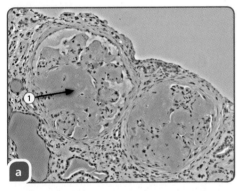

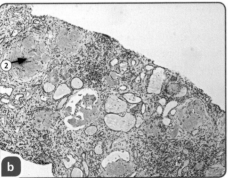

Figure 6.6 Renal biopsy of a patient with amyloidosis. (a) ① Deposits of amyloid in the glomeruli (H&E stain). (b) ② The deposits stain pink with Congo red. Courtesy of Dr Stephen Sampson.

affected patients this is in the setting of overt myeloma, but in most patients the underlying plasma cell clone occurs at low frequency in the bone marrow, or is undetectable.

Amyloid A amyloidosis

This is caused by deposition of the serum amyloid A protein, which is an acute phase reactant. Therefore AA amyloidosis is a complication of chronic inflammatory conditions in which the concentration of this protein is increased for a prolonged time, usually years. Examples include chronic infections, connective tissue disease and hereditary fever syndromes such as familial Mediterranean fever.

Cryoglobulinaemia

Certain immunoglobulins precipitate in the cold (forming a cryoprecipitate), so are known as cryoglobulins. This property is linked to their tendency to deposit in tissues, including the glomerulus, and set up an inflammatory response.

Three types of cryoglobulin (known as cryoglobulinaemia when in the circulation) are recognised (**Table 6.4**).

- Type 1 cryoglobulinaemia has a monoclonal component only; it may complicate myeloma or other clonal B-cell disorders
- Type 2 (also known as mixed) cryoglobulinaemia has a monoclonal component, usually IgM, which has rheumatoid factor activity, i.e. it binds to IgG; the resulting cryoprecipitate therefore has both monoclonal (IgM) and polyclonal (IgG) components
- Type 3 cryoglobulinaemia has a polyclonal component only; it may be seen in chronic inflammatory conditions

Type 2 cryoglobulinaemia

This is the most common cryoglobulinaemia. There is an associated underlying hepatitis C infection in many patients. Presentation is variable; there may be a purpuric rash, arthralgia or hepatic and renal involvement. Renal involvement takes the form of nephritic

Cryoglobulinaemias			
Aspect	Type 1 cryoglobulinaemia	Type 2 cryoglobulinaemia (mixed)	Type 3 cryoglobulinaemia
Components	Monoclonal immunoglobulin only (can be any class)	Monoclonal (usually IgM) and polyclonal IgG	Polyclonal IgG
Underlying conditions	Myeloma, other clonal B-cell disorders	Hepatitis C, idiopathic	Chronic inflammatory conditions (e.g. Sjögren's syndrome)
Rheumatoid factor	Absent	Present (monoclonal)	Present (polyclonal)
Complement consumption	No	Yes	Yes
Renal involvement	Rare	Common	Rare
Ig, immunoglobulin.			

Table 6.4 Comparison of cryoglobulinaemias

syndrome, nephrotic syndrome or rapidly progressive glomerulonephritis.

The diagnostic approach depends upon demonstration of the cryoglobulin and its consequences for complement activation in the clinical settings outlined in the previous paragraph. Demonstration and analysis of the cryoglobulin requires that a blood sample is kept warm in a thermos flask (to avoid premature precipitation of the protein) whilst sent to the laboratory. Other investigations show high concentrations of rheumatoid factor and marked consumption of complement via the classical pathway (activation via immune complexes). A biopsy of skin and/or kidney is required if there is doubt about the diagnosis and will show:

- leucocytoclastic vasculitis in the skin, i.e. vasculitis characterised by the presence of neutrophils and debris from disintegrating neutrophil nuclei

- a type 1 mesangiocapillary glomerulonephritis (see page 191) in the kidney, often with deposits of cryoglobulin in the capillary loops

> **Type 2 cryoglobulinaemia is strongly indicated by a pattern of complement consumption** that indicates activation via the classical pathway, i.e. a low or even unmeasurable concentration of C4, with a lesser reduction in concentration of C3.

Underlying hepatitis C infection is treated. The acute manifestations of the cryoglobulinaemia itself may be managed with high-dose corticosteroids, other forms of immunosuppression and plasma exchange. If the underlying condition can be treated, the outlook is good, with most patients making a full recovery (although there may be residual chronic renal damage).

Diabetic nephropathy

Diabetic nephropathy is a microvascular complication of type 1 and type 2 diabetes mellitus. In diabetes, chronic hyperglycaemia damages endothelial cells to cause:

- Macrovascular damage, resulting in stroke, ischaemic heart disease and peripheral vascular disease

- Microvascular damage, leading to nephropathy (glomerular damage), retinopathy (damage to retinal vessels) and neuropathy (nerve damage)

The damage accumulates gradually over many years and is exacerbated by poor control of hyperglycaemia. The systemic nature of diabetes means that it is unusual to find significant isolated diabetic nephropathy in the absence of other microvascular complications, for example diabetic retinopathy. Furthermore, it often coexists with macrovascular complications involving the kidney, such as renal artery stenosis (see page 281).

Epidemiology

Nephropathy eventually affects up to a third of both type 1 and 2 diabetic patients. Up to one quarter of patients on renal replacement programmes in Western Europe have diabetic nephropathy, reflecting the high prevalence of type 2 diabetes.

There is some evidence that better glycaemic and blood pressure control is reducing the incidence of diabetic nephropathy in both types of diabetes.

Aetiology and pathogenesis

In diabetic nephropathy, three major changes occur:

- thickening of the capillary basement membrane
- excessive production of extracellular matrix
- scarring of the glomeruli (glomerulosclerosis)

Sometimes there is sclerotic expansion of glomerular matrix in a nodular pattern, the Kimmelstiel-Wilson lesion (**Figures 6.7** and **6.8**).

These three changes permit small amounts of protein to cross the filtration membrane, i.e. they result in microalbuminuria. This is albumin excretion at 30–300 mg/24 h, which is too low to be revealed by dipstick testing (see below). Over time, it progresses to overt proteinuria. A decline in renal excretory function occurs later in the disease.

The changes above represent involvement of the glomeruli. With increasing glomerulosclerosis there is a corresponding increase

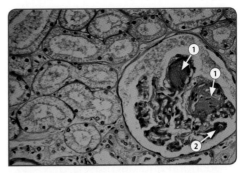

Figure 6.8 H&E section showing single glomerulus with two nodular sclerosing (Kimmelstiel-Wilson) lesions ① with diffuse mesangial expansion ②.

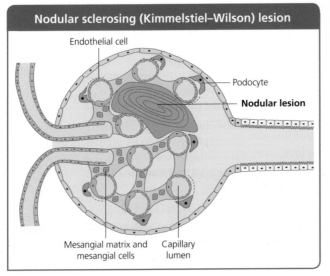

Figure 6.7 Nodular sclerosing (Kimmelstiel–Wilson) lesion of diabetic nephropathy

Nodular sclerosing (Kimmelstiel–Wilson) lesion

Endothelial cell

Podocyte

Nodular lesion

Mesangial matrix and mesangial cells

Capillary lumen

in tubulointerstitial fibrosis and atrophy. Tubular involvement in diabetes also manifests as hyporeninaemic hypoaldosteronism (also known as type 4 renal tubular acidosis; see page 289) which presents as hyperkalaemia.

In type 1 diabetes, the median time to development of nephropathy is 15 years. The length of time required for type 2 diabetes to produce significant nephropathy is unclear, because of its ill-defined time of onset. Rarely, patients with type 2 diabetes may have overt nephropathy at diagnosis.

Progressive diabetic nephropathy both causes and exacerbates hypertension.

Microalbuminuria

Albumin excretion in the urine is quantified by measurement of an albumin:creatinine ratio (ACR) or protein:creatinine ratio. Microalbuminuria is defined by an ACR > 2.5 mg/mmol in men and >3.5 mg/mmol in women. This is below the threshold detectable with dipstick urinalysis, which is why all patients with diabetes require annual determination of urinary ACR.

Proteinuria and decreased GFR

Proteinuria is defined as an ACR > 30 mg/mmol or a protein-positive dipstick result. As the disease progresses, proteinuria increases and may reach the range associated with the nephrotic syndrome. Simultaneously, GFR decreases (after having been increased initially in a phase of hyperfiltration that is not clinically relevant); ultimately, this results in end-stage renal failure.

Clinical features

Early diabetic nephropathy is asymptomatic. As it progresses, renal function deteriorates and chronic kidney disease develops (see Chapter 4). Associated hypertension is common. Ultimately renal deterioration reaches an irreversible phase, when it manifests with the clinical features of end-stage renal failure (see Chapter 4).

Infections

Hyperglycaemia and glycosuria favour the growth of microorganisms. In the urinary tract, in addition to lower tract infections, this susceptibility can manifest as pyelonephritis, papillary necrosis or rare complications such as emphysematous pyelonephritis (upper urinary tract infection with gas-forming organisms) and xanthogranulomatous pyelonephritis (a destructive chronic inflammatory process) (see page 293).

Diagnostic approach

A clinical diagnosis is usually made without histological confirmation in patients who have had diabetes for many years (even only a few years in type 2 diabetes), and who develop an increase in urinary albumin in the setting of microvascular complications elsewhere, usually retinopathy. Atypical features prompt renal biopsy, because another coincidental renal pathology is always possible (see below).

Investigations

Regular quantification of proteinuria, usually accomplished by determination of albumin:creatinine ratio, is an essential part of routine diabetic monitoring. Diabetic control and diabetic complications in other organs are monitored as usual.

Biopsy

Renal biopsy is usually carried out only if there are atypical features, such as:

- a very short natural history (months rather than years)
- absence of other microvascular complications
- the presence of haematuria.

Another pathology may be found, but diabetic nephropathy itself manifests as a diffuse or nodular (see **Figure 6.7**) accumulation of material in the mesangium.

Management

Good control of both blood glucose and blood pressure is essential in all patients with diabetes but especially those with an ACR that is indicative of microvascular complications. Guidelines suggest a target of < 130/80 mmHg in type 2 diabetes with kidney, eye or cerebrovascular damage. In type I diabetes the target is < 135/85 mmHg unless there is albuminuria or features of the metabolic syndrome, in which case it is < 130/80 mmHg. Treatment for hypertension includes use of an angiotensin-converting enzyme inhibitor or an angiotensin II receptor blocker; a combination of drugs from these two classes may provide additional benefit but at the risk of an increase in complications such as acute kidney injury and hyperkalaemia.

> **Engaging the patient in self-management is paramount to improving outcome in diabetes.** This can be fostered by:
>
> - clear and positive communication
> - addressing the patient's concerns
> - referring the patient to support groups
> - promoting self-monitoring and recording of blood glucose levels and blood pressure

When diabetic nephropathy progresses to end-stage renal failure, management is as for any other patient group (see pages 114–122 and 168–173). Provided severe macrovascular disease, in particular coronary artery disease, is ruled out options include renal transplantation, or in the younger patient with type 1 diabetes, kidney–pancreas transplantation.

Prognosis

The high incidence of vascular complications means that patients with diabetes often do poorly on renal replacement therapy. In addition to the usual complications of macrovascular disease (e.g. stroke, ischaemic heart disease and peripheral vascular disease), the poor state of their blood vessels means that there are often difficulties in obtaining satisfactory access for haemodialysis.

Thrombotic microangiopathies

The thrombotic microangiopathies are a rare group of conditions that have in common injury to the microcirculation. They are characterised by endothelial damage and deposition of thrombi in capillaries, including those making up the glomeruli. The resulting strands of fibrin cause shear injury to the red blood cells, with the production of schistocytes – fragmented red blood cells (**Figure 6.9**), and a microangiopathic haemolytic anaemia – a significant fall in haemoglobin concentration due to the fragmentation and destruction of red blood cells.

Aetiology

There are three groups of conditions: haemolytic–uraemic syndrome, thrombotic thrombocytopenic purpura and a miscellaneous group of conditions that may cause a thrombotic microangiopathy.

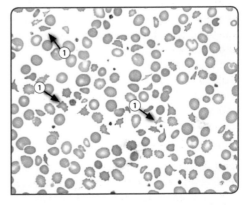

Figure 6.9 Peripheral blood film showing multiple examples of schistocytes ①. Courtesy of Dr Elizabeth Rhodes.

Haemolytic–uraemic syndrome

This represents the co-occurrence of acute kidney injury and microangiopathic haemolytic anaemia. The cause may be congenital or acquired.

- Congenital haemolytic–uraemic syndrome is usually the result of a deficiency of control proteins of the alternative pathway of complement activation; this is also known as atypical haemolytic–uraemic syndrome
- Acquired haemolytic–uraemic syndrome is usually caused by verotoxin-producing strains of *Escherichia coli*, although other bacteria (e.g. *Shigella*) and some viruses can be responsible

The acquired type may be seen in epidemic form after exposure to a common source, for example bean sprouts or meat contaminated with *E. coli*.

Thrombotic thrombocytopenic purpura

In this condition, there is microangiopathic haemolytic anaemia in association with more widespread pathology, which can include acute kidney injury, central nervous system involvement and pyrexia. Some cases are congenital; they are the result of a deficiency of ADAMTS13, an enzyme that cleaves large-molecular-weight forms of von Willebrand's factor. The acquired form is caused by development of autoantibodies to this enzyme, for unknown reasons.

Miscellaneous microangiopathies

A number of different processes leading to endothelial injury cause microangiopathic haemolytic anaemia and varying degrees of organ involvement. These include:

- accelerated hypertension
- drugs, notably calcineurin inhibitors such as ciclosporin and tacrolimus
- malignancy
- pregnancy
- infection

- autoimmune conditions such as the antiphospholipid antibody syndrome.

Clinical features and investigations

Renal involvement takes the form of acute kidney injury or a nephritic picture. Nervous system involvement usually manifests as fluctuating encephalopathy.

The congenital forms of haemolytic–uraemic syndrome and thrombotic thrombocytopenic purpura are usually recurrent.

Serial estimations of platelet count and lactate dehydrogenase are useful in monitoring the activity of the haemolytic process. Specialised assays exist for the various deficiencies in the congenital forms. Renal biopsy is not usually required.

Management

In haemolytic–uraemic syndrome associated with verotoxin-producing micro-organisms the use of antibiotics is avoided because they cause further release of the toxin. Abnormal activation of the alternative pathway of complement in atypical haemolytic–uraemic syndrome can be controlled with eculizumab, a monoclonal antibody to the complement component C5; however, this drug is extremely expensive. It is unclear whether eculizumab is helpful in verotoxin-associated haemolytic–uraemic syndrome.

Plasma exchange with an appropriate replacement fluid is indicated in thrombotic thrombocytopenic purpura. It both removes any causative autoantibody and replaces ADAMTS13.

Management of thrombotic microangiopathies is otherwise supportive, with treatment of any predisposing condition if possible. The outlook for the recurrent forms is often poor; for example, atypical haemolytic–uraemic syndrome usually recurs in a transplanted kidney (this is an indication for eculizumab).

Answers to starter questions

1. A palpable purpuric rash indicates an underlying vasculitis, whereas a non-palpable one does not. Vasculitis may be relatively benign and confined to the skin, but may also be the presentation of potentially serious systemic disease, such as Henoch–Schönlein purpura, ANCA-associated vasculitis, or cryoglobulinaemia, which are common causes of secondary glomerular disease in this setting.

2. Coughing up blood (i.e. haemoptysis) can be a symptom of a number of serious diseases such as lung cancer or pulmonary embolus. However, if there is also progressive renal dysfunction and blood and protein in the urine (i.e. a rapidly progressive glomerulonephritis), this suggests a disease such as a small vessel vasculitis or anti-glomerular basement membrane disease. If these conditions are not diagnosed and treated promptly they may cause irreversible loss of kidney function.

3. Hepatitis C infection commonly causes a type 2 cryoglobulinaemia, which is due to a monoclonal IgM rheumatoid factor with specificity for polyclonal IgG. This produces large amounts of circulating immune complexes. Its key manifestations are cutaneous vasculitis, which presents with a palpable purpuric rash, and a mesangiocapillary glomerulonephritis, a particular pattern of glomerular disease associated with blood and protein in the urine, and various degrees of renal failure

4. Diabetes is the single most common cause of end-stage renal failure in Western Europe, and is responsible for about a quarter of all cases. Treatment of end-stage renal failure with dialysis is very expensive, costing £25,000–£30,000 per patient per year. The best way to reduce the incidence of renal failure in diabetic patients is by good control of blood pressure and blood sugar.

5. Verotoxin-producing strains of *Escherichia coli* are a known cause of haemolytic–uraemic syndrome, a microangiopathy which damages the microcirculation, including the glomerulus, thus causing acute kidney injury. Cases have been documented where children were infected after contact with cows.

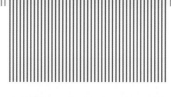

Chapter 7
Electrolyte disorders

Starter questions

Answers to the following questions are on pages 248–249.

1. How are urine and serum osmolality used to determine the cause of hyponatraemia?
2. Why do potassium levels need to be kept within such a narrow range?
3. What is the difference between 'dehydration' and 'volume depletion'?
4. What is the role of calcium gluconate in the treatment of hyperkalaemia?

Introduction

Electrolytes are salts that conduct an electrical current when separated into positively and negatively charged ions in solution. The major physiologically significant ions in body fluids, including blood, are:

- sodium (Na^+)
- potassium (K^+)
- calcium (Ca^{2+})
- phosphate (PO_4^{3-})
- magnesium (Mg^{2+})
- bicarbonate (HCO_3^-)

These play vital roles in many physiological processes, including muscle and neurological functions, fluid balance and acid–base balance (**Table 7.1**).

For tissues to function normally, the ratio of concentrations in the intracellular and extracellular compartments must be maintained for each electrolyte, i.e. the concentration gradient across the cell membrane must be kept unchanged. Therefore maintenance of plasma electrolyte concentrations is an essential aspect of homeostasis. It is achieved by several mechanisms regulated by the kidneys and hormones such as aldosterone and parathyroid hormone (PTH) (see page 31).

Physiological ions: concentrations and functions

Ion	Intracellular concentration (mmol/L)	Extracellular concentration (mmol/L)	Principal functions (not exhaustive)
Sodium: Na^+	10	140	Cell membrane potential, maintenance of blood volume
Potassium: K^+	140	4	Cell membrane potential
Calcium: Ca^{2+}	0.0001	2.5	Cell membrane potential, enzyme co-factor, signal transduction
Phosphate: PO_4^{3-}	50	1	Energy metabolism (ATP), buffering, nucleic acid synthesis
Magnesium: Mg^{2+}	5–20	1	Enzyme cofactor, cell membrane potential
Bicarbonate: HCO_3^-	10	24	Buffering
Chloride: Cl^-	4	100	Fluid balance, acid/base balance, cell membrane potential

Table 7.1 The most common physiological ions and their normal total concentrations and functions

Serum osmolality is an estimate of the number of osmotically active particles in the serum, and is measured in mOsm/kg. Electrolytes exert osmotic pressure, so they influence the movement of water. The body keeps extracellular osmolality within a narrow range, 275–295 mOsm/kg, because concentrations outside this range significantly alter the movement of water into or out of cells via osmosis.

Electrolyte disorders are imbalances in the plasma concentrations of ionised salts of, for example, sodium, potassium and calcium. Causes include:

- loss of body fluids (e.g. as a result of vomiting, diarrhoea or prolonged sweating)
- use of certain medications (e.g. diuretics that alter renal handling of electrolytes)
- renal impairment
- endocrine abnormalities

Treatment of electrolyte disorders depends on the cause. It may include removal of the precipitating factor, such as a particular drug; replacement of deficient electrolytes with oral or intravenous supplementation; and restoration of normal fluid balance.

Osmolality is proportional to the number of **particles per kilogram of plasma,** expressed as mOsm/kg.

Osmolarity is proportional to the number of **particles per litre of plasma.** It is affected by changes in water content, temperature and pressure.

Calculated osmolarity = 2[Na^+] + 2[K^+] + [glucose] + [urea]

Case 6 Cough, fever and shortness of breath

Presentation

Ajay Patel, aged 74 years, presents to the emergency department with a 3-day history of fever, cough and shortness of breath. His past medical history includes hypertension, for which he takes ramipril, and diet-controlled diabetes. In triage, he is found to have the following:

- respiratory rate 30 breaths/min
- oxygen saturation 88% on air
- blood pressure 130/80 mmHg
- heart rate 103 beats/min
- temperature 38.7°C

He is immediately transferred to the resuscitation area and seen by the registrar.

Case 6 *continued*

Initial interpretation

The high respiratory rate, low oxygen saturation, high heart rate and high temperature identify acute illness, with signs of the systemic inflammatory response syndrome. Therefore Mr Patel is moved to a high-dependency setting for close monitoring.

> A diagnosis of **systemic inflammatory response syndrome** is made when ≥2 of the following are present:
>
> - temperature > 38°C or < 36°C
> - respiratory rate > 20 breaths/min or $P_a\text{CO}_2$ < 4.3 kPa
> - heart rate > 90 beats/min
> - total white cell count < 4 × 10^9/L or > 12 × 10^9/L

History

Mr Patel reports feeling generally unwell for the last week. His cough and shortness of breath came on gradually, and he has had rigors (episodes of shaking or shivering associated with increased temperature) intermittently for 24 h. He has been bringing up green sputum, and his wife says he has been intermittently confused. He has been managing to drink well but has lost his appetite over the past 3 days. He denies vomiting and diarrhoea. Mr Patel's wife tried to persuade him to visit the general practitioner 2 days ago, but he refused to go because he 'doesn't like doctors'.

Interpretation of history

The short history suggests an acute process is present. A cough producing

Pneumonia and hyponatraemia

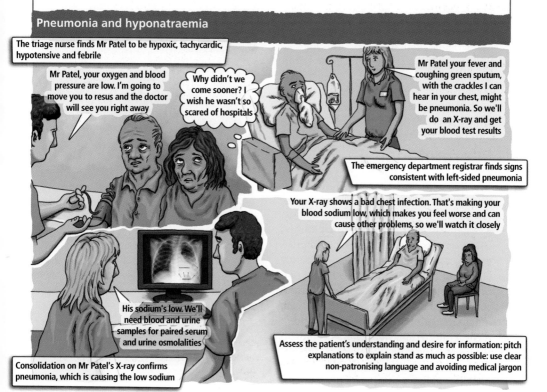

The triage nurse finds Mr Patel to be hypoxic, tachycardic, hypotensive and febrile

Mr Patel, your oxygen and blood pressure are low. I'm going to move you to resus and the doctor will see you right away

Why didn't we come sooner? I wish he wasn't so scared of hospitals

Mr Patel your fever and coughing green sputum, with the crackles I can hear in your chest, might be pneumonia. So we'll do an X-ray and get your blood test results

The emergency department registrar finds signs consistent with left-sided pneumonia

Your X-ray shows a bad chest infection. That's making your blood sodium low, which makes you feel worse and can cause other problems, so we'll watch it closely

His sodium's low. We'll need blood and urine samples for paired serum and urine osmolalities

Consolidation on Mr Patel's X-ray confirms pneumonia, which is causing the low sodium

Assess the patient's understanding and desire for information: pitch explanations to explain stand as much as possible: use clear non-patronising language and avoiding medical jargon

Case 6 continued

green sputum is the result of a bacterial respiratory tract infection; the fever and rigors, which reflect a systemic inflammatory response, further support this. The shortness of breath is a consequence of impaired gas exchange in the affected lung area.

The intermittent confusion could be delirium, a disorder of thought, perception and consciousness. This can be caused by infection, particularly in the elderly, or by an electrolyte abnormality such as hyponatraemia.

Mr Patel's loss of appetite is probably a result of the underlying infection. If it had been present for longer, e.g. weeks to months, a more sinister cause would have to be considered (e.g. malignancy).

Examination

Mr Patel has moist mucous membranes and warm peripheries; and his capillary refill time (the time taken for colour to return) after pressure is applied to cause skin blanching is <2s. Jugular venous pressure (JVP) is not raised, and heart sounds are normal. On auscultation, crackles are audible over the upper part of the right chest. There is no ankle swelling.

Interpretation of findings

Right-sided crackles with a productive cough in the context of fever support a diagnosis of right-sided pneumonia. Other serious conditions that could present like this include lung malignancy (although fever would be less likely) and bronchiectasis (bronchial dilation associated with thickening of the mucosa, mucus plugging and chronic infection). A chest radiograph would help to confirm the underlying lung pathology.

There are no clinical signs of volume depletion (cool peripheries, dry mucous membranes, low JVP, prolonged capillary refill time or hypotension). There are also no signs of fluid overload (raised JVP, bibasal crackles or peripheral oedema); however, peripheral vasdilation (evidenced by warm peripheries and a rapid capillary refill time) may be present as part of the systemic inflammatory response.

Investigations

Blood tests show that Mr Patel is hyponatraemic (sodium 126 mmol/L), with slightly increased urea and creatinine concentration at the upper limit of normal (**Table 7.2**). White cell count (WCC) and C-reactive protein (CRP) concentration are increased.

Blood and urine are taken at the same time to measure serum and urinary osmolalities. These results are used to determine the underlying cause of hyponatraemia (see **Table 7.4**). The results show that serum

Ajay Patel's blood and urine test results		
Test	Result	Normal range
Sodium (mmol/L)	126	135–146
Potassium (mmol/L)	3.4	3.5–5.5
Urea (mmol/L)	7.8	2.5–6.7
Serum creatinine (μmol/L)	109	50–110
C-reactive protein (mg/L)	138	<5
White cell count (cells/L)	17.7×10^9	$4–11 \times 10^9$
Neutrophils (cells/L)	15.4×10^9	$2.0–7.5 \times 10^9$
Urine osmolality (mOsm/kg)	496	300–900*
Serum osmolality (mOsm/kg)	260	275–296
*Extreme conditions 50–1200		

Table 7.2 Blood and urine test results for Ajay Patel

Case 6 *continued*

osmolality is low and urine osmolality is high, relative to serum osmolality.

The chest radiograph shows right upper lobe consolidation, an area of opacification due to filling of airspaces with fluid, which can occur as a result of infection (**Figure 7.1**).

Diagnosis

The following findings point towards right upper lobe pneumonia:

- cough producing green sputum, with fevers and rigors
- signs of systemic inflammatory response syndrome
- a focal area of crackles on lung auscultation
- increased WCC and CRP
- right upper zone consolidation on the chest radiograph

Although Mr Patel's serum sodium is low, he is clinically euvolaemic, i.e. his

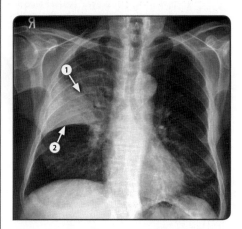

Figure 7.1 Chest radiograph for Ajay Patel showing infective consolidation in the right upper lobe ①, bounded inferiorly by the horizontal fissure ②, i.e. lobar pneumonia.

total body fluid content is normal and he is not over- or under-hydrated. This is demonstrated by his moist mucous membranes, normal JVP and capillary refill time, and lack of peripheral oedema. He may, however, have relative hypovolaemia due to vasodilation. His hyponatraemia is associated with high urine osmolality and low serum osmolality, which suggests avid reabsorption of water by the kidney. The syndrome of inappropriate antidiuretic hormone (ADH) secretion secondary to pneumonia is the most likely cause of the hyponatraemia.

Hyponatraemia is usually an incidental finding as in Mr Patel's case. When hyponatraemia is severe, patients may present with symptoms resulting directly from it, for example lethargy, decreased consciousness, seizures and coma.

Having been given supplemental oxygen for his low oxygen saturation and started on intravenous fluids, Mr Patel is started on intravenous antibiotics for severe community-acquired pneumonia. With sepsis he is at risk of developing hypotension, so his normal antihypertensive medication (ramipril) is withheld.

With this treatment, the observations normalise. Mr Patel's symptoms of cough, shortness of breath, fever and confusion improve quickly, and his sodium increases to within the normal range over the next few days.

A urine sample is sent for a pneumococcal antigen test, and the result is positive. Sputum culture grows *Streptococcus pneumoniae*. These findings confirm that Mr Patel has pneumococcal pneumonia.

Case 7 Increased serum potassium

Presentation

Jane MacLean, who is 64 years old, has a history of type 2 diabetes, for which she takes metformin and gliclazide. She had a myocardial infarction 2 years ago. Since then, she has developed symptoms of cardiac failure, including shortness of breath on exertion and swelling around the ankles.

Her symptoms progressed despite treatment with ramipril, bisoprolol and furosemide. She became unable to walk her dog up the hill without making multiple stops. Therefore her cardiologist started her on spironolactone 3 weeks ago.

She attended her GP for blood tests last week; her potassium concentration was found to be 7.1 mmol/L. Therefore she has been urgently referred to the emergency department.

Initial interpretation

Increased potassium may be an artefactual finding when analysis of a blood sample is delayed. However, a true serum potassium > 6.5 mmol/L is a medical emergency that requires immediate treatment.

Mrs MacLean is on optimal treatment for heart failure. However, her potassium level has become dangerously high since starting spironolactone, a potassium-sparing diuretic.

Further history

Mrs MacLean's answers to further questions reveal that she was due to have her blood electrolytes checked 1 week after starting spironolactone, but she missed

Spironalactone and hyperkalaemia

Mrs MacLean's cardiologist has prescribed her spironolactone for her heart failure. A week later her GP, Dr Syed, orders a urea and electrolytes blood test to check her potassium and kidney function

Three weeks later, Dr Syed receives a phone call from the pathology lab informing her that Mrs MacLean's potassium level is dangerously high

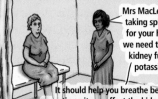

Mrs MacLean, as you're taking spironolactone for your heart failure, we need to watch your kidney function and potassium levels

It should help you breathe better, but sometimes it can affect the kidneys, so we'll see you in a week for these blood tests

Hello. I understand Jane MacLean (DOB 9-11-54, hospital number 9864024) is registered at your practice. Her bloods from this morning show a potassium of 7.1 mmol/L, sodium is 138 mmol/L, urea 4.5 mmol/L and creatinine 118 μmol/L

Hmm, she must have missed two phlebotomy appointments, even though I called and left messages. I hope she's alright. Could just be a haemolysed sample if it sat around...

Hello Mrs MacLean, this is Dr Syed from the Maple Tree Practice

Hello, is everything alright?

I'm afraid your blood test shows that you have very high potassium. You'll need to go to the emergency department to check this and possibly receive treatment. In the meantime, stop your spironolactone and your ramipril

Well...I could go tomorrow, but I've plans tonight and I feel fine...?

No, I'm afraid this is a potential emergency. This could be very dangerous for your heart

We're going to repeat your blood tests and do an ECG immediately

I feel like a pin cushion...okay, fine, but I hope I can go home later on

I hope so, too, but we really need to get your potassium levels under control

Dr Syed immediately telephones Mrs MacLean. Both spironolactone and ramipril can contribute to hyperkalaemia

The triage nurse takes bloods for repeat U&Es and performs an ECG to show the medical team urgently

the appointment because she was on holiday. She reports feeling more tired than usual over the past couple of days, and has not been out for her regular walks, but she has no other symptoms. She takes no potassium-containing medications but eats a diet rich in fruit and uses a salt substitute with meals because she is concerned about her blood pressure.

Some drugs have predictable adverse effects necessitating careful monitoring. One such drug is spironolactone, which causes hyperkalaemia. Other examples are thiazide diuretics which cause hyponatraemia and angiotensin-converting enzyme (ACE) inhibitors, which can cause hyperkalaemia and increase creatinine concentration.

Examination

On examination, Mrs MacLean looks well. She has:

- blood pressure 148/79 mmHg
- heart rate 81 beats/min
- oxygen saturation 99% on room air
- respiratory rate 16 breaths/min

Normal heart sounds and fine bibasal crackles are heard on chest auscultation. Mrs MacLean's abdomen is soft and non-tender. She has mild pedal oedema.

Interpretation of findings

The examination findings are consistent with mild cardiac failure.

- Bibasal crackles result from the presence of fluid in the alveoli; another cause is pulmonary fibrosis (but in this case the crackles would persist even once the fluid overload is treated

- Mild pedal oedema is a consequence of accumulation of fluid in dependent tissues

Mrs MacLean's tiredness is probably related to her heart failure: cardiac output is reduced, resulting in impaired supply of blood to the tissues, including skeletal muscle. It could also be a non-specific effect of the hyperkalaemia.

Investigations

Blood tests are repeated in the emergency department to confirm hyperkalaemia. The results are:

- sodium 138 mmol/L
- potassium 7.4 mmol/L
- urea 4.5 mmol/L
- creatinine 118 μmol/L

Electrocardiography (ECG) shows peaked T waves, broad QRS complexes and flat P waves (**Figure 7.2**).

Diagnosis

The most likely cause for the hyperkalaemia is the combined use of an ACE inhibitor and spironolactone. It may have been exacerbated by a high-potassium diet; Mrs MacLean has been using a salt substitute and this contains potassium chloride.

Spironolactone inhibits the action of aldosterone by competing for intracellular receptors at the collecting duct (Figure 1.22). This decreases the reabsorption of sodium and water and prevents potassium excretion. By blocking the renin–angiotensin–aldosterone system, ACE inhibitors such as ramipril (which Mrs Maclean takes) impair aldosterone secretion, thereby promoting potassium retention.

Hyperkalaemia is often asymptomatic and only found incidentally. However, it can produce symptoms related to cardiac

Case 7 *continued*

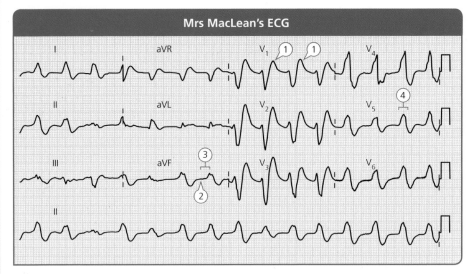

Mrs MacLean's ECG

Figure 7.2 The 12-lead electrocardiogram (ECG) for Jane MacLean showing the typical changes of hyperkalaemia: ① tall, tented T waves; ② small or absent P waves; ③ long PR interval; ④ prolonged and bizarre QRS complex.

or skeletal muscle dysfunction, including weakness, fatigue, palpitations and chest pain. It is possible that Mrs MacLean's fatigue is partly caused by her hyperkalaemia.

Mrs MacLean is attached to a cardiac monitor, and an intravenous cannula is inserted. She is started on intravenous calcium gluconate which stabilises the myocardium and an insulin–dextrose infusion to drive potassium into cells (the effect of insulin) while preventing hypoglycaemia (additional dextrose). The ECG is repeated and serum electrolytes are rechecked after this initial treatment to ensure that potassium concentration is decreasing.

While the potassium level is high, ramipril is withheld and spironolactone is stopped. Mrs MacLean is also advised to follow a low-potassium diet and to stop using the salt substitute. Once her serum potassium concentration has normalised, she is discharged.

She sees her cardiologist as an outpatient regarding further management of the heart failure, and her furosemide dose is increased to compensate for the cessation of spironolactone. She is also referred to a supervised exercise programme to build up her exercise tolerance; she finds this extremely beneficial.

Hyponatraemia

Hyponatraemia is defined as a serum sodium concentration < 135 mmol/L, which is normally associated with a reduction in serum osmolality. It occurs when there is an excess of total body water compared with total body sodium, and becomes clinically significant when plasma sodium concentration is < 125 mmol/L or when sodium concentration decreases rapidly (> 20 mmol/L in 24 h).

> **Plasma sodium concentration can be artefactually low if circulating levels of lipids or proteins are very high.** Plasma is normally 93% water, the remainder being proteins and lipids. Dissolved constituents of plasma are expressed as the concentration in the total blood volume even though many, like sodium, are soluble in only the aqueous phase. If water occupies a reduced percentage of total volume because more lipids and proteins are present, the sodium concentration will appear lower than it actually is (pseudohyponatraemia).

Epidemiology and aetiology

Hyponatraemia is the commonest electrolyte abnormality in hospital in-patients, affecting up to 30% of this population. The elderly are particularly susceptible because of altered water metabolism, an impaired thirst mechanism, impaired renal function and the increased use of salt-depleting drugs, such as thiazide diuretics, in these patients.

Hyponatraemia may be caused by sodium loss, water retention or a combination of both. It is typically classified according to both plasma osmolality and volume status.

When classified according to plasma osmolality (**Figure 7.3**), hyponatraemia may be isotonic, hypertonic or hypotonic. In isotonic and hypertonic hyponatraemia total body sodium concentration is normal, but measured sodium concentration is decreased.

- In isotonic hyponatraemia, excess lipid or protein in the plasma causes a fall in the plasma water fraction (which contains sodium). This results in a reduction in the measured sodium concentration, but no change in plasma water sodium concentration or osmolality
- In hypertonic hyponatraemia, there is a decrease in measured sodium due to the presence of osmotically active particles in the serum, which cause water to shift from the intracellular to extracellular compartment. This has a dilutional effect on sodium.

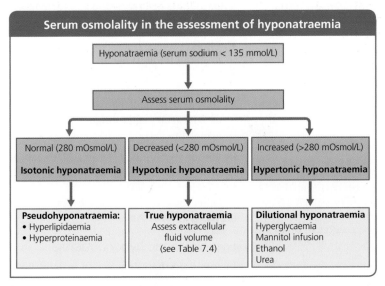

Figure 7.3 Use of serum osmolality in the assessment of hyponatraemia.

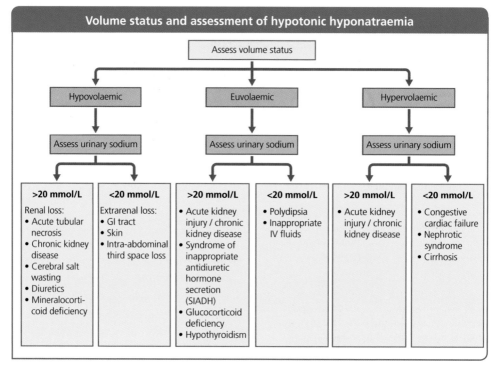

Figure 7.4 Use of volume status in the assessment of hyponatraemia. Determining the patient's volume status and evaluating the urinary sodium concentration helps establish the cause of hyponatraemia. GI, gastrointestinal; IV, intravenous; SIADH, syndrome of inappropriate antidiuretic hormone secretion.

Hypotonic hyponatraemia can be viewed as true hyponatraemia and classified according to volume status as (**Figure 7.4**):

- **euvolaemic**, i.e. with normal body fluid volume
- **hypovolaemic**, i.e. with decreased extracellular fluid volume
- **hypervolaemic**, i.e. with excess extracellular fluid volume

This classification is useful, because knowledge of the volume status is required for identification of the cause of hyponatraemia (**Table 7.3**) and guides treatment decisions.

Plasma sodium content does not equate to total body sodium content. It is more common for hyponatraemia to result from the dilution of plasma sodium by retained water, rather than sodium loss. This occurs in oedematous states, in which total body sodium is increased whatever the serum sodium concentration.

Euvolaemic hyponatraemia

This is a relative excess of water compared with sodium. The excess water is not clinically apparent, because it is mainly intracellular.

The most common cause is syndrome of inappropriate ADH secretion, in which the sodium level is lowered by either:

- the abnormal release of ADH from the posterior pituitary gland
- or by abnormal resetting of the osmostat, the regulatory centres that control osmolality of extracellular fluid, with the release of ADH at an inappropriately low plasma osmolality

By either mechanism, excess ADH causes excess water reabsorption in the renal tubules (see page 38).

Other causes of euvolaemic hyponatraemia are listed in **Table 7.3**.

Hypovolaemic hyponatraemia

In this type there is a deficit in total body

Hyponatraemia: causes, associations and clinical features			
Type of hyponatraemia	Causes	Associations	Clinical features
Euvolaemic	Syndrome of inappropriate ADH secretion	Malignancy: small-cell lung cancer, lymphoma, sarcoma, mesothelioma, thymoma, pancreatic carcinoma	Euvolaemia: absence of features of volume depletion or fluid overload
		Pulmonary disease: pneumonia, active tuberculosis, abscess, empyema	
		Neurological disease: head injury, infection, neoplasm, intracranial disease	
		Trauma	
		Drugs (e.g. antidepressants, carbamazepine, MDMA or 'ecstasy')	
	Primary polydipsia	Psychiatric conditions	
	Hypotonic intravenous fluids	Hospitalisation	
	Rare causes: severe hypothyroidism, glucocorticoid deficiency; decreased sodium intake		
	Abnormal resetting of the osmostat so serum osmolality is maintained at a lower set point	Old age	
		Pregnancy	
Hypovolaemic	Renal sodium loss	Diuretics	Symptoms and signs of volume depletion (e.g. thirst, low JVP, postural hypotension)
		Mineralocorticoid deficiency	
		Renal tubular disorders	
		Cerebral salt wasting	
	Extrarenal sodium loss	Diarrhoea	
		Vomiting	
		Excessive sweating	
Hypervolaemic	Failure to excrete sodium load	Advanced renal failure	Peripheral oedema
			Ascites
	Response to states of decreased effective circulating volume	Congestive cardiac failure	Raised JVP
		Cirrhosis	Pulmonary oedema
		Nephrotic syndrome	
		Severe hypoalbuminaemia (e.g. due to malnutrition)	

ADH, antidiuretic hormone; JVP, jugular venous pressure

Table 7.3 Causes of hyponatraemia, and their associations and clinical features

sodium and total body water, with the sodium deficit greater than the water deficit. Loss of extracellular fluid volume results in a compensatory increase in ADH secretion that increases reabsorption of water in the collecting duct.

Hypervolaemic hyponatraemia

This is an excess in total body water and total body sodium, with a greater water excess relative to sodium. It is characterised by fluid overload with hyponatraemia and excessive ADH, and occurs in patients with:

- advanced heart failure; arterial under-filling occurs as a result of decreased cardiac output and dilation of the splanchnic bed. This triggers a baroreceptor response resulting in activation of the renin–angiotensin–aldosterone system and release of noradrenaline (norepinephrine) and ADH
- Advanced renal failure caused by the inability to correctly excrete appropriate amounts of sodium and water
- Cirrhosis: there is, particularly splanchnic, vasodilation. This results in release of vasoconstrictors, including ADH, which promote retention of water

Clinical features

Hyponatraemia is usually asymptomatic. Even if it is severe it can be well tolerated if it has developed gradually, because the body is able to adapt. The most significant clinical features result from its effect on the brain: most patients with symptomatic hyponatraemia have mild brain oedema.

In chronic hyponatraemia, the brain compensates for the decrease in serum sodium concentration by moving osmotically active electrolytes out of brain cells to promote water loss and thereby mitigate cerebral oedema. If plasma sodium decreases acutely this adaptation does not occur, therefore changes in osmotic pressure drive water into cells, resulting in:

- cerebral oedema
- coma
- brainstem herniation

Symptoms are non-specific and include nausea, headache, fatigue, confusion, and in severe cases, seizures and coma.

Diagnostic approach

A diagnosis of hyponatraemia is made by measuring plasma sodium concentration (**Figure 7.3**). It is often an incidental finding, but it should be suspected in certain presentations, such as confusion, particularly in elderly patients on multiple medications.

A thorough history of past and present illness may point towards the underlying cause of hyponatraemia. A drug history is vital: various medications cause SIADH, and certain diuretics induce renal sodium loss. Assessment of intravascular volume status is key, because the results are used to guide management (**Figure 7.4**). Examination is carried out to detect signs of potential causes of hyponatraemia, such as congestive cardiac failure, renal failure, cirrhosis, pulmonary and neurological infection and malignancy (see **Table 7.3**).

Investigation of hyponatraemia	
Test	**Rationale**
Urea, creatinine and electrolytes	To confirm hyponatraemia and assess renal function and potassium concentration
Thyroid function tests	To exclude thyroid dysfunction, particularly hypothyroidism, as a cause of hyponatraemia
Blood glucose	To exclude hyperglycaemia as a cause of hypertonic hyponatraemia
Serum osmolality	To establish whether hyponatraemia is associated with increased, decreased or normal osmolality; true physiologically significant hyponatraemia is hypotonic (see Table 7.3)
Urine osmolality	To help ascertain the cause of hyponatraemia ■ Low osmolality (< 100 mmol/kg H_2O) suggests excessive water intake ■ Low osmolality and volume depletion occur in cerebral salt-wasting caused by CNS disease (e.g. subarachnoid haemorrhage); SIADH is associated with euvolaemia and high urinary osmolality
Urinary sodium concentration	To assess the ability of the kidneys to conserve sodium

CNS, central nervous system; SIADH, syndrome of inappropriate antidiuretic hormone secretion.

Table 7.4 Blood and urine tests used routinely in the investigation of hyponatraemia

Investigations

Blood and urine tests

Table 7.4 shows the blood and urine tests that are used in the assessment of a patient with hyponatraemia.

Dilutional hyponatraemia

Most patients with hyponatraemia have low plasma osmolality, because of the osmotic effect of the low sodium. Hyponatraemia in the context of hyperosmolality suggests a diagnosis of dilutional hyponatraemia caused by additional osmotically active substances such as glucose, mannitol and ethanol, or urea in advanced CKD, which draw free water from the intracellular space into the extracellular space. This is not true hyponatraemia, because the serum osmolality is normal or increased, rather than decreased and total body sodium is normal. Dilutional hyponatraemia corrects with restoration of normoglycaemia or removal of the additional osmotically active substance.

Pseudohyponatraemia

Normal serum osmolality (isosomolality) suggests the presence of pseudohyponatraemia, an artefactual hyponatraemia resulting from high levels of lipids or proteins in the blood.

Imaging

A chest radiograph may be indicated to exclude congestive cardiac failure, pneumonia or lung malignancy, which can be associated with hyponatraemia. CT of the head may be warranted for patients with altered mental status, either to rule out cerebral pathology or to search for a cause if cerebral salt wasting is considered. This latter condition is seen particularly in the case of subarachnoid haemorrhage, and is thought to be due to the release of natriuretic peptides from the brain, plus systemic hypertension causing a pressure natriuresis.

Management

Management of hyponatraemia with increased serum osmolality (> 295 mOsm/kg) is focused on treating the cause. If serum osmolality is low (< 275 mOsm/kg), management is guided by volume status. To avoid neurological complications such as central pontine myelinolysis, plasma sodium concentration is not allowed to increase by more than 8 mmol/L in 24 h.

> **The predicted increase in sodium that will be produced by a given volume of a particular fluid** can be calculated by the use of formulae available online.

> **Central pontine myelinolysis is a neurological condition caused by damage to the myelin sheath of nerve fibres in the brainstem, usually the pons.** It occurs when hyponatraemia is corrected too rapidly, and results from fluid shifts in response to changes in extracellular osmolality. Symptoms include paraparesis, quadriparesis, dysphagia, dysarthria, altered consciousness and 'locked-in syndrome'.

Hypovolaemic hyponatraemia

Management is focused on restoring normovolaemia and replacing the sodium deficit.

- Diuretics are stopped
- Intravenous 0.9% NaCl is given to address the volume deficit

The amount of sodium required to achieve the desired plasma concentration is calculated:

$$\text{Na required (Na deficit)} = 0.6 \times \text{body weight} \times [\text{desired Na}^+ - \text{actual Na}^+]$$

where sodium required is in mmol, body weight is in kg, and desired and actual sodium concentrations are in mmol/L.

Euvolaemic hyponatraemia

Management requires the following:

- Diuretics and medications that induce SIADH are stopped
- Mineralocorticoid deficiency or hypothyroidism is identified and treated
- Fluid is restricted to 1–1.5 L/day

The tetracycline demeclocycline is considered if there is no response to fluid restriction. It is thought to interfere with the signalling cascade initiated by the binding of ADH to its receptor.

Vasopressor receptor antagonists (vaptans) may be used under the direction of an endocrinologist or nephrologist.

Hypervolaemic hyponatraemia

This is managed with:

- fluid restriction to 1 L/day
- sodium restriction (total body sodium is usually increased)
- diuretics and, when indicated, potassium replacement

Neurological complications

Hypertonic saline (3%) is reserved for seizures or other life-threatening neurological complications of hyponatraemia. It is only used in in a setting in which close monitoring is provided, such as intensive care.

Prognosis

Hyponatraemia is an independent risk factor for mortality in patients who have been admitted to hospital, i.e. mortality is raised regardless of comorbidities. The reason for this is incompletely understood; however, hyponatraemia may cause organ dysfunction, thereby contributing to mortality indirectly.

Prognosis depends on how quickly hyponatraemia has developed, and the underlying cause. If the onset has been rapid, it is more likely to be associated with cerebral oedema and other neurological complications, such as seizures and coma. Hyponatraemia caused by severe pneumonia or malignancy has a poorer prognosis than that caused by medications, which can be withdrawn.

Hypernatraemia

Hypernatraemia is defined as a serum sodium concentration > 145 mmol/L. In most cases, the cause is a decrease in total body water relative to sodium. It is usually clinically significant only if the concentration is > 155 mmol/L or if the increase has been rapid (> 20 mmol/L in 24 h).

Hypernatraemia is a common electrolyte disorder. Infants and the elderly are particularly susceptible. Most cases result from limited access to water, an impaired thirst mechanism or a condition causing increased fluid loss.

Epidemiology

Hypernatraemia is mainly encountered in hospitals, affecting up to 5% of inpatients. The incidence in the community and on admission to hospital is low. Those most at risk of hypernatraemia include infants, the elderly, the critically ill, people with altered mental status and those with hypothalamic lesions affecting thirst, where homeostatic mechanisms are more likely to be impaired.

Aetiology

Causes of hypernatraemia are listed in **Table 7.5**. It usually arises from water loss with inadequate fluid replacement, rather than sodium gain. Normally, increased plasma tonicity caused by increased sodium concentration results in thirst. This prompts the intake of fluids, the water content of which dilutes the plasma and thereby normalises its sodium concentration.

The commonest causes of hypernatraemia are inability to access water, inadequate drinking as a consequence of impaired thirst mechanisms and increased fluid loss, e.g. diarrhoea and vomiting. A less common but serious cause is diabetes insipidus, in which hypernatraemia is a result of:

- decreased ADH secretion, causing central (or cranial) diabetes inspidus
- renal resistance to ADH, causing nephrogenic diabetes insipidus

Nephrogenic diabetes insipidus is congenital or acquired (see **Table 7.5**) and central diabetes

Hypernatraemia: mechanisms and causes		
Mechanism	**Causes**	
Pure free water loss (dehydration)	Inadequate water intake	Inability to access water
		Impaired thirst
		Altered mental status
		Neurological disease (e.g. dementia)
	Diabetes insipidus	Central (decreased ADH secretion)
		Nephrogenic (renal tubular resistance to ADH):
		■ Congenital
		■ Acquired:
		– Some drugs: e.g. lithium,
		– amphotericin B, demeclocycline
		– Hypercalcaemia
Hypotonic fluid loss (loss of water and electrolytes)	Dermal losses	Burns
		Sweating
	Gastrointestinal losses	Non-secretory diarrhoea, laxatives
		Vomiting
		Fistulae
	Urinary losses	Diuretics (loop and thiazide diuretics)
		Osmotic diuresis (e.g. hyperglycaemia, mannitol)
		Acute tubular necrosis (diuretic phase)
Hypertonic sodium gain	Iatrogenic	Hypertonic saline (e.g. 3% sodium chloride)
		Nasogastric or nasojejunal feeding
		Sodium-containing intravenous medications
		Hypertonic intravenous sodium bicarbonate (e.g. 8.4%)
		Hypertonic dialysis
	Excess salt ingestion	Inadvertent
		Deliberate poisoning
		Saltwater drowning
	Hyperaldosteronism	Primary (Conn's syndrome, i.e. aldosterone-secreting adenoma)
		Increased glucocorticoid (Cushing's disease or syndrome)
		Ectopic adrenocorticotrophic hormone (e.g. in small-cell lung cancer)

ADH, antidiuretic hormone.

Table 7.5 Underlying mechanisms and causes of hypernatraemia

insipidus is idiopathic or results from brain tumours, cranial surgery or brain trauma.

Clinical features

Symptoms depend on the degree of hypernatraemia, and include:

■ thirst
■ weakness
■ lethargy
■ irritability
■ tremor
■ ataxia
■ confusion
■ seizures and
■ coma

Confusion and coma generally occur only if sodium is > 155 mmol/L. Signs of volume depletion (see Figure 3.7) may also be present, i.e.:

- tachycardia
- hypotension
- dry mucous membranes
- decreased skin turgor
- cool peripheries
- prolonged capillary refill time
- low jugular venous pressure

Diagnostic approach

Hypernatraemia is diagnosed when the sodium concentration of the blood is found to be increased. Although there are no specific symptoms, it should be suspected in a patient presenting with signs of volume depletion. A normal blood sodium concentration excludes hypernatraemia.

During the history, the patient is assessed for inadequate water intake or excessive loss of water, for example as a result of vomiting, diarrhoea or large losses from the gastrointestinal tract via a fistula or stoma. Sources of sodium excess are also sought, although this is a rare contributing factor. Intravascular volume is assessed because there may be volume depletion as well as dehydration (**Figure 7.5**; see also page 72).

> **'Dehydration' and 'volume depletion' are often used interchangeably but refer to different physiological states that can coincide or occur independently.** Dehydration describes a loss of total body water, resulting in hypertonicity, whereas volume depletion refers to a reduction in the effective circulating volume in the intravascular space.

Investigations

Investigations will define the extent of hypernatraemia and help determine its cause.

Blood tests

These confirm the diagnosis of hypernatraemia, assess its severity and identify the underlying causes:

- serum urea, creatinine and electrolytes to determine serum sodium concentration and assess renal function
- a bone profile to exclude hypercalcaemia, which can cause nephrogenic diabetes insipidus

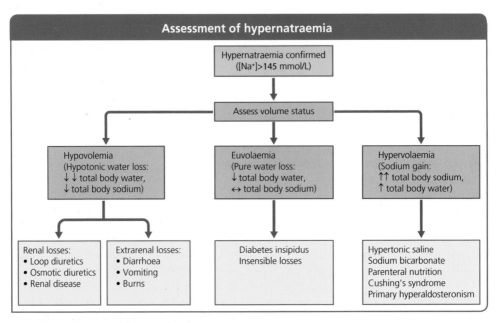

Figure 7.5 Assessment of hypernatraemia.

- serum osmolality to determine plasma tonicity
- full blood count to exclude infection and anaemia
- glucose concentration to exclude hyperosmolar hyperglycaemic state, a medical emergency that is associated with type 2 diabetes and can result in severe dehydration
- arterial or venous blood gases to exclude acid–base disorders, particularly if there is a history of prolonged vomiting

Urine tests

The following tests help determine the underlying cause of the hypernatraemia:

- Urine osmolality: under normal circumstances, the kidneys respond to hypernatraemia by excreting maximally concentrated urine, so urinary osmolality is high (usually > 800 mOsmol/kg); this compensation occurs with extrarenal fluid losses, for example in cases of vomiting, diarrhoea and burns
  - Isotonic urine can occur with hypernatraemia caused by diuretics
  - Hypotonic urine is produced in central or nephrogenic diabetes insipidus
- Urine sodium concentration: this is measured to assess renal excretion of sodium

Management

Management is focused on prevention of ongoing water loss. This may require stopping diuretics, treating diarrhoea or giving antiemetics to prevent vomiting.

Water deficit is calculated to guide fluid replacement:

$$\text{Water deficit} = \text{total body water} \times (\text{Serum [Na}^+]/140)-1$$

where water deficit is in litres, total body water is body weight (kg) × 0.6 in men or × 0.5 in women, and sodium concentration is in mmol/L.

The aim is to replace one third of the water deficit in the first 24 h, alongside replacing ongoing fluid losses and providing maintenance requirements. Correcting sodium too rapidly can cause cerebral oedema.

Fluid should be replaced by mouth, or if the patient is unable to drink, via nasogastric tube. If intravenous fluid replacement is required, fluid is replaced with alternating bags of 0.5% dextrose with 0.18% saline, and 0.9% saline. Serum sodium is checked every 12–24 h and not allowed to decrease by > 8 mmol/L in any 24-h period.

Prognosis

This depends on the severity of the hypernatraemia and its speed of onset. In elderly patients, severe hypernatraemia is associated with mortality of up to 70%, although this may reflect the severity of other comorbidities rather than hypernatraemia itself. As with hyponatraemia, hypernatraemia is an independent risk factor for mortality.

Hypokalaemia

Hypokalaemia is defined as a serum potassium concentration < 3.5 mmol/L. Potassium is the most abundant intracellular ion. The potassium gradient between the intracellular and extracellular compartments is vital for the maintenance of cell membrane resting potentials. Therefore normal potassium homeostasis is essential for cellular function (see page 43).

Potassium homeostasis depends mainly on renal secretion from the collecting duct, which is under the control of aldosterone. Potassium entry into cells is also regulated by various factors, as shown in **Figure 7.6**.

Hypokalaemia is classified as mild, moderate or severe (**Table 7.6**); most cases are in the mild category. This classification can help guide treatment.

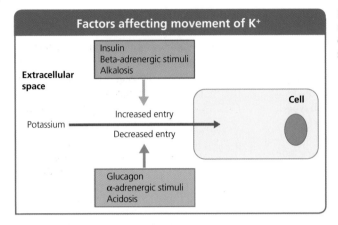

Figure 7.6 Factors controlling movement of potassium from the extracellular to the intracellular space.

Table 7.6 Clinical features of hypokalaemia

Severity	Potassium concentration (mmol/L)	Clinical features
Mild	3.1–3.5	Usually asymptomatic
Moderate	2.5–3	Lethargy
		Generalised weakness, muscle pain
		Constipation
Severe	< 2.5	Marked muscle weakness and ascending paralysis
		Respiratory failure as a result of weakness of respiratory muscles
		Ileus resulting from weakness of gut wall muscles
		Paraesthesia
		Tetany

Epidemiology

It is one of the most common electrolyte disorders in patients admitted to hospital. Up to 20% of in-patients have hypokalaemia with a potassium concentration < 3 mmol/L, and up to 5% have potassium < 2.5 mmol/L. Hypokalaemia is also common in the community, with the results of some studies showing a 3% prevalence. People taking diuretics, and those with anorexia nervosa or alcoholism, are particularly at risk.

Aetiology

Hypokalaemia occurs secondary to:

■ inadequate intake of potassium

■ increased excretion of potassium
■ a shift of potassium from the extracellular to the intracellular space

Most cases are caused by increased renal loss as a result of the use of drugs that inhibit tubular reuptake of potassium, endocrine abnormalities or inherited tubular defects (**Table 7.7**).

Clinical features

The symptoms of hypokalaemia are non-specific, and many patients with mild hypokalaemia are asymptomatic. Moderate hypokalaemia results in lethargy, generalised weakness, muscle pain and constipation. At potassium concentrations below

Hypokalaemia: mechanisms and causes	
Mechanism	Causes
Increased loss	**Renal loss** ■ Use of certain drugs (e.g. diuretics, carbonic anhydrase inhibitors, penicillins), liquorice (mimics effect of aldosterone) ■ Renal tubular toxins ■ Endocrine e.g. aldosterone excess ■ Renal tubular defects ■ Bicarbonaturia ■ Magnesium deficiency **Gastrointestinal loss** ■ Diarrhoea ■ Vomiting ■ Intestinal fistulae ■ Laxative abuse ■ Villous adenoma ■ Pyloric stenosis ■ Bowel preparation for surgery or colonoscopy
Decreased intake	Inadequate potassium replacement while on intravenous fluids Total parenteral nutrition Poor diet and malnutrition Anorexia nervosa
Extracellular to intracellular potassium shift	Acute alkalosis (potassium absorbed and hydrogen ions secreted) Insulin treatment Catecholamines and β-adrenergic agonists Theophylline Caffeine Familial hypokalaemic periodic paralysis Thyrotoxicosis Chloroquine intoxication
Other	Chronic peritoneal dialysis Plasmapheresis

Table 7.7 Underlying mechanisms and causes of hypokalaemia

2.5 mmol/L, severe neuromuscular complications can occur (see **Table 7.6**).

All patients with hypokalaemia are at risk of cardiac arrhythmias, even those with a mild deficiency. However, arrhythmias are more likely to occur in those with underlying cardiac disease. The arrhythmogenic effect of hypokalaemia is attributed to prolonged ventricular depolarisation, slowed conduction within the conducting system and abnormal pacemaker activity. The resultant arrhythmias are primarily tachyarrhythmias such as ventricular tachycardia and ventricular fibrillation, which can be life-threatening.

> **Each 0.3 mmol/L reduction in serum potassium reflects 100 mmol/L of total body deficit.** Alkalosis in a patient on diuretics usually indicates a total body potassium deficit; the potassium loss favours an intracellular shift of hydrogen ions, producing an extracellular alkalosis.

Diagnostic approach

Hypokalaemia is diagnosed when blood test results show a low serum potassium concentration. Because it can be asymptomatic, it is often an incidental finding. It is suspected in patients presenting with vague symptoms such as lethargy and weakness, and those taking diuretics, as well as any patient presenting with a cardiac arrhythmia.

The cause may be suspected from the presentation, for example vomiting, diarrhoea or anorexia. It is essential to take a detailed drug history and to ask about non-prescribed medications, such as laxatives, because these are common causes of hypokalaemia.

Investigations

Investigations are aimed at defining the degree of hypokalaemia, determining its cause, and detecting other associated electrolyte disturbances.

Blood tests

The following blood tests are used in the assessment of hypokalaemia:

■ urea and electrolytes, to confirm hypokalaemia and determine serum sodium concentration and renal function
■ chloride concentration, to help differentiate between causes of hypokalaemia, particularly when acid–base disorders are present

- magnesium concentration, because hypomagnesaemia and hypokalaemia often coexist
- arterial or venous blood gases, because acid–base disorders can be associated with hypokalaemia
- digoxin concentration, if the patient is taking digoxin

Patients who are known or suspected to take digoxin (a cardiac medication used in the management of heart failure and atrial fibrillation) should have their serum digoxin concentration checked. Digoxin acts by inhibiting the Na^+–K^+ATPase pump. Careful dosing is required to prevent toxicity (which causes arrhythmias) because it has a narrow therapeutic window. Hypokalaemia results in enhanced binding of digoxin to the pump and therefore results in toxicity.

Urine tests

The urinary potassium concentration will confirm whether hypokalaemia is the result of excessive urinary potassium loss. This is typically encountered with diuretic use. However, once common causes have been excluded rare conditions should be considered, e.g. renal tubular acidosis and hereditary renal tubulopathies (e.g. Bartter's syndrome).

Low urinary potassium suggests poor potassium intake, intracellular shift or gastrointestinal loss.

Specialised tests

Unexplained hypokalaemia (hypokalaemia with a cause not revealed by the history or by blood and urine tests) requires specialised tests to identify the cause. Plasma aldosterone:renin ratio is determined in the investigation of primary hyperaldosteronism, which is considered in patients with unexplained hypokalaemia and hypertension. Patients with hypokalaemia and clinical signs of steroid excess, for example weight gain (particularly in the abdominal area), facial puffiness, striae and proximal myopathy, undergo a dexamethasone suppression test for Cushing's syndrome.

Typical ECG changes in hypokalaemia include the following (**Figure 7.7**):

- flattened or inverted T waves, representing abnormal ventricular repolarisation
- ST depression, representing changes to the resting potential in myocardial cells
- Prominent U waves, which represent repolarisation of Purkinje fibres

Management

Management of hypokalaemia comprises prevention of ongoing potassium losses and replenishment of stores (**Table 7.8**). Underlying causes (e.g. drugs, diet, diarrhoea and vomiting) are addressed where possible. Laxatives and diuretics are stopped and, if required, a potassium-sparing agent prescribed. Diarrhoea and vomiting are managed with fluid replacement, and anti-motility drugs (e.g. loperamide) and anti-emetics are used if appropriate.

Oral potassium supplements are given if serum potassium is between 2.5 and 3.5 mmol/L; intravenous replacement is given if serum potassium is ≤2.5 mmol/L, the patient is unable to tolerate oral medications or has symptomatic hypokalaemia.

Supplements are used cautiously in patients with renal impairment: the risk of iatrogenic hyperkalaemia must be remembered.

> **Potassium has an irritant effect, and can damage small veins when infused at high concentrations.** Therefore it is infused into a large peripheral vein or a central vein. Up to 20 mmol/h can be given; the total amount infused should not exceed 200 mmol/day.

Prognosis

This depends entirely on the cause. Hypokalaemia secondary to reversible conditions such as diarrhoea or diuretic use is easily treatable. In contrast, hypokalaemia secondary to genetic tubular defects has little potential for complete resolution.

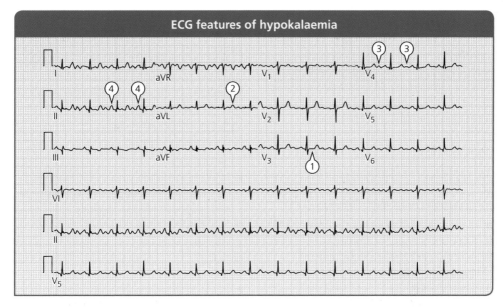

ECG features of hypokalaemia

Figure 7.7 Electrocardiographic features of hypokalaemia. (1), ST depression; (2), small-amplitude T waves; (3), U wave after the T wave (usually in leads V_4–V_6); (4), large P wave with prolonged PR interval.

Hypokalaemia: management	
Management aim	**Treatment**
Identify and stop ongoing losses	Discontinue diuretics and/or laxatives
	Consider a potassium-sparing diuretic if diuretics are required
	Treat diarrhoea or vomiting
	Control hyperglycaemia (causes an osmotic diuresis)
Replenish stores	Oral replacement is preferable, and supplements are given if potassium is < 3.5 mmol/L
	Consider intravenous potassium replacement in patients: ■ with serum potassium < 2.5 mmol/L ■ unable to tolerate oral supplements ■ with symptomatic hypokalaemia

Table 7.8 Management of hypokalaemia

Hyperkalaemia

Hyperkalaemia is defined as a serum potassium concentration > 5.5 mmol/L. It is: categorised as:

■ Mild: serum potassium 5.5–5.9 mmol/L
■ Moderate: serum potassium 6–6.4 mmol/L
■ Severe: serum potassium ≥ 6.5 mmol/L

Patients with acute or chronic kidney disease are particularly at risk because of their reduced renal potassium excretion, and many cases are associated with medication use. Severe hyperkalaemia can result in life-threatening cardiac arrhythmias and is therefore a medical emergency (see Chapter 13).

Epidemiology

Hyperkalaemia affects 1–10% of patients admitted to hospital. Those at extremes of age (premature babies and the elderly), are most at risk because of their low glomerular filtration rate, and in the elderly, reduced renal blood flow and polypharmacy.

Aetiology

The causes of hyperkalaemia can be grouped according to the mechanisms by which they increase potassium levels (**Table 7.9**):

- decreased renal potassium excretion
- increased potassium intake
- intracellular to extracellular shift of potassium

Clinical features

Symptoms of hyperkalaemia are non-specific and include weakness and fatigue. Cardiac arrhythmias are the most clinically important sequelae; patients may present with palpitations or chest pain, which require urgent management.

> Severe hyperkalaemia is a medical emergency requiring urgent management. There is a significant risk of cardiac arrest.

Diagnostic approach

The diagnosis of hyperkalaemia is based on the finding of high serum potassium concentration. Its symptoms are non-specific, so it is often detected incidentally when blood tests are done for another reason. Hyperkalaemia is considered in patients presenting with symptoms of weakness, fatigue and palpitations. It should always be excluded in patients with an arrhythmia or renal impairment.

A thorough history is vital to identify sources of potassium and check for the use of potassium-sparing drugs. Features of corticosteroid deficiency are also sought to ensure that hypoadrenalism (Addison's disease) is not missed.

If a finding of increased serum potassium concentration is unexpected, for example in a patient with normal renal function who is not taking any drugs that could cause hyperkalaemia, the possibility of pseudohyperkalaemia is considered. This can be the result of the release of potassium from red blood cells when they lyse, which can occur:

- when blood has been stored for too long before analysis
- while blood is being taken, for example because of a prolonged tourniquet time or difficulty collecting the sample
- if a sample is shaken vigorously

If a result is thought to be spurious, the test is repeated.

> A rapid serum potassium concentration can be obtained by running a sample of blood through a blood gas machine, most of which measure serum electrolyte concentrations.

Investigations

The following blood tests are useful in the assessment of hyperkalaemia:

- urea and electrolytes, to confirm hyperkalaemia and assess renal function
- full blood count, to exclude anaemia and infection
- arterial or venous blood gas, to determine arterial pH and plasma bicarbonate levels; the results may enable exclusion of metabolic acidosis, which can be associated with hyperkalaemia
- glucose concentration, if the patient has known or suspected diabetes
- digoxin level, if the patient is taking digoxin
- plasma cortisol, if hypoadrenalism (Addison's disease) is suspected
- serum creatine kinase, if rhabdomyolysis (extensive breakdown of muscle often complicated by acute kidney injury; see Chapter 3) is suspected

Electrocardiographic changes typical of hyperkalaemia reflect severity (**Table 7.10**; see also **Figure 7.2**).

Hyperkalaemia: mechanisms and causes	
Mechanism	Causes
Decreased renal potassium excretion	Decreased GFR in acute and chronic kidney disease
	Drugs ■ Potassium-sparing diuretics acting on the distal tubule (e.g. amiloride) ■ High-dose trimethoprim (amiloride-like action) ■ Inhibition of the renin-angiotensin-aldosterone system (e.g. by beta-blockers, angiotensin-converting enzyme inhibitors, angiotensin II receptor blockers, spironolactone)
	Mineralocorticoid deficiency ■ Hypoadrenalism (Addison's disease) ■ Type 4 renal tubular acidosis
	Genetic disorder ■ Pseudohypoaldosteronism
Increased potassium intake	Dietary excess
	Salt substitutes
	Potassium supplements
	Intravenous fluids containing potassium
	Upper gastrointestinal bleeding
Intracellular to extracellular shift of potassium	Metabolic acidosis
	Use of certain drugs, for example: ■ Digoxin ■ Ciclosporin ■ Methotrexate ■ Theophylline
	Cell lysis ■ Tumour lysis syndrome ■ Rhabdomyolysis ■ Haemolysis ■ Burns ■ Trauma
	Insulin deficiency
	Genetic disorder ■ Hyperkalaemic periodic paralysis
	Artefact ■ Haemolysis (e.g. difficulty collecting sample, prolonged tourniquet time, shaking of tube) ■ Excessive cooling of sample ■ Delay in analysis of sample ■ Leucocytosis or thrombocytosis ■ Contamination of sample (e.g. sample taken from arm receiving fluids containing potassium)

Table 7.9 Underlying mechanisms and causes of hyperkalaemia

Management

The aim of management is to prevent any adverse cardiac effects of hyperkalaemia and to bring the serum potassium concentration down to within the normal range. Dietary potassium intake is limited. For full discussion of the management of hyperkalaemia, see page 321.

Renal replacement therapy

In rare instances this is required for patients with renal impairment who are not already

Hyperkalaemia: ECG changes	
Severity	Features
Mild hyperkalaemia: potassium 5.5–6.5 mmol/L	Tall tented T waves representing abnormal repolarisation
	Short QT interval as a result of shortening of the repolarisation phase
Moderate hyperkalaemia: potassium 6.5–7.5 mmol/L	Prolonged PR interval representing a decreased rate of atrial and ventricular depolarisation
	Wide QRS complex representing intraventricular conduction delay
Severe hyperkalaemia: potassium ≥ 7.5 mmol/L	Loss of P waves as a result of sinoventricular conduction, when the sinoatrial node generates an impulse that is conducted to the atrioventricular node without atrial contraction
	Progressive widening of the T wave and loss of the ST segment
	Replacement of the QRST waves with a diphasic sine wave, which is a preterminal event, unless immediate treatment is started

Table 7.10 Electrocardiographic changes in hyperkalaemia

on renal replacement therapy, and for intractable hyperkalaemia.

Prognosis

Transient hyperkalaemia with a defined cause has a good prognosis: full resolution is expected with correction of the underlying cause. Recurrent episodes may occur in patients with persistent risk factors for hyperkalaemia, for example CKD. Prognosis is much worse in severe hyperkalaemia, because life-threatening cardiac sequelae are more likely, and when onset of hyperkalaemia is sudden, because this also increases the risk of life-threatening arrhythmias. Patients with chronic hyperkalaemia appear to adapt to be able to tolerate serum potassium concentrations that are much higher than normal.

Hypocalcaemia

Hypocalcaemia is a corrected serum calcium concentration < 2.25 mmol/L. It is a common finding among in-patients, and is more prevalent with increasing severity of illness. Hypocalcaemia is also encountered in primary care; vitamin D deficiency is the commonest cause in this setting.

Because maintenance of extracellular calcium concentration is essential for normal functioning of excitable tissues, the typical symptoms of hypocalcaemia result from changes in neuromuscular excitability. Chronic hypocalcaemia is often asymptomatic, but acute hypocalcaemia usually precipitates severe symptoms that necessitate admission to hospital for rapid treatment.

Epidemiology

Hypocalcaemia is encountered in both primary and secondary care, and affects patients of all ages. Studies have shown a prevalence of roughly 25% of patients admitted to hospital and 88% of those receiving intensive care.

Values for calcium concentrations must be corrected when albumin concentrations are abnormal. A large proportion of calcium is transported in the blood bound to albumin; only free ionised calcium is biologically active. This means that in a patient with hypoalbuminaemia, an abnormally high serum calcium concentration may appear to be normal if the corrected value for calcium concentration is not used. The corrected calcium is usually calculated by the laboratory but can also be determined by using the following equation:

$$\text{Corrected } [Ca^{2+}] = \text{measured } [Ca^{2+}] + \left\{(40 - [alb]) \times 0.2\right\}$$

where alb is albumin.

Aetiology

The commonest causes of hypocalcaemia are vitamin D deficiency and impaired vitamin D metabolism, hypoparathyroidism following surgery to the thyroid or parathyroid glands, renal failure and hypomagnesaemia (**Table 7.11**).

Clinical features

Symptoms usually correlate with severity of hypocalcaemia and the speed at which it has developed. Mild hypocalcaemia is usually asymptomatic. Symptoms are related to neuromuscular irritability, and include paraesthesia, muscle cramps, carpopedal spasm (spasm of the muscles of the hands or feet; see **Figure 7.8b**), tetany, laryngeal stridor and convulsions.

Signs of hypocalcaemia include Chvostek's sign and Trosseau's sign (**Figure 7.8**).

- Chvostek's sign is tested for by tapping the facial nerve at the angle of the jaw; the result is positive when facial muscles on the same side contract momentarily as a result of neuromuscular excitability (see **Figure 7.8a**)
- Trosseau's sign is tested for by placing a blood pressure cuff around the patient's upper arm, inflating to a pressure above systolic blood pressure and holding the cuff in position for 3 min; this occludes blood flow through the brachial artery, and without blood flow, neuromuscular irritability caused by hypocalcaemia results in spasm of hand and forearm muscles because of latent tetany (see **Figure 7.8b**)

Hypocalcaemia: causes	
Cause	Key fact(s)
Acquired hypoparathyroidism: parathyroid destruction	Most commonly the result of thyroid or parathyroid surgery
	Can also occur with radiotherapy and infiltration (metastases, sarcoidosis, amyloidosis)
Acquired hypoparathyroidism: reduced secretion of PTH	Occurs with hypomagnesaemia and drugs that decrease PTH secretion (e.g. cinacalcet)
Congenital hypoparathyroidism	Caused by parathyroid agenesis
Hereditary hypoparathyroidism	May occur as part of several rare genetic conditions (e.g. autoimmune polyglandular syndrome type 1)
PTH resistance (pseudohypoparathyroidism)	Inherited forms characterised by tissue resistance to PTH
	Also caused by hypomagnesaemia
Vitamin D deficiency	Common in the general population, especially in those with low exposure to ultraviolet light
	Common in CKD because of impaired conversion of 25-hydroxyvitamin D to 1,25-dihydroxyvitamin D
Vitamin D resistance	Hereditary vitamin D-resistant rickets is a rare condition caused by a mutation in the vitamin D receptor; it presents in early childhood
Alkalosis (e.g. resulting from prolonged hyperventilation)	Precipitates a decrease in ionised calcium and a functional hypocalcaemia
Drugs	Cinacalcet, a calcimimetic, inhibits PTH release
	Chemotherapeutic agents such as cisplatin cause hypomagnesaemic hypocalcaemia
	Bisphosphonates suppress osteoclast activity, which can result in hypocalcaemia
Acute pancreatitis	Hypocalcaemia can result from precipitation of calcium soaps in the abdominal cavity
Hyperphosphataemia	Phosphate binds calcium readily, which can result in hypocalcaemia
Osteoblastic metastases	Certain cancers (e.g. prostate cancer and breast cancer) can cause osteoblastic metastases; these are associated with increased bone formation and avid calcium uptake

CKD, chronic kidney disease; PTH, parathyroid hormone.

Table 7.11 Causes of hypocalcaemia

Clinical features of hypocalcaemia

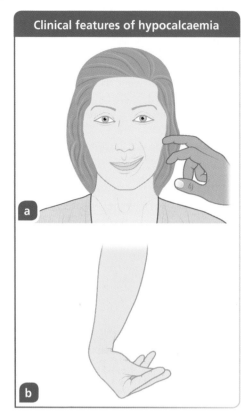

Figure 7.8 Clinical features of hypocalcaemia. (a) Chvostek's sign is a feature of facial nerve hyperexcitability. (b) Trosseau's sign of latent tetany is elicited by compressing the brachial artery with a blood pressure cuff; in the hypocalcaemic patient, this induces muscle spasm in the hand.

Diagnostic approach

Hypocalcaemia is diagnosed when a low corrected value for serum calcium concentration is found on blood tests. Patients with mild hypocalcaemia or those who have developed hypocalcaemia slowly can be asymptomatic, so the finding of hypocalcaemia may be incidental. Patients with acute or severe hypocalcaemia can present with symptoms of neuromuscular excitability that suggest a diagnosis of hypocalcaemia. For this group, urgent assessment and management are required because of the risk of tetany, seizures and cardiac arrhythmias.

Investigations

Investigations are directed towards determining the effects of hypocalcaemia, and determining its cause. They include blood tests, ECG and imaging.

Blood tests

The blood tests listed in **Table 7.12** should be performed on all patients with hypocalcaemia. If pancreatitis is suspected, serum amylase or lipase concentration should also be measured. Urea, creatinine and electolytes are measured primarily to exclude renal impairment, which causes altered calcium homeostasis. Albumin measurement is required to exclude artefactual hypocalcaemia, which occurs when hypoalbuminaemia results in decreased total calcium without any effect on physiologically-active, ionised calcium. In practice, most laboratories provide a corrected calcium result; however, this is less accurate in cases of extreme hypocalcaemia. Renal phosphate excretion is stimulated by PTH so phosphate is low in non-parathyroid-related hypocalcaemia and high in PTH deficiency. Hyperphosphataemia can itself cause hypocalcaemia. PTH measurement also helps distinguish between causes of hypocalcemia; PTH concentration is:

- high if the parathyroid glands are functioning normally
- inappropriately normal or low if they are not

Electrocardiography

In hypocalcaemia, ECG changes include the following (**Figure 7.9**):

- prolonged QT interval, primarily as a result of ST segment prolongation; this is proportional to the degree of hypocalcaemia
- arrhythmias, e.g. ventricular tachycardia and ventricular fibrillation

The T wave is usually unaffected, or mildly reduced in amplitude, because hypocalcaemia does not affect repolarisation.

Investigation of hypocalcaemia: blood tests	
Test	**Rationale**
Urea, creatinine and electrolytes	To exclude renal impairment, and therefore impaired calcium homeostasis
	To exclude disorders of sodium and potassium balance
Albumin	To distinguish true hypocalcemia, a reduction in ionised calcium, from artefactual hypocalcaemia
Phosphate	To help distinguish between causes of hypocalcaemia
Vitamin D	To exclude vitamin D deficiency as a cause of hypocalcaemia
Alkaline phosphatase	Increased alkaline phosphatase can be associated with osteomalacia resulting from vitamin D deficiency
Magnesium	To exclude hypomagnesaemia as a cause of hypocalcaemia
PTH	To help distinguish between causes of hypocalcaemia by indicating parathyroid gland function
PTH, parathyroid hormone.	

Table 7.12 Blood tests used routinely in the investigation of hypocalcaemia

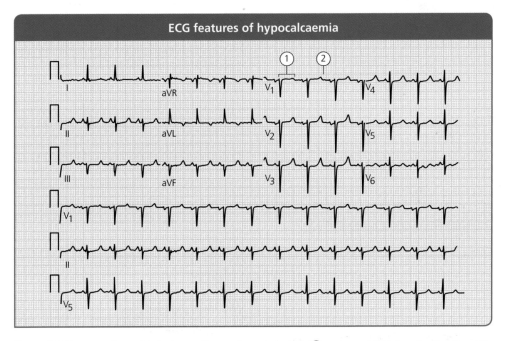

ECG features of hypocalcaemia

Figure 7.9 Electrocardiographic features of hypocalcaemia include ① prolonged QT interval with a long ST segment and ② small T waves.

Imaging

This may be considered to confirm certain diagnoses. Possible studies include radiography and CT.

- Radiography of weight-bearing bones (i.e. pelvis, pubic rami, femoral neck and proximal ribs) is carried out if osteomalacia or rickets is suspected, to look for pathognomonic Looser's zones; these are transverse lucencies that run perpendicular to the surface of the bone and represent incomplete stress fractures
- A CT scan of the chest, abdomen and pelvis may be indicated if malignancy (causing osteoblastic metastases) is suspected

Management

Treatment of hypocalcaemia varies depending on its severity, speed of onset and clinical features. Hypocalcaemia requires urgent treatment if the patient is symptomatic or if the corrected calcium concentration is < 1.9 mmol/L, because the risk of complications such as tetany, seizures and cardiac dysrhythmias is increased.

Medication

For mild, asymptomatic hypocalcaemia (serum corrected calcium > 1.9 mmol/L), calcium supplements are given, along with vitamin D if vitamin D deficiency is present.

If the patient is symptomatic or has a serum corrected calcium concentration < 1.9 mmol/L, urgent replacement is required. First, 10 mL of 10% calcium gluconate is given intravenously over at least 5 minutes. Its effect is short-lived, so it is followed by 40 mL of 10% calcium gluconate in 500 mL of 0.9% saline or 5% dextrose over 24 h. The infusion rate is adjusted up to three or four times a day, until the concentration is within the normal range.

> Intravenous calcium has a sclerosant effect; it induces an inflammatory response that eventually leads to fibrosis. This can occur if it extravasates, i.e. passes out of the vein and into surrounding tissue. Therefore calcium is administered via as large a vein as possible to avoid extravasation.

If hypoparathyroidism is present, 25-hydroxyvitamin D in the form of vitamin D_2 (ergocalciferol) or vitamin D_3 (cholecalciferol) is ineffective, because PTH is needed for the conversion of vitamin D to its active form, 1,25-dihydroxyvitamin D (see page 42). In such cases, alfacalcidol or calcitriol is used (see page 113).

Hypomagnesaemic hypocalcaemia is treated with intravenous magnesium replacement alone. This treatment removes the effect of hypomagnesaemia on PTH secretion and PTH resistance (see **Table 7.11**).

Prognosis

Clinical features usually resolve with normalisation of plasma calcium levels. Chronic hypocalcaemia may lead to osteomalacia because of inadequate mineralisation of bone.

Hypercalcaemia

Hypercalcaemia is defined as a serum calcium concentration > 2.6 mmol/L. It occurs when the rate of the release of calcium into the bloodstream is greater than the rate of its renal excretion or deposition in bone.

This disorder is found both in the community and among hospitalised patients. Primary hyperparathyroidism and malignancy account for about 90% of cases.

Epidemiology

The commonest cause is primary hyperparathyroidism, which has a prevalence of up to 25 cases per 100,000 in the worldwide adult population and is more common in women.

Hypercalcaemia is fairly common in hospital in-patients, predominantly because of the high prevalence of malignancy. It affects up to 30% of patients with cancer.

Aetiology

Hypercalcaemia results from:

- reduced calcium excretion
- increased calcium absorption
- calcium shift between body compartments

It is commonly a consequence of disorders of PTH; causes are classified as PTH-mediated (**Table 7.13**) and non–PTH-mediated (**Table 7.14**). Secondary hyperparathyroidism is included in **Table 7.13** for completeness, but this is associated with a low or normal calcium concentration.

PTH-mediated hypercalcaemia: pathophysiology and clinical features		
Cause	Pathophysiology	Clinical features
Primary hyperparathyroidism	Excessive PTH secretion by parathyroid gland causes excessive resorption of calcium from bone	Symptoms of hypercalcaemia (see below) Osteopenia
Secondary hyperparathyroidism (causes hypercalcaemia when prolonged, merging into tertiary hyperparathyroidism)	Excessive PTH production due to chronic hyperphosphataemia, hypocalcaemia and impaired vitamin D production in CKD	Renal osteodystrophy Cardiovascular calcification Soft tissue calcification Symptoms of CKD (see page 162)
Tertiary hyperparathyroidism	Excessive PTH production following prolonged secondary hyperparathyroidism Characterised by parathyroid gland hypertrophy and autonomous PTH secretion	Symptoms of hypercalcaemia Renal osteodystrophy Cardiovascular calcification Soft tissue calcification Symptoms of CKD (see page 162) Persists after renal transplantation

CKD, chronic kidney disease; PTH, parathyroid hormone.

Table 7.13 Causes of parathyroid hormone-mediated hypercalcaemia, and their pathophysiology and clinical features

Clinical features

The clinical features of hypercalcaemia depend on the underlying cause, the severity of the biochemical abnormality, the rate at which it develops and the chronicity. Mild but chronic hypercalcaemia produces symptoms related to calcium deposition in tissues (joint pain) and increased renal calcium excretion (renal stones), whereas more severe or acute onset hypercalcaemia results in clinical features caused by the following (Table 7.15).

- nephrogenic diabetes insipidus, i.e. polyuria and nocturia
- increased calcium-induced gastrin release in the stomach, resulting in dyspepsia
- abnormal neuromuscular and cardiac function as a result of an increased threshold for depolarisation within excitable tissues (e.g. weakness, lethargy and cardiac arrhythmias)
- neuropsychiatric effects (e.g. depression)

Diagnostic approach

Hypercalcaemia is diagnosed when blood test results show increased serum calcium concentration. This may be an incidental finding in an asymptomatic patient, or an anticipated finding in a patient presenting with a set of symptoms suggesting hypercalcaemia.

A crucial part of the investigation of hypercalcaemia is establishing the underlying cause. This may be apparent from the history, for example excessive use of calcium supplements, or the examination, for example the finding of a mass, suggesting malignancy. However, it also entails further blood tests, ECG and imaging.

Investigations

A number of investigations are required to determine the cause of hypercalcaemia and to assess for complications.

Blood tests

In the investigation of hypercalcaemia, the possible blood tests are:

- corrected calcium concentration, to confirm hypercalcaemia
- serum urea, creatinine and electrolytes, to exclude renal impairment and other electrolyte disorders

Non-PTH-mediated hypercalcaemia: pathophysiology and clinical features

Cause	Pathophysiology	Clinical features
Malignancy ■ Breast cancer ■ Lung cancer ■ Myeloma ■ Lymphoma	Osteolytic metastases with release of osteoclast-activating factors Tumour secretion of parathyroid hormone-related protein Tumour secretion of 1,25-dihydroxyvitamin D	Symptoms associated with underlying malignancy Symptoms of hypercalcaemia Pathological fractures (in cases of osteolytic metastases)
Use of thiazide diuretics (increased renal absorption)	Decreased renal calcium excretion	Hypercalcaemia more likely to occur if increased bone resorption or primary hyperparathyroidism already present
Vitamin D intoxication	Excessive intestinal absorption of calcium and excessive renal reabsorption of calcium	Clinical features of hypercalcaemia Cardiovascular and soft tissue calcification if chronic
Use of calcium-containing drugs	Increased intestinal absorption of calcium	Clinical features of hypercalcaemia
Granulomatous disease ■ Sarcoidosis ■ Tuberculosis ■ Crohn's disease	Excessive production of 1,25-dihydroxyvitamin D as a result of presence of 1α-hydroxylase in macrophages and giant cells that form the granuloma	Clinical features of hypercalcaemia Symptoms associated with underlying disease
Familial hypocalciuric hypercalcaemia	Inactivating mutations in the calcium-sensing receptor gene, resulting in hyposensitivity to calcium, hypercalcaemia and low renal calcium excretion	Autosomal dominant inheritance Hypercalcaemia often asymptomatic PTH not suppressed Normal renal function
Miscellaneous	Thyrotoxicosis, prolonged immobilisation leading to increased bone resorption	Clinical features of underlying disease

PTH, parathyroid hormone.

Table 7.14 Causes of non-parathyroid hormone-mediated hypercalcaemia, and their pathophysiology and clinical features

- phosphate, to help differentiate between causes of hypercalcaemia
- albumin, to enable calculation of the corrected calcium concentration
- alkaline phosphatase, because an increased concentration in the context of hypercalcaemia suggests bony metastases, thyrotoxicosis or sarcoidosis
- PTH, to help differentiate between causes of hypercalcaemia
- thyroid function tests, to exclude thyrotoxicosis
- full blood count, to exclude anaemia and infection
- myeloma screen (if myeloma is suspected), i.e. serum protein electrophoresis, immunoglobulins and erythrocyte sedimentation rate, along with urinary Bence Jone protein, to exclude myeloma as a cause of hypercalcaemia

Serum calcium concentration is best checked by using a sample obtained without the use of a tourniquet. Use of a tourniquet causes haemoconcentration, i.e. increased concentration of cells and proteins, including calcium-carrying albumin, in the blood; this can lead to a falsely increased calcium concentration when the sample is analysed.

Electrocardiography

Hypercalcaemia can cause a shortening of the QT interval.

Imaging

In patients with hypercalcaemia, radiography of the chest is carried out to look for evidence of malignancy, for example,

System or organ	Complication	Clinical features	Mechanism
Hypercalcaemia: complications and their clinical features			
Biliary tract	Gallstones	Right upper quadrant pain, nausea, vomiting, fever resulting from cholecystitis	Calcium precipitation in bile
Pancreas	Pancreatitis	Epigastric pain radiating to the back, nausea, vomiting, systemic inflammatory response syndrome	Activation of digestive enzymes within pancreatic acinar cells
Muscle	Impaired function	Muscle weakness	Increased threshold for depolarisation within muscle cells
Bones and joints	Chondrocalcinosis	Joint pain, swelling and redness	Deposition of calcium salts in connective tissue
	Pathological fractures	Bone pain	Altered bone metabolism
Central nervous system	Impaired function	Lethargy, anxiety, depression, confusion, drowsiness, coma	Altered nerve conduction in central nervous system
Heart	Impaired function	Bradycardia, arrhythmia, short QT interval	Altered membrane potentials and cardiac conduction
Kidneys	Renal stones	Loin pain, nausea, vomiting	Increased urinary calcium excretion
	Nephrogenic diabetes insipidus	Thirst and polyuria	Impaired urine concentration
	Volume depletion	Thirst, tachycardia, hypotension, cool peripheries, prolonged capillary refill time	Increased renal excretion of water and sodium
	Renal failure	Nausea, anorexia, lethargy, hyperkalaemia, metabolic acidosis	Decreased glomerular filtration rate as a result of volume depletion
			Renal tract obstruction caused by stones
Gastrointestinal tract	Impaired function	Nausea, vomiting, anorexia	Centrally mediated because of altered neurological function
		Constipation	Impaired peristalsis, volume depletion
		Dyspepsia	Increased gastrin production
		Abdominal pain	Sluggish peristalsis, constipation, renal stones

Table 7.15 Complications of hypercalcaemia, and their clinical features

respiratory primary malignancy or metastases, and sarcoidosis, for example hilar lymphadenopathy. In cases of hyperparathyroidism, signs of bone demineralisation may also be present. Further imaging, for example CT, to exclude malignancy may also be required.

Management

The aims are to lower the serum calcium concentration to a safe level and treat the cause of hypercalcaemia. Attempts to lower serum calcium, using intravenous fluids and medications, are made in any patient with a corrected calcium > 3 mmol/L, unless this is long-standing and the patient is completely asymptomatic. Drugs that contain calcium, for example Calcichew D_3 (a combination of calcium carbonate and vitamin D_3) or induce hypercalcaemia, for example thiazide diuretics, are stopped.

Medication

Choice of medications depends on the severity of the biochemical abnormality and the response to treatment. For example, mild hypercalcaemia may respond to treatment with fluids only, whereas more severe hypercalcaemia requires medication.

Intravenous fluids

Patients with hypercalcaemia usually have volume depletion caused by nephrogenic diabetes insipidus and inadequate fluid intake. This is corrected by administration of 0.9% saline. Calciuresis is promoted by ensuring a urine output of 200 mL/h.

Furosemide

Oral or intravenous furosemide increases urine flow and promotes calciuresis. However, it is used with caution because of potential effects on fluid balance (hypovolaemia) and electrolyte derangements (e.g. hypokalaemia). Regular assessment of volume status is essential to avoid hypovolaemia.

Bisphosphonates

If serum calcium remains high despite 24 h of adequate intravenous fluid therapy, a bisphosphonate, for example pamidronate or zoledronic acid, is given. Serum calcium should begin to decrease after 24–48 h; however, it takes 4–5 days for the peak effect to be apparent.

Cinacalcet

This drug mimics the effect of calcium on tissues by activating the calcium-sensing receptor on cell membranes. It is therefore called a 'calcimimetic'. Cinacalcet may be considered for patients with CKD and secondary or tertiary hyperparathyroidism. Note that secondary hyperparathyroidism is not associated with hypercalcaemia.

Surgery

Parathyroidectomy may be required for patients with chronic hypercalcaemia secondary to primary or tertiary hyperparathyroidism.

Prognosis

This depends largely on the cause. For example, significant hypercalcaemia caused by hyperparathyroidism can be effectively treated with a parathyroidectomy. Conversely, hypercalcaemia resulting from an untreatable metastatic malignancy is associated with poor survival. In CKD with tertiary hyperparathyroidism, chronic hypercalcaemia associated with hyperphosphataemia, results in vascular calcification. This contributes significantly to the high rate of cardiovascular morbidity and mortality in patients with renal disease.

Hypophosphataemia

Hypophosphataemia is a serum phosphate concentration < 0.8 mmol/L. It is found in up to 5% of patients admitted to hospital but is more common in the critically ill, of whom it can affect up to 80%.

- Mild to moderate hypophosphataemia (0.3–0.7 mmol/L) is usually asymptomatic and is often detected incidentally
- Severe hypophosphataemia (< 0.3 mmol/L) can result in non-specific symptoms such as muscular weakness and altered mental status

Aetiology

Causes of hypophosphataemia include the following (**Table 7.16**):

- inadequate intake or decreased intestinal absorption of phosphate
- increased renal excretion of phosphate
- redistribution of phosphate from the extracellular space to the intracellular space

Clinical features

Symptoms of hypophosphataemia depend on the severity and duration of phosphate depletion. Mild hypophosphataemia (0.5–0.7 mmol/L) is usually asymptomatic. However, severe hypophosphataemia (< 0.3 mmol/L) can have clinically significant effects. These result from impaired cellular function as a result of decreased formation of essential phosphate-containing compounds such as

Hypophosphataemia: mechanisms and causes	
Mechanism	Causes
Inadequate intake or decreased intestinal absorption	Vitamin D deficiency
	Phosphate binders
	Enteral nutrition with inadequate phosphate
	Parenteral nutrition with inadequate phosphate
Increased renal excretion	Primary hyperparathyroidism
	Phosphate-wasting syndromes, e.g. Fanconi's syndrome (congenital/acquired proximal tubulopathy results in decreased reabsorption of glucose, amino acids, bicarbonate, phosphate)
Redistribution	Respiratory alkalosis: stimulates phosphofructokinase and formation of phosphate glycolytic intermediaries, thereby driving phosphate into cells
	Recovery phase of diabetic ketoacidosis: increased phosphate uptake into phosphate-deplete tissues
	Refeeding syndrome: increased phosphate uptake into phosphate-deplete tissues
Other	Alcohol withdrawal: multifactorial

Table 7.16 Mechanisms underlying and causes of hypophosphataemia

adenosine triphosphate (ATP) and 2,3-diphosphoglycerate. Depletion of ATP affects all cell types, particularly the most metabolically active, i.e. those in the brain and muscles.

Common consequences include:

- rhabdomyolysis, which results in muscle weakness
- impaired neurological function, which causes confusion, seizures and coma
- haemolysis and impaired white blood cell function

Because 2,3-diphosphoglycerate acts to decrease the affinity of oxygen for haemoglobin, a decrease shifts the oxyhaemoglobin dissociation curve to the left. This results in decreased oxygen delivery to the tissues.

Management

Management is focused on preventing or treating conditions in which hypophosphataemia may occur, and replacing phosphate. In mild to moderate hypophosphataemia, oral supplementation is used. However, in severe or symptomatic hypophosphataemia, intravenous replacement is required.

> **Careful monitoring is required when administering intravenous phosphate replacement,** because of the risk of electrolyte disorders, such as hypocalcaemia, and cardiac arrhythmias.

Hyperphosphataemia

Hyperphosphataemia is an increased serum phosphate concentration, i.e. >1.4 mmol/L. It occurs infrequently in the general population but is common in individuals with CKD, affecting up to 70% of this group. Incidence increases with age because of the increased prevalence of CKD in the elderly.

Aetiology

The commonest cause is CKD (**Table 7.17**), in which hyperphosphataemia results from impaired renal phosphate excretion. It also occurs:

Hyperphosphataemia: mechanisms and causes	
Mechanism	**Causes**
Increased phosphate intake	Phosphate-rich total parenteral nutrition
	Excessive use of phosphate enemas
Increased phosphate absorption in gastrointestinal tract and renal tract	Vitamin D intoxication
Decreased phosphate excretion	Acute kidney injury
	Chronic kidney disease
	Hypoparathyroidism
	Pseudohypoparathyroidism
Shift of phosphate from intracellular to extracellular space	Tumour lysis syndrome
	Rhabdomyolysis
	Haemolysis
Artefactual hyperphosphataemia	Haemolysis of blood sample
	Paraproteinaemia (because of interference with laboratory techniques)

Table 7.17 Mechanisms underlying and causes of hyperphosphataemia

- with increased phosphate intake, for example when phosphate-rich total parenteral nutrition (TPN) is used
- under circumstances in which phosphate moves from the intracellular space to the extracellular space, for example in states of cell breakdown such as rhabdomyolysis, when intracellular contents are released into the circulation

Clinical features

Hyperphosphataemia is usually asymptomatic but can result in clinically significant sequelae. Because of inhibition of 1-hydroxylation of 25-hydroxyvitamin D_3 (25-hydroxycholecalciferol) in the kidney, hyperphosphataemia can lead to a decrease in activation of vitamin D (see page 43); this, in turn, can cause hypocalcaemia.

Phosphate may combine with calcium and precipitate in soft tissues, particularly when hyperphosphataemia is long-standing, as in CKD. This can affect solid organs, cardiac tissue and muscle. Prolonged hyperphosphataemaia also promotes vascular calcification.

Increased uptake of phosphate by vascular smooth muscle cells induces an osteochondrogenic phenotypic change, resulting in mineralisation of the extracellular matrix. This results in arteriosclerosis and increased blood pressure.

Phosphate concentrations are affected by calcium homeostasis. Vitamin D increases phosphate uptake in the gut. PTH mobilises phosphate from bone but is also phosphaturic, so some excess phosphate is excreted.

Management

Management is directed towards the underlying cause, when possible, for example by changing the composition of TPN in TPN-associated hyperphosphataemia and by following a low-phosphate diet in CKD. Oral calcium salts and polymers such as sevelamer are given to bind phosphate in the gut and reduce its absorption (see page 112).

Hypomagnesaemia

Hypomagnesaemia is a serum magnesium concentration < 0.7 mmol/L. Plasma magnesium concentrations are maintained between 0.7 and 1.2 mmol/L. They are affected by dietary intake, renal handling and gastrointestinal absorption. Hypomagnesaemia occurs in less than 2% of the general population, but up to 20% of hospital in-patients. It is more common in the intensive care setting, affecting up to 60% of patients, and in hospital inpatients with alcoholism, affecting up to 30%.

Mild hypomagnesamia, i.e. serum magnesium 0.5–0.7 mmol/L, is usually asymptomatic. However, severe hypomagnesaemia (< 0.3 mmol/L) is a medical emergency because of the potential for cardiac arrhythmias.

Hypomagnesaemia is usually associated with other electrolyte abnormalities, particularly hypokalaemia and hypocalcaemia. Factors such as diuretic use and diarrhoea can cause both hypomagnesaemia and hypokalaemia. Hypomagnesaemia can also increase renal potassium loss directly and it can cause hypocalcaemia by impairing PTH release and promoting skeletal uptake of calcium in exchange for magnesium release.

Aetiology

Usually the cause is magnesium deficiency due to:

- malnutrition or malabsorption
- parathyroid disorders
- chronic alcoholism and alcohol withdrawal
- chronic diarrhoea
- long-term use of proton pump inhibitors
- renal disorders that impair magnesium reabsorption (e.g. acute tubular necrosis, renal tubular acidosis and post-obstructive diuresis)
- use of certain drugs (e.g. diuretics, cisplatin)
- chronic mineralocorticoid excess

Magnesium is the fourth most abundant cation in the body. It is:

- a cofactor for many enzyme processes using ATP and nucleic acid metabolism
- mostly present in bone, muscle and other soft tissues; about 1–2% is present in extracellular fluid
- involved in regulation of PTH secretion

Clinical features

Symptoms of hypomagnesaemia are nonspecific. They include:

- decreased appetite
- weakness and lethargy
- vomiting
- tetany
- agitation
- delirium
- ataxia, tremor and convulsions
- cardiac arrhythmias

These are largely the result of altered neuromuscular function, effects on cardiac electrophysiology and the propensity to cause hypokalaemia and hypocalcaemia.

Investigations

Serum magnesium, protein, calcium, phosphate and potassium, are measured to confirm hypomagnesaemia and exclude coexisting electrolyte abnormalities.

Electrocardiographic changes include:

- prolonged QTc interval
- tall T waves
- ST depression
- atrial and ventricular ectopic beats
- atrial tachyarrhythmias
- torsade de pointes

Management

Mild, asymptomatic hypomagnesaemia (> 0.5 mmol/L) is managed with oral magnesium salts. Severe (< 0.5 mmol/L) or symptomatic hypomagnesaemia requires intravenous replacement with magnesium sulphate.

Hypermagnesaemia

Hypermagnesaemia is a serum magnesium concentration > 1 mmol/L. It is uncommon but occurs in up to 15% of in-patients, usually due to decreased magnesium excretion as a result of renal failure. Other causes of hypermagnesaemia include ingestion of medications containing magnesium and TPN.

Clinical features

Hypermagnesaemia is usually asymptomatic until serum magnesium concentration exceeds 2 mmol/L. Neuromuscular symptoms occur because hypermagnesaemia results in blockage of neuromuscular transmission;

these include loss of deep tendon reflexes, weakness, paraesthesia, paralysis, respiratory depression and seizures. Cardiac conduction is also affected, leading to depressed sinoatrial node activity and atrial fibrillation. Cardiac arrest can occur if serum magnesium exceeds 6 mmol/L.

Investigations

Key investigations include:

- serum magnesium to confirm the presence of hypermagnesaemia
- serum potassium and calcium, because hyperkalaemia and hypercalcaemia often coexist with hypermagnesaemia
- thyroid function tests and early morning cortisol if hypermagnesaemia is recurrent, to exclude hypothyroidism and adrenal insufficiency, which can cause a mild increase in serum magnesium
- ECG to exclude cardiac arrhythmias

Management

Hypermagnesaemia is prevented in patients who are at risk, for example those with renal impairment and receiving magnesium supplements, by monitoring serum magnesium concentration and withdrawing supplements when it has normalised.

If hypermagnesaemia is symptomatic with cardiac effects or respiratory depression, treatment is required. This may include one or more of the following:

- intravenous calcium gluconate 10% (10 mL intravenously over 30 s) in a high-dependency setting with ECG monitoring, to antagonise the effect of hypermagnesaemia
- loop diuretics (if urine output is normal) co-prescribed with intravenous fluid (e.g. 0.9% saline) to enhance renal magnesium loss
- dialysis in patients with renal impairment and severe symptomatic hypermagnesaemia (> 4 mmol/L) or with cardiac or neuromuscular symptoms (regardless of concentration)
- enemas to improve gastrointestinal clearance
- cessation of any medications containing magnesium (e.g. laxatives or antacids)

Answers to starter questions

1. Serum and urine osmolality help identify the cause of hyponatraemia because the difference between them indicates the site and nature of the underlying pathophysiological disturbance. Decreased serum osmolality with increased urine osmolality implies excess water absorption in the kidney and suggests a diagnosis of the syndrome of inappropriate anti-diuretic hormone secretion (SIADH). Increased serum osmolality indicates the presence of additional osmotically active substances such as glucose, mannitol, ethanol and urea in advanced chronic kidney disease. Low urine osmolality and low serum osmolality suggests water intoxication; this is a rare condition caused by the administration or consumption of water at a rate which exceeds the kidneys' ability to eliminate the water load.

2. The difference between intra-and extracellular potassium concentration determines a cell's resting potential, i.e. its ability to conduct electrical signals as action potentials. Abnormal potassium concentrations therefore disrupt excitable tissues and can result in dangerous neuromuscular and cardiac complications, such as heart arrhythmias.

Answers *continued*

3. Dehydration describes a loss of total body water resulting in hypertonicity, whereas volume depletion is a reduction in the volume of the extracellular space, including the effective circulating volume in the intravascular space. This is an important distinction, because treating dehydration only requires the administration of water (if given intravenously then 5% glucose is used), whereas treatment of volume depletion requires water plus solutes (usually given as 0.9% sodium chloride).

4. Calcium gluconate helps stabilise the membrane of cardiac myocytes against undesirable depolarisation. It therefore 'protects' the heart from arrhythmias. In treating hyperkalaemia, intravenous calcium gluconate is given for this immediate protective effect, while longer lasting measures are instituted.

Chapter 8
Acid–base disorders

Starter questions

Answers to the following questions are on page 267.

1. How does calculation of the anion gap help to establish the cause of a metabolic acidosis?
2. When can a venous, rather than arterial, blood gas be useful in assessing acid-base balance?
3. How does the respiratory system compensate for metabolic abnormalities?
4. Why does metabolic activity generate acid?
5. Why is acidosis associated with heavy breathing? When is it not associated with this?

Introduction

Changes in plasma pH alter the structure and function of macromolecules, and the efficiency of biochemical reactions. The body therefore has multiple buffering systems to keep plasma pH close to the optimal level of 7.35–7.45 (see page 45). Acid–base disorders occur when these systems are overwhelmed by an underlying pathological process that has one of two origins:

- Respiratory, e.g. when CO_2 is retained in the blood by respiratory failure
- Metabolic, e.g. increased production of ketone bodies in diabetic ketoacidosis

These processes cause either an increase or decrease in plasma pH:

- Acidosis is a decrease in plasma pH (< 7.35)
- Alkalosis is an increase in plasma pH (> 7.45)

Acid–base disorders are categorised according to whether they are either respiratory or metabolic, and cause either acidosis or alkalosis.

In a healthy person, small disturbances in plasma pH are corrected by compensatory mechanisms (see page 46). Acid–base disturbances with a respiratory cause are partially compensated (plasma pH is partially corrected) by normal metabolic compensatory mechanisms, and disturbances with a metabolic cause are compensated via the respiratory system (Chapter 1 pages 46–49, **Figure 8.1**).

Intermediate and final products of many metabolic processes are acidic (e.g. carbon dioxide, various organic and inorganic acids) therefore acidosis is seen more frequently than

alkalosis. A mild degree of acidosis is often found in common diseases such as chronic obstructive pulmonary disease (where it is respiratory in origin) and chronic kidney disease (metabolic in origin).

The fundamental principle of managing acid–base disorders is to address the underlying cause; it is rare that direct correction of the acidosis or alkalosis is indicated.

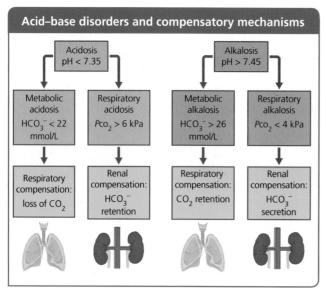

Figure 8.1 Acid–base disorders and their physiological compensatory mechanisms. Respiratory compensation for metabolic acid–base disturbances occurs quickly (minutes to hours), whereas renal compensation takes several days to reach its maximal effect.

Case 8 No passage of urine for over 24 h

Presentation

Donald Brooks, who is 90 years old, presents to the emergency department having not passed urine for over 24 h.

Initial interpretation

Passing no urine for 24 hours (anuria) suggests acute kidney injury (AKI; see Chapter 3). AKI has pre-renal, renal and post-renal causes, but the presence of anuria suggests an obstruction (a post-renal cause). In a man of this age a prostatic cause is most probable. Asking Mr Brooks about any acute illnesses over the past few days (e.g. severe diarrhoea

and vomiting that could have caused prerenal AKI), any new drugs that could have caused intrinsic renal AKI or a history of prostatic symptoms (e.g. nocturia, hesitancy, terminal dribbling) to suggest postrenal AKI will help determine the cause of his anuria.

Further history

Mr Brooks has had increasing difficulty passing urine for several months. Over the past few days, he has passed minimal amounts of urine and has passed nothing for 24 h. He complains of lower abdominal discomfort and feeling generally unwell.

Case 8 *continued*

Post-renal AKI: emergency presentation

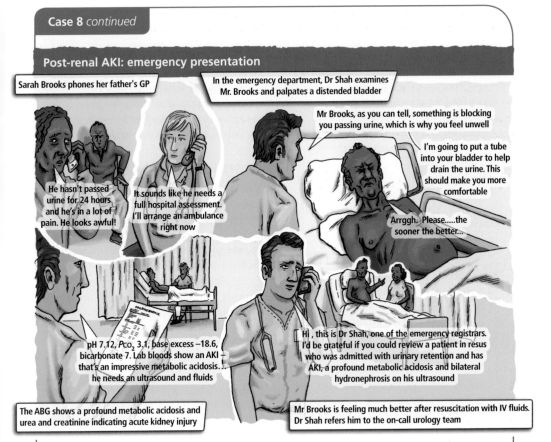

Sarah Brooks phones her father's GP

In the emergency department, Dr Shah examines Mr. Brooks and palpates a distended bladder

He hasn't passed urine for 24 hours and he's in a lot of pain. He looks awful!

It sounds like he needs a full hospital assessment. I'll arrange an ambulance right now

Mr Brooks, as you can tell, something is blocking you passing urine, which is why you feel unwell

I'm going to put a tube into your bladder to help drain the urine. This should make you more comfortable

Arrggh. Please.....the sooner the better...

pH 7.12, Pco₂ 3.1, base excess −18.6, bicarbonate 7. Lab bloods show an AKI – that's an impressive metabolic acidosis. he needs an ultrasound and fluids

Hi , this is Dr Shah, one of the emergency registrars. I'd be grateful if you could review a patient in resus who was admitted with urinary retention and has AKI, a profound metabolic acidosis and bilateral hydronephrosis on his ultrasound

The ABG shows a profound metabolic acidosis and urea and creatinine indicating acute kidney injury

Mr Brooks is feeling much better after resuscitation with IV fluids. Dr Shah refers him to the on-call urology team

Examination

On examination, Mr Brooks is drowsy but easily rousable. He is also slightly tachypnoeic, breathing at 20 breaths per minute. He is warm and well perfused; on auscultation his chest is clear and his heart sounds are normal. His abdomen is soft. There is suprapubic tenderness and a suprapubic mass that is dull to percussion. A digital rectal examination shows a smoothly enlarged prostate.

Interpretation of findings

Drowsiness has various causes, including sepsis and acidaemia. The tachypnoea could reflect:

- a primary respiratory problem, for example pneumonia
- a cardiac problem, for example congestive cardiac failure or acute coronary syndrome

- a physiological response to sepsis, hypovolaemia or acidaemia

These will be excluded by the history, examination and investigation findings. The history of decreased urine output with examination findings of a suprapubic mass (indicating a palpable bladder) suggest that the cause of Mr Brooks's presentation is an obstructive uropathy. Obstructions can affect any part of the urinary tract, but the palpable bladder indicates that this is a bladder outflow problem most likely to be due to the prostate: either benign hypertrophy or prostate cancer (although cancer is unlikely because of the smooth enlargement). An urethral stricture is another much less likely possibility.

Investigations

Blood tests, including an assessment of renal function and acid–base status, are routine investigations in cases of suspected AKI and the results are shown in **Table 8.1**.

Because a suprapubic mass was palpable, a bladder scan is carried out. There is > 1 L of urine in Mr Brooks's bladder.

The baseline creatinine concentration of 113 μmol/L 4 months ago was only just above the upper limit of the normal range. This means there was a significant decrease in glomerular filtration rate at this time that might be chronic. The most recent urea and creatinine test results show that there has been an acute deterioration in renal function.

The blood gas results show:

- Metabolic acidosis (low pH and low bicarbonate). The bicarbonate has been used up buffering the retained acid products of metabolism
- Respiratory compensation (low P_{CO_2}). Acidosis increases respiration, meaning more CO_2 has been expired ('blown off') than usual. This helps restore the ratio of CO_2 to bicarbonate, with the intention of correcting the blood pH

After the bladder scan, a catheter is inserted into Mr Brooks's bladder and 1.5 L of urine is drained. A subsequent ultrasound scan of the renal tract shows bilateral hydronephrosis, i.e. dilatation of the pelvicalyceal system (the renal pelvis and calyces) caused by the outflow of urine from below the renal pelvis being obstructed. It also shows bilateral hydroureter (dilatation of the ureters, due to obstruction to the flow of urine down the ureter).

Diagnosis

The increase in Mr Brooks' serum urea and creatinine concentrations confirms the presence of AKI. A metabolic acidosis has occurred because the kidneys are unable to excrete waste acids, allowing them to build up in the blood. Bilateral hydronephrosis and hydroureter point towards an obstruction distal to the ureters. The enlarged prostate detected on examination suggests the obstruction is due to prostatic hypertrophy which, from the history, has been present for some time. This has caused a build-up of urine, and therefore pressure, on both sides of the urinary tract, causing damage to the kidneys at the level of the nephron. The overall picture is of AKI with a postrenal cause. Mr Brooks is referred to the urology team, who confirm that the post-renal AKI is due to acute-on-chronic urinary retention secondary to prostatic hypertrophy.

Donald Brooks's blood test results		
Test	Result	Normal range
Urea and electrolytes		
Sodium	134 mmol/L	135–145
Potassium	5.9 mmol/L	3.3–5.3
Urea	24.6 mmol/L	2.5–7.5
Creatinine	376 μmol/L (113 μmol/L 4 months ago)	58–110
Arterial blood gases (on room air)		
pH	7.12	7.35–7.45
P_aCO_2	3.1 kPa	4.7–6.0
P_aO_2	10.3 kPa	> 10
Base excess	-18.6 mmol/L	± 2
Bicarbonate	7 mmol/L	22–26
Lactate	2.4 mmol/L	0.7–2.1

P_aCO_2, arterial partial pressure of carbon dioxide; P_aO_2, arterial partial pressure of oxygen.

Table 8.1 Blood test results for Donald Brooks

Case 9 2 days of vomiting

Presentation

Michael Parks, a 21-year-old student, is referred to the emergency department by his GP, with a 2-day history of nausea and vomiting. He is unable to keep any fluids or food down and is feeling very unwell. He says his flatmate has recently been unwell with similar symptoms. He has no diarrhoea or abdominal pain.

Initial interpretation

Michael has a 2-day history of vomiting without diarrhoea or abdominal pain. His flatmate being unwell with similar symptoms suggests that he has an infection.

The vast majority of gastrointestinal symptoms secondary to an infection (e.g. norovirus) settle without any particular intervention. However, the fact that Mi-

chael feels unwell enough to attend the emergency department suggests that this is more serious.

Further history

Michael has no other medical problems and is normally fit and well. He has not recently been abroad or eaten any unusual foods so his symptoms are unlikely to be due to travel-related or food-borne infections.

Examination

On examination, Michael has:

- a blood pressure of 97/50 mmHg
- a heart rate of 110 bpm
- a respiratory rate of 9 breaths/min
- oxygen saturation of 96% on room air

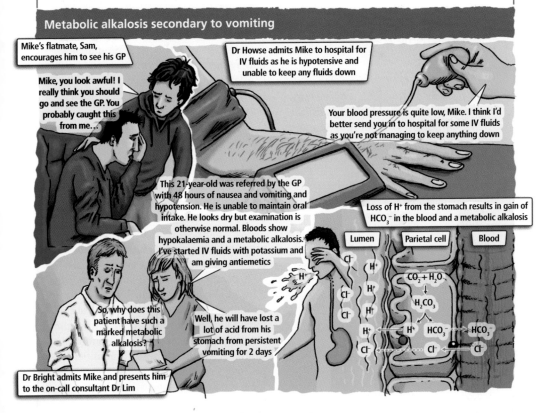

Metabolic alkalosis secondary to vomiting

Case 9 *continued*

He has decreased skin turgor and dry mucous membranes. His abdomen is soft and non-tender, and his bowel sounds are normal.

Interpretation of findings

Michael is mildly hypotensive and tachy-cardic, with a low respiratory rate and normal oxygen saturation on room air. This suggests that he has lost a significant amount of fluid, but that any resulting reduced tissue perfusion has not led to an acidosis, which would have increased his respiratory rate.

Decreased skin turgor, i.e. a pinched fold of skin over the upper chest that takes longer to relax back to normal, and dry mucous membranes, for example a dry tongue, are clinical signs of volume deple-tion (see Figure 3.7). Given that Michael has had no diarrhoea and his abdomen is soft and non-tender, it appears that his lower gastrointestinal tract is not signifi-cantly affected by the infection.

Investigations

Blood tests, including urea and electro-lytes and arterial blood gas analysis, are carried out to assess renal function and acid–base status; the results are shown in **Table 8.2**.

Breathing affects the acidity of the blood, because carbon dioxide is acidic when dissolved in plasma. Therefore changes in respiratory rate affect plasma pH:

- hyperventilation 'blows off' carbon dioxide, increasing the blood's pH. It is a normal response to a metabolic acidosis

- hypoventilation is a compensatory response to alkalosis. Carbon dioxide is retained, lowering the plasma pH

Michael Parks's blood test results

Test	Result	Normal range
Urea and electrolytes		
Sodium	135 mmol/L	135–145
Potassium	2.9 mmol/L	3.3–5.3
Urea	9.3 mmol/L	2.5–7.5
Creatinine	85 µmol/L	58–110
Arterial blood gases on room air		
pH	7.49	7.35–7.45
P_aco_2	6.9 kPa	4.7–6.0
P_ao_2	11 kPa	(>10)
Base excess	5 mmol/L	± 2
Bicarbonate	35 mmol/L	22–26
Lactate	1.4 mmol/L	0.7–2.1

P_ao_2, arterial partial pressure of oxygen; P_aco_2, arterial partial pressure of carbon dioxide.

Table 8.2 Blood test results for Michael Parks

Diagnosis

Two days of vomiting with no diarrhoea and recent contact with a friend with similar symptoms suggest that Michael has acquired a 'vomiting bug' such as norovirus.

The increased pH and high bicarbonate concentration confirm a metabolic alkalo-sis. The arterial partial pressure of carbon dioxide (P_aco_2) has increased as a conse-quence of respiratory compensation as the body attempts to decrease pH back to normal, i.e. increase the concentration of hydrogen ions by reducing the respiratory rate. This prevents loss of carbon dioxide, increases P_aco_2 and decreases blood pH.

It is unusual for vomiting to result in a metabolic alkalosis, but it is seen if the vomiting is prolonged because of the sus-tained loss of hydrochloric acid from the stomach. Michael is given intravenous flu-ids (0.9% sodium chloride) and antiemet-ics, and his vomiting stops. He rapidly feels much better and is discharged the following day.

Diagnosis of acid–base disorders

Acid–base disorders are diagnosed by measuring the changes in plasma pH, partial pressure of carbon dioxide, bicarbonate and base excess (**Table 8.3**), typically with a blood gas machine. These measurements also show the changes that take place as the body attempts to restore plasma pH to the optimal level of 7.35–7.45.

The Davenport diagram (**Figure 8.2**) is a useful conceptual tool for summarising the changes in pH, bicarbonate and carbon dioxide, and the effects of compensation (although it is not used much in clinical practice). A more clinically useful stepwise method for interpreting blood gas results is shown in **Table 8.4**.

Multiple disorders

In many cases more than one acid–base disorder is present, giving a 'mixed picture'. In these cases, interpretation of the blood gas results requires consideration of the clinical context. For example, a patient with acute kidney injury and a metabolic acidosis could have a concurrent pneumonia with inadequate respiratory compensation, resulting in a respiratory acidosis.

Acid–base abnormalities: key features			
Normal value or abnormality	Blood pH	P_{CO_2}	Bicarbonate concentration
Normal value	7.35–7.45	4.7–6 kPa	22–26 mmol/L
Metabolic acidosis	Decreased	Decreased	Decreased
Metabolic alkalosis	Increased	Normal or increased	Increased
Respiratory acidosis	Decreased	Increased	Normal (acutely) Increased (chronically)
Respiratory alkalosis	Increased (can be normal chronically)	Decreased	Normal (acutely) Decreased (chronically)

P_{CO_2}, partial pressure of carbon dioxide.

Table 8.3 Key features of acid–base abnormalities

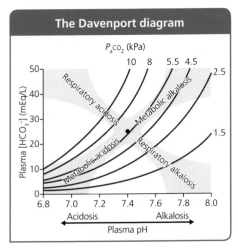

The Davenport diagram

P_aCO_2 (kPa)

Figure 8.2 The Davenport diagram aids diagnosis of acid–base disorders. Plasma pH, bicarbonate concentration and the arterial partial pressure of carbon dioxide (P_aCO_2) are plotted. The latter two are direct determinants of pH, and their proportions indicate whether the cause is metabolic or respiratory. By plotting a set of values on the diagram, it is easy to determine the primary acid–base abnormality and the level of compensation, which gives some indication of the duration of the underlying problem. The black dot in the centre marks normal values.

Interpretation of blood gas results		
Step	Question	Rationale
1	What is the pH?	Is there an acidosis or an alkalosis?
2	What is the P_{CO_2}?	Is it causing the problem or compensating for the problem? ■ Acidosis and low P_{CO_2}: metabolic acidosis with respiratory compensation is likely ■ Acidosis with high P_{CO_2}: respiratory acidosis is present
3	What is the bicarbonate concentration?	A primarily metabolic disturbance is likely if there is: ■ acidosis with low bicarbonate ■ alkalosis with high bicarbonate
4	What is the base excess?	The base excess measures all bases, not purely bicarbonate ■ Negative base excess reflects the presence of excess acid ■ High base excess reflects an increased bicarbonate level
5	What does the base picture suggest?	If the problem is primarily metabolic, the bicarbonate and base excess help to confirm this If the problem is respiratory, the bicarbonate and base excess help determine how acute or chronic the derangement is because the bicarbonate buffer takes effect over days ■ Respiratory acidosis with normal bicarbonate and base excess is likely to be acute, because the bicarbonate buffer has not had time to act ■ Respiratory acidosis with increased bicarbonate and base excess is likely to be chronic ■ Respiratory acidosis with low bicarbonate suggests a combined respiratory and metabolic acidosis
6	What is the oxygen?	Low P_{O_2} with normal P_{CO_2}: type 1 respiratory failure is present. This results from a problem with oxygenation Low P_{O_2} with increased P_{CO_2}: type 2 respiratory failure is present. This results from inadequate ventilation In type 2 respiratory failure, low P_{O_2} can be the result of both poor oxygenation and poor ventilation

P_{CO_2}, partial pressure of carbon dioxide; P_{O_2}, partial pressure of oxygen.

Table 8.4 A stepwise method for interpreting blood gas results

Metabolic acidosis

Metabolic acidosis is a blood pH < 7.35 with a bicarbonate concentration < 22 mmol/L. Normal, physiological compensation is via the respiratory system: there is an increase in respiratory rate as the body tries to remove carbon dioxide from the blood via the lungs ('blowing off' CO_2). Metabolic acidosis occurs in several clinical conditions, but is a particularly common finding in acutely unwell patients. It either presents alone, as pure metabolic acidosis, or in conjunction with another acid–base disorder.

Aetiology

Metabolic acidosis results from:

■ generation of excess acid that overwhelms compensatory mechanisms, e.g. in acute kidney injury, diabetic ketoacidosis and lactic acidosis
■ loss of bicarbonate, e.g. in diarrhoea
■ accidental or intentional ingestion of excess acid, e.g. ethylene glycol (the primary ingredient of anti-freeze), salicylates (drug overdose) or methanol

Clinical features

The general clinical features of acid–base disorders, including metabolic acidosis, are shown in **Table 8.5**. The features of metabolic acidosis are non-specific and vary depending on the underlying cause. For example, a patient with metabolic acidosis secondary to septic shock resulting from urinary sepsis will be pyrexial with tachycardia, hypotension and suprapubic tenderness, whereas a patient with metabolic acidosis due to diabetic ketoacidosis will be hyperventilating and smelling of ketones.

Patients with metabolic acidosis compensate by hyperventilating. Their breaths are deep and sighing in nature, known as Kussmaul's respiration.

Diagnostic approach

Diagnosis of metabolic acidosis is based on blood gas results. The history and examination findings, together with the results of additional blood tests and imaging studies, will point towards the cause.

Metabolic acidosis is classified according to the anion gap. This indicates the amount of unmeasured anions (not chloride or bicarbonate) present, and is used to determine the underlying cause (**Table 8.6**). If the anion gap is raised then the unmeasured anions will be from either endogenous sources (renal failure, diabetic ketoacidosis, lactic acidosis) or exogenous sources (toxins). The anion gap is calculated using the following equation:

$$\text{anion gap} = [Na^+ + K^+] - [Cl^- + HCO_3^-]$$

Normally, the anion gap is 8–17 mmol/L.

Investigations

Arterial or venous blood gases results show:

- decreased pH (< 7.35)
- decreased bicarbonate concentration (< 22 mmol/L)

Acid–base disorders: clinical features				
Category	Metabolic acidosis	Metabolic alkalosis	Respiratory acidosis	Respiratory alkalosis
General	Fatigue	Restlessness followed by lethargy	Lethargy	Lethargy
Central nervous system	Headache	Confusion Irritability	Drowsiness Confusion Headache	Dizziness Confusion Syncope Seizures
Neuromuscular	Twitching Hypotonia Decreased reflexes	Tremors Muscle cramps Paraesthesia (tingling) of extremities	Muscle weakness Hyper-reflexia	Tetany Paraesthesia (tingling) of extremities
Cardiovascular	Low blood pressure Warm, flushed skin (vasodilation)	Tachycardia	Tachycardia Bounding pulse Warm, flushed skin (vasodilation)	None
Respiratory	Kussmaul's respiration Breathlessness	Compensatory hypoventilation	Hypoventilation (if a cause of respiratory acidosis) Hyperventilation (stimulated by hypercapnia)	Deep hyperventilation Chest tightness
Gastrointestinal	Decreased appetite Nausea and vomiting	Nausea and vomiting Diarrhoea	None	None

Table 8.5 General clinical features of acid–base disorders. Each disorder also has more specific features that depend on the underlying cause

Normal- or high-anion-gap metabolic acidosis: causes

Type of metabolic acidosis	Causes
Normal anion gap	Gastrointestinal bicarbonate loss: ■ Diarrhoea ■ Ileostomy ■ Ureterosigmoidostomy Renal bicarbonate loss: ■ Proximal renal tubular acidosis Decreased renal excretion of hydrogen ions: ■ Distal renal tubular acidosis Hypoaldosteronism
High anion gap	Renal failure Lactic acidosis Ketoacidosis: ■ Diabetic ketoacidosis ■ Inborn errors of metabolism ■ Starvation Ingestion of excess acid: ■ Methanol ■ Ethylene glycol ■ Ethanol ■ Salicylates ■ Paraldehyde

Table 8.6 Causes of metabolic acidosis with a normal or high anion gap. A low anion gap is most commonly seen when serum albumin (a negatively-charged protein) is low, because other negatively charged ions such as chloride and bicarbonate are retained

■ decreased partial pressure of carbon dioxide ($P\text{co}_2$)

Urea and electrolytes and chloride blood tests are taken to calculate the anion gap. Lactate and blood glucose are measured to exclude lactic acidosis and diabetic ketoacidosis respectively (usually done on an arterial sample for blood gas measurement). Drug levels are measured if an overdose is suspected, e.g. with salicylates or consumption of toxins.

Radiological imaging does not help diagnose metabolic acidosis, but can confirm the underlying cause.

For example, in metabolic acidosis resulting from sepsis secondary to pneumonia, the diagnosis of pneumonia is made with a chest X-ray. Intra-abdominal sepsis (e.g. secondary to bowel perforation) is diagnosed with an erect chest X-ray (to detect air under the diaphragm) and a CT of the abdomen.

Management

Management of metabolic acidosis depends on the underlying cause. For example:

■ if they have volume depletion, fluid resuscitation is started
■ if the patient has sepsis, antibiotics and IV fluids are given
■ if they have acute kidney injury, the cause is sought and addressed

The patient may need to be transferred to a high-dependency setting for closer monitoring and early senior review arranged.

Medication

Intravenous sodium bicarbonate is rarely required, but is given in certain types of metabolic acidosis, including:

■ life-threatening acidosis (pH < 7 and bicarbonate concentration < 10 mmol/L), to replenish the bicarbonate–carbonic anhydrase buffering system
■ renal failure and treatment of severe hyperkalaemia
■ salicylate intoxication, to promote excretion of salicylic acid

Chronic mild metabolic acidosis (pH >7.25), for example in chronic kidney disease, is treated with oral sodium bicarbonate.

Ensure that the patient's lung function is adequate before giving bicarbonate. The bicarbonate will generate additional carbon dioxide that the patient should be able to excrete via the lungs to avoid respiratory failure. For example, a patient with severe COPD will not be able to excrete the additional carbon dioxide rapidly enough, causing it to accumulate.

Metabolic alkalosis

Metabolic alkalosis is a plasma pH >7.45 caused by a loss of acid or an increase in bicarbonate. Like metabolic acidosis it is a common finding in hospital inpatients and its presence is associated with increased mortality. The compensation for metabolic alkalosis is a decreased respiratory rate in order to retain carbon dioxide, although the effect of this is small.

Aetiology

The causes of metabolic alkalosis are summarised in **Table 8.7**. Metabolic alkalosis is initiated by the loss of hydrogen ions or gain of base in the extracellular fluid (**Figure 8.3**). In response to an increase in serum bicarbonate concentation, the kidneys increase bicarbonate excretion which results in correction of metabolic alkalosis. For metabolic alkalosis to be maintained, additional factors that inhibit renal excretion of bicarbonate must be present. These are chloride depletion (the most important), potassium depletion, extracellular fluid volume depletion and decreased GFR (**Table 8.8**).

During chloride depletion (e.g. due to loss of chloride-rich gastric secretions or renal losses secondary to loop or thiazide diuretics)

Metabolic alkalosis: causes	
Mechanism	**Causes**
Loss of acid from extracellular fluid	Renal losses: ■ Diuretics ■ Mineralocorticoid excess (e.g. Cushing's syndrome or Conn's syndrome) ■ Potassium depletion Gastrointestinal losses: ■ Vomiting ■ Gastric aspiration (e.g. via nasogastric tube)
Addition of base to extracellular fluid	Milk–alkali syndrome (excessive consumption of milk and alkali to treat dyspeptic symptoms) Use of certain drugs: ■ Bicarbonate supplementation (oral or intravenous) ■ Penicillins Massive blood transfusion (because the associated citrate anticoagulant is a weak base)

Table 8.7 Causes of metabolic alkalosis

the kidney reabsorbs more bicarbonate (in place of chloride) alongside sodium and potassium to maintain the electroneutrality

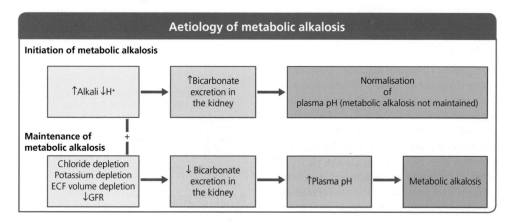

Figure 8.3 Aetiology of metabolic alkalosis. Once metabolic alkalosis has been initiated, additional factors that result in impaired renal excretion of bicarbonate must be present for it to be maintained. ECF, extracellular fluid; GFR, glomerular filtration rate.

Metabolic alkalosis: maintenance	
Mechanism	Causes
Chloride depletion	Gastrointestinal losses: ■ Vomiting ■ Villous adenoma Use of certain drugs ■ Diuretics Cystic fibrosis
Potassium depletion	Renal tubular disorders: ■ Bartter's syndrome Use of certain drugs: ■ Laxatives Hyperaldosteronism (Cushing's or Conn's syndrome): ■ Primary ■ Secondary
Decreased extracellular fluid volume	True volume depletion Decreased effective circulating volume (e.g. cardiac failure, cirrhosis) Diuretics
Decreased GFR	Causes of AKI or CKD

Table 8.8 Maintenance of metabolic alkalosis

of the extracellular fluid; this also increases the bicarbonate concentration in the blood. Potassium depletion results in intracellular shifts of H+ in exchange for K^+, causing an intracellular acidosis. In the kidney this causes potassium reabsorption, H^+ secretion and a net gain of bicarbonate. Potassium depletion also stimulates renal ammoniagenesis, during which bicarbonate is generated (see page 51). Volume depletion and a subsequent decrease in renal perfusion stimulates the renin–angiotensin–aldosterone system resulting in increased renal reabsorption of sodium and water, and secretion of H+ into the tubular lumen. This is associated with systemic bicarbonate gain via the HCO_3^-/Cl^- cotransporter on the basolateral membrane. A fall in GFR results in decreased filtration of bicarbonate at the glomerulus.

Clinical features

As with metabolic acidosis, the clinical features depend on the underlying cause. General features are shown in **Table 8.5**.

Tingling, paraesthesia, tetany and convulsions are caused by the increased pH reducing free calcium in the blood. Many causes of metabolic alkalosis are associated with volume depletion, so patients often have hypotension, decreased urine output and low jugular venous pressure. Respiratory compensation is limited by the drive to prevent hypoxia, so an increase in Pco_2 to > 7 kPa is rare.

Diagnostic approach

Diagnosis of metabolic alkalosis is based on blood gas analysis (**Table 8.3**). The history, examination findings and additional blood tests and imaging are used to indicate possible causes. For example, a history of diuretic use, particularly thiazides, can cause mild metabolic alkalosis.

Investigations

Urinary chloride is used to distinguish between causes of metabolic alkalosis.

■ Low urinary chloride (< 10 mmol/L) indicates volume depletion (e.g. as a result of vomiting)
■ Normal (10–20 mmol/L) or increased (> 20 mmol/L) urinary chloride indicates euvolaemia or hypervolaemia. Causes of metabolic alkalosis in this context include severe potassium deficiency, excess aldosterone and Bartter's syndrome

Recent diuretic use increases urinary chloride levels, preventing chloride from being used to diagnose metabolic alkalosis. However, as the diuretic effect wears off, urinary chloride concentration will fall.

Management

The underlying cause of metabolic alkalosis is sought and addressed, for example by stopping diuretics or removing a villous adenoma. Most cases associated with chloride deficiency and volume depletion respond to intravenous fluids containing sodium chloride (0.9% saline). Potassium supplementation is given if the serum concentration is low.

Prognosis

Prognosis largely depends on the cause; if easily reversible the prognosis will improve with removal of the cause (e.g. metabolic alkalosis with chloride depletion due to diuretics will respond to them being stopped). If due to a chronic problem, e.g. metabolic alkalosis with chloride depletion due to cystic fibrosis, it is more difficult to control. Generally, the higher the pH, the greater the associated mortality rate (up to 80% with pH >7.65).

Respiratory acidosis

Respiratory acidosis is an increase in P_{CO_2} above 6 kPa (hypercapnia) caused by alveolar hypoventilation. It is common in patients with chronic obstructive pulmonary disease (COPD), chest wall deformities or neuromuscular abnormalities.

Respiratory acidosis is either acute or chronic:

- acute respiratory acidosis presents with low pH, increased P_{CO_2} and normal bicarbonate concentration
- chronic respiratory acidosis presents with low pH, increased P_{CO_2} and elevated bicarbonate concentration

Aetiology

Respiratory acidosis is caused by the retention of CO_2, which results from various pathologies (Table 8.9).

Acute respiratory acidosis is caused by a sudden ventilatory failure that increases P_{CO_2}, usually as a result of an acute complication to an underlying disorder (e.g. pneumonia in COPD, paralysis in myasthenia gravis). Chronic respiratory acidosis is caused by an underlying chronic condition that results in the hypercapnia (e.g. stable COPD). Partial compensation for this results in the retention of bicarbonate.

Hypercapnia causes peripheral and cerebral vasodilation, increased intracerebral pressure and the stimulation of ventilation.

Clinical features

The clinical features of respiratory acidosis include (see Table 8.5):

- dyspnoea
- flushed appearance
- warm peripheries
- tachycardia and bounding (large volume) pulse
- headache
- confusion
- altered consciousness

Diagnostic approach

A diagnosis of respiratory acidosis is based on arterial blood gas analysis. The history and examination, along with additional blood tests and imaging, point towards the cause. For example, a patient with a respiratory acidosis secondary to an infective exacerbation of COPD will present with cough, increased sputum volume and purulence, tachypnoea, increased work of breathing, low oxygen saturations, wheeze and focal crackles on auscultation of the chest. Their chest radiograph will show hyperventilation and, possibly, consolidation and their blood test results will show increased white cell count and C-reactive protein concentration.

Investigations

Blood gases show pH < 7.35, increased P_{CO_2} (> 6 kPa) and usually low P_{O_2} (< 10.6 kPa).

Respiratory acidosis: causes		
Mechanism	**Time course**	**Cause**
Airway obstruction	Acute	Upper airway obstruction (e.g. foreign body aspiration, hypopharyngeal obstruction due to decreased consciousness)
		Acute exacerbation of chronic obstructive pulmonary disease
		Bronchospasm (e.g. severe asthma)
	Chronic	Chronic obstructive pulmonary disorder
		Vocal cord paralysis
		Tumour of vocal cords or larynx
Alveolar disease	Acute	Pulmonary oedema
		Pneumonia
		Acute respiratory distress syndrome
	Chronic	Pulmonary fibrosis
Pleural disease	Acute	Pneumothorax
Central respiratory centre depression	Acute	Drugs: opiates, benzodiazepines, anaesthetics
		CNS or cervical cord trauma
	Chronic	Drugs: chronic use of opiates or benzodiazepines
		Brain tumour
Neuromuscular disorders	Acute	Guillian Barre Syndrome
		Myaesthenic crisis
		Tetanus
		Status epilepticus
		Neurotoxins: organophosphates, snake venom, botulinum toxin
		Use of muscle relaxants
	Chronic	Myaesthenia gravis
		Motor neurone disease
		Myopathies
		Muscular dystrophy
		Poliomyelitis
		Diaphragmatic splinting (e.g. in obesity or gross ascites where diaphragmatic movement is limited)
		Diaphragmatic paralysis
Structural chest wall abnormalities	Acute	Flail chest (a section of the chest wall that moves independently following broken ribs)
	Chronic	Severe kyphosis
Metabolic causes	Acute	Catabolic states (e.g. malignant hyperthermia)
Iatrogenic causes	Acute	Misplaced endotracheal tube during mechanical ventilation
		Inadequate ventilation of intubated patients

Table 8.9 Causes of respiratory acidosis

If the respiratory acidosis persists over days, metabolic compensation occurs. The Henderson–Hasselbalch equation shifts to the right (see page 46), resulting in increased renal excretion of acid and a subsequent increase in plasma bicarbonate concentration (26 mmol/L).

Chest X-rays are carried out to look for signs of pneumonia, pneumothorax, pulmonary oedema and hyperinflation (the latter found in COPD and asthma). Blood tests such as white cell count and C-reactive protein measurement help diagnose or exclude an infection.

Management

The underlying cause of respiratory acidosis is treated. For example:

- antibiotics are given for pneumonia
- diuretics and nitrates are given for pulmonary oedema
- nebulised bronchodilators and steroids are given for asthma and COPD
- any pneumothorax is decompressed

Some patients require ventilatory support with non-invasive ventilation or endotracheal intubation and mechanical ventilation, depending on the underlying pathology.

Prognosis

Prognosis depends on the cause. For example, respiratory acidosis in a patient with acute asthma is a sign of a life-threatening attack, whereas in a patient with COPD or chest wall deformities it is chronic and is not a sign of acute severe disease.

Respiratory alkalosis

Respiratory alkalosis is a decrease in Pco_2 (< 4.7 kPa), caused by alveolar hyperventilation. This reduces the ratio of Pco_2 to bicarbonate, which results in a high blood pH (> 7.45). Increased respiratory rate is often an early sign of critical illness; respiratory alkalosis is therefore a non-specific feature in critically unwell patients. Respiratory alkalosis is either acute or chronic:

- in acute respiratory alkalosis: P_aco_2 is low, plasma pH is alkalaemic and serum bicarbonate concentration is normal
- in chronic respiratory alkalosis: P_aco_2 is low, pH is normal or mildly alkalaemic and serum bicarbonate concentration is low

Aetiology

Respiratory alkalosis results from an increased respiratory drive, which has a number of causes (**Table 8.10**). If sufficiently severe or longstanding, some of these causes (e.g. pneumonia, pulmonary oedema, pneumothorax), will eventually lead to ventilatory failure and, therefore, respiratory acidosis.

In earlier stages, however, respiratory alkalosis occurs due to an increased respiratory rate.

In chronic respiratory alkalosis there is partial compensation as the kidney increases the excretion of bicarbonate. This reduces the blood pH to normal or near-normal levels in chronic patients.

Clinical features

Hyperventilation causes a decrease in ionised calcium, which results in paraesthesia of the extremities and lips, chest tightness, dyspnoea and tetany (see **Table 8.5**). An acute decrease in carbon dioxide levels provokes cerebral vasoconstriction and causes neurological symptoms such as dizziness, confusion, syncope and seizures.

> Cerebral vasoconstriction caused by respiratory alkalosis also results in decreased intracerebral pressure. Ventilator-induced hyperventilation is used in the management of head injuries to reduce intracranial pressure.

Respiratory alkalosis: causes		
Mechanism	Time course	Cause
Respiratory causes	Acute	Pneumonia
		Pulmonary oedema
		Acute pleural effusion
		Pneumothorax
		Right-to-left shunts
	Chronic	Interstitial lung disease
		High altitude
		Right-to-left shunts
Central nervous system causes	Acute	Pain
		Anxiety and panic disorders
		Fever
		Encephalitis
		Meningitis
		Trauma
	Chronic	Stroke
Endocrine causes	Chronic	Pregnancy
		Hyperthyroidism
Use of certain drugs	Acute	Catecholamines
	Chronic	Salicylates
		Progesterone
Other	Acute	Sepsis
		Anaemia
		Metabolic acidosis
		Hepatic failure
	Chronic	Anaemia
		Metabolic acidosis
		Hepatic failure

Table 8.10 Causes of respiratory alkalosis

Diagnostic approach

The diagnosis of respiratory alkalosis is based on blood gas analysis. History and examination findings, along with the results of blood tests and imaging, will indicate the cause.

Investigations

Arterial blood gas results in respiratory alkalosis typically show:

- Increased pH (can be normal if chronic)
- Decreased $P_a\text{co}_2$
- Normal (acute) or decreased (chronic) bicarbonate concentration

Management

Management of respiratory alkalosis depends on the underlying cause. Addressing the respiratory alkalosis alone is unlikely to be successful if the precipitant is not removed. For example, an anxious, hyperventilating patient who is in pain is unlikely to improve until their pain is relieved. Similarly, a tachypnoeic patient with a bacterial chest infection will not improve without appropriate antibiotics and resolution of the infection.

Answers to starter questions

1. The anion gap is an estimation of the concentration of anions not usually measured in serum (routinely, only bicarbonate and chloride are measured). It helps determine the cause of metabolic acidosis, because if it is raised there are a relatively limited number of sources for the unmeasured anions: either endogenous (renal failure, diabetic ketoacidosis, lactic acidosis) or exogenous (toxins such as ethylene glycol or methanol).

2. Venous blood gas samples correlate well with arterial samples for most parameters of acid-base balance. Venepuncture is less painful and carries fewer potential side effects than arterial puncture. Venous samples are not useful when an accurate Po_2 measure is needed (it is variable because of varying oxygen extraction by the tissues) and are therefore generally not used in the assessment of respiratory problems.

3. The lungs compensate for metabolic abnormalities because carbon dioxide is acidic in solution and the amount exhaled can be adjusted to need. No matter what the metabolic cause of a change in pH, it is initially compensated for by the body's bicarbonate buffering system:

$$\text{Bicarbonate } (HCO_3^-) + H^+ \Leftrightarrow \text{Carbonic acid } (H_2CO_3) \Leftrightarrow CO_2 + H_2O$$

This means that pH can be maintained by controlling H^+ excretion in the urine and CO_2 exhalation by the lungs. For example, in a metabolic acidosis, hyperventilation occurs to lower the blood acid load and increase pH. In metabolic alkalosis, hypoventilation occurs to retain CO_2 and decrease blood pH.

4. Metabolic activity generates acid because the products of aerobic cellular respiration (CO_2) and anaerobic respiration (lactic acid) are both acidic. This must be continually compensated for by the body's buffer systems and by the excretion of CO_2 in the lungs and H^+ in the urine.

5. Severe acidosis is associated with deep and strenuous breathing, called Kussmaul breathing, in order to 'blow off' acid via CO_2 exhalation. This type of hyperventilation occurs in diabetic ketoacidosis, when a diabetic patient's inability to metabolise sugar leads to excessive fat catabolism and keto acid production. Kussmaul breathing does not occur in acidosis if this is sufficiently compensated or if there is central respiratory depression (e.g. due to opiates).

Chapter 9
Hypertension and renovascular disease

Starter questions

Answers to the following questions are on page 284.

1. How has the bite of the South American pit viper *Bothrops jararaca* helped in the treatment of hypertension?
2. Why does the pulse pressure, the difference between systolic and diastolic pressure, tend to widen with age and in people with chronic kidney disease?
3. How can abdominal auscultation help diagnose the cause of a patient's high blood pressure?
4. What might be causing hypertension in a patient presenting with panic attacks, sweating and pallor?
5. How can severe hypertension cause visual disturbances?

Introduction

Hypertension (chronic abnormally high blood pressure) is a common problem and a major risk factor for atherosclerosis, the accumulation of fatty deposits in arterial walls. In turn, atherosclerosis is a key cause of ischaemic heart disease and stroke, major causes of death worldwide. Ischaemic heart disease alone causes a third of all deaths globally and hypertension is believed to be responsible for at least 50% of these.

Because of its role in regulating salt and water balance, the kidney is an important organ in the genesis of hypertension. It is also a key site of the harmful effects of hypertension (see next section), both in terms of the main body of the organ and in terms of the effect on its blood supply (renovascular disease; page 281).

Although hypertension is usually a chronic condition it can enter an accelerated phase (see page 279) that is a medical emergency. Finally, there are some specific issues involved when controlling hypertension in pregnancy and diabetes page 283).

Hypertension and renal disease

Hypertension and renal disease are closely interlinked: hypertension can be the cause or the result of the renal disease, and vice versa. Consequently hypertension is an extremely common finding in most forms of renal disease. The effects of hypertension on the kidney are:

■ Damage to the renal arteries. Hypertension is a major risk factor for atherosclerosis, which affects the large renal arteries obstructing blood flow. In smaller renal arteries, hypertension leads to fibromuscular hyperplasia of the arterial wall and subsequent narrowing of the lumen. The result of both these effects on large and small arteries is a decrease in perfusion of the kidney which stimulates renin release (see Chapter 1, page 35).
■ Transmission of raised systemic blood pressure to the glomerulus, although partially mitigated by renal autoregulation, eventually leads to collapse and fibrosis

of the glomerular tuft. High pressure in the tubulointerstitial compartment causes tubular atrophy and interstitial fibrosis. These combined effects cause further disturbance of the microcirculation within the kidney triggering renin release and, as the damage causes progressive renal impairment, progressive salt and water retention.
■ As outlined above, the effects of hypertension on the kidney increase renin release and favour salt and water retention. Both these mechanisms drive a further increase in hypertension, setting up a potential vicious circle of uncontrolled high blood pressure and further renal damage.

The above considerations emphasise that good control of hypertension has a key role in halting or slowing the decline in renal function that occurs in chronic kidney disease. Therefore management of hypertension is a vital component of the care of the renal patient.

Case 10 An incidental finding of hypertension

Presentation

Malcolm Williams, who is 33 years old, goes to see his general practitioner (GP) to complain of headaches, which he has had on and off over the past few weeks.

Initial interpretation

There are a number of recognised headache syndromes, such as migraine and tension-type headaches. Furthermore, there are 'red flag' headache-related

Case 10 *continued*

symptoms that must be sought and ruled out because of their association with serious underlying pathology. The most important red flag symptoms are:

- early morning headache or associated vomiting may indicate raised intracranial pressure
- associated neurological features (e.g. seizures, focal signs or symptoms)
- symptoms suggesting other serious disease (e.g. giant cell arteritis, glaucoma)

Hypertension is rarely a cause of headache; however blood pressure should always be measured.

Further history

Malcolm confirms he has none of the red flag symptoms listed above. He says he has previously been well, with no serious illnesses. He does recall noticing that his urine has been darker than usual at the same time that he has had the occasional cold.

Examination

Examination of Malcolm's heart and lungs is normal. No abnormalities are found on palpating and auscultating the abdomen, and there are no gross neurological signs.

At 184/124 mmHg, Malcolm's blood pressure is very high (normal is < 140/90 mmHg). Examination of his optic fundus demonstrates haemorrhages, exudates and optic disc oedema (**Figure 9.1**). Dipstick urinalysis shows the presence of both blood and protein.

Interpretation of findings

It is likely that Malcolm's very high blood pressure is causing his headaches. Hypertension is usually asymptomatic, but Malcolm's blood pressure is

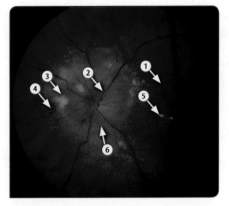

Figure 9.1 Fundoscopy image for Malcolm Williams, showing features of all four grades of hypertensive retinopathy. Stage 1: 'silver wiring' ① and arterial attenuation. Stage 2: arteriovenous nipping ②. Stage 3: 'cotton wool spots' ③ and flame haemorrhages ④. Stage 4: hard exudates ⑤ and optic disc oedema ⑥.

high enough to trigger intracranial pain receptors.

His headaches do not have features of tension headaches (constant dull band-like ache) or migraine (accompanying visual aura, vomiting). The absence of red flag symptoms means that there is no reason to suspect raised intracranial pressure or other neurological disease.

The findings of fundoscopy and urinalysis are signs associated with accelerated hypertension. Very high sustained blood pressure damages the delicate vessels of the retina. Similarly, it seems likely that the hypertension has damaged the glomeruli in Malcom's kidneys, causing leakage of blood and protein into the urine, i.e. haematuria and proteinuria, respectively. Alternatively or additionally there may be an underlying renal problem causing the hypertension.

Hypertension is usually managed in primary care. However, the signs of hypertensive retinopathy and presumptive hypertensive nephropathy warrant urgent referral to either a nephrologist or hypertension specialist for evaluation.

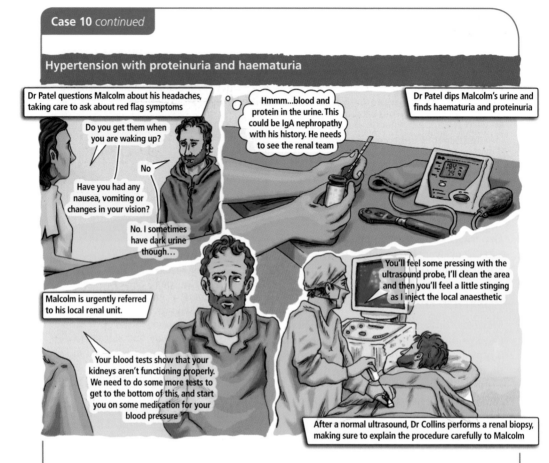

Case 10 *continued*

Hypertension with proteinuria and haematuria

Dr Patel questions Malcolm about his headaches, taking care to ask about red flag symptoms

Do you get them when you are waking up?

No

Have you had any nausea, vomiting or changes in your vision?

No. I sometimes have dark urine though...

Hmmm...blood and protein in the urine. This could be IgA nephropathy with his history. He needs to see the renal team

Dr Patel dips Malcolm's urine and finds haematuria and proteinuria

Malcolm is urgently referred to his local renal unit.

Your blood tests show that your kidneys aren't functioning properly. We need to do some more tests to get to the bottom of this, and start you on some medication for your blood pressure

You'll feel some pressing with the ultrasound probe, I'll clean the area and then you'll feel a little stinging as I inject the local anaesthetic

After a normal ultrasound, Dr Collins performs a renal biopsy, making sure to explain the procedure carefully to Malcolm

Investigations

Malcolm is seen that day in his local renal unit. The results of blood tests show a moderate degree of renal impairment; estimated glomerular filtration rate is 54 mL/min/1.73 m². Evidence of borderline left ventricular hypertrophy is found on electrocardiography: the height of the tallest R wave added to the depth of the deepest S wave in the frontal (V) leads is 45 mm. A renal ultrasound scan is arranged, and shows normal-sized kidneys with no abnormal features.

Diagnosis

Malcolm's ECG result suggests that his hypertension is actually long-standing: the left ventricle has increased its muscle mass in response to the increased peripheral vascular resistance, and this takes time. At this stage it is unclear whether the high blood pressure itself has caused damage to the kidneys, and therefore a decreased GFR, or whether there is an underlying renal problem that has caused his high blood pressure; both might be happening.

Although Malcolm's blood pressure must be controlled, there are none of the features that would suggest admission and intravenous therapy is needed (see **Table 9.6**). He is started on oral treatment with nifedipine as a modified release preparation. The modified release preparation of nifedipine acts for a few hours; the dose can therefore be adjusted frequently by the medical team to obtain a controlled reduction of blood pressure. He attends weekly appointments as an outpatient; ramipril, an angiotensin-converting enzyme inhibitor, is added in after a few days, and the modified release nifedipine is changed to the long-acting preparation, because once the acute phase is past the longer action of this preparation (24 h) gives smoother control of blood pressure.

Over the next few weeks, Malcolm's blood pressure normalises with treatment. However, his renal function does not improve, and the haematuria and proteinuria persist. This increases the probability that he has an underlying renal condition, and a renal biopsy is required to diagnose this.

The normal size of his kidneys, as shown on ultrasound, means that it is safe to perform a renal biopsy. This shows that Malcolm has immunoglobulin A nephropathy, which explains the dark urine (visible haematuria) he has noticed during upper respiratory tract infections (see page 188).

With treatment, Malcolm's blood pressure remains well controlled, and his headaches resolve. He requires indefinite renal follow up because of his underlying kidney problem, which was the cause of his hypertension.

> **To minimise the risk of bleeding,** blood pressure must be reduced to < 160/90 mmHg before carrying out a renal biopsy.

Case 11 Proteinuria and hypertension

Presentation

Ashok Patel, a 57-year-old man originally from India, has been found by his GP to have proteinuria on routine screening. He has been referred to the local renal unit, where he is seen by the consultant, Dr Chalmers.

Initial interpretation

Asymptomatic urinary abnormalities, i.e. the detection of blood or protein on dipstick urinalysis, are common reasons for referral to nephrology outpatient departments. Further investigation is essential because these findings may be the initial presentation of serious underlying disease, including renal tract malignancy (blood) or significant renal disease (blood and/or protein).

Further history

Five years ago, Mr Patel was diagnosed with type 2 diabetes mellitus; so far, this has been managed with dietary changes alone. Two years ago, his blood pressure was found to be increased on 24-h monitoring (145/95 mmHg), and he was started on ramipril 2.5 mg/day.

Mr Patel has taken the tablets regularly, but he has found it difficult to stick to his diet. Routine retinal screening, which he has undergone every year, has shown evidence of early diabetic retinopathy for which no specific treatment has been required. He has no other significant past medical history and is a non-smoker.

His mother is still alive; she is 82 years old. His father died in his sixties of myocardial infarction. He has three siblings, two of whom have also been diagnosed with type 2 diabetes mellitus.

Case 11 *continued*

Examination

Dr Chalmers examines Mr Patel and finds that he is obese; his body mass index is 31.5 kg/m² (the healthy range is 18.5–24.9 kg/m²). No peripheral oedema is present. Measured in the clinic, his blood pressure is 156/94 mmHg. There are no other abnormalities.

Interpretation of findings

The absence of peripheral oedema means that Mr Patel's proteinuria is not sufficient to lead to nephrotic syndrome, i.e. the triad of heavy proteinuria, oedema and low serum albumin concentration (see page 176). Lesser degrees of proteinuria would be typical of early diabetic nephropathy in this clinical setting. Although a single clinic blood pressure measurement provides limited information, Mr Patel's blood pressure is clearly too high; an appropriate target for him as a diabetic is < 130/80 mmHg.

Mr Patel has a strong family history (father, siblings) of type 2 diabetes. People of South Asian origin are at higher risk of type 2 diabetes than the general population. They are also more likely to develop complications of diabetes: Mr Patel's father died in his sixties, probably as a result of accelerated coronary artery disease due to diabetes, and Mr Patel himself already has evidence of diabetic retinopathy and nephropathy. In addition to his diabetes, other significant risk factors for vascular disease are his raised body mass index and blood pressure. Fortunately, he is a non-smoker; smoking is the strongest risk factor.

Investigations

Dr Chalmers sends urine samples for quantification of the proteinuria, and he

Ashok Patel blood test results

Test	Result	Normal range or target
Urine albumin:creatinine ratio	56 mg/mmol	< 3 mg/mmol
Serum creatinine	75 µmol/L	50–110 µmol/L
Serum albumin	37 g/L	35–50 g/L
Haemoglobin A1c	63 mmol/mol	< 48 mmol/mol

Table 9.1 Blood test results for Ashok Patel

arranges blood tests (**Table 9.1**). He also arranges a renal ultrasound (US) scan, which shows normal-sized kidneys and no sign of pathology. Although the need for US in this clinical context can be debated, it would certainly be required if renal biopsy were planned.

Diagnosis and management

The increased albumin:creatinine ratio confirms significant proteinuria. This value will serve as a baseline for future measurements in the monitoring of Mr Patel's kidney function.

The normal serum creatinine concentration indicates that excretory renal function is normal; this means that the probable underlying diabetic nephropathy is still at an early stage. Serum albumin is also normal, which is also consistent with early diabetic nephropathy; later in the natural history proteinuria may increase to amounts sufficient to cause nephrotic syndrome. The raised haemoglobin A1c shows that Mr Patel's glycaemic control has been poor over the past 3 months (see page 89).

Dr Chalmers feels that there is enough evidence to make a diagnosis of diabetic nephropathy as the cause of the proteinuria, without the need for renal biopsy.

Case 11 *continued*

The key measures are to reduce blood pressure and improve glycaemic control.

Dr Chalmers explains the position to Mr Patel, emphasising the need for him to take responsibility for altering his lifestyle and losing weight; if he succeeds at this, his blood pressure, as well as his diabetes, will be easier to control. Meanwhile, Dr Chalmers advises the GP to increase the dose of ramipril to the maximum, and to add in other agents, if necessary, to reach the target blood pressure.

Mr Patel has found it hard to stick to his diet. However, the discovery of protein in his urine as a result of his diabetes has alarmed him; he has a young family and wants to live to see them grow up. He resolves to try to take more exercise, cut down his salt intake and generally improve his diet.

Hypertension

Blood pressure is a continuous variable, and the exact definition and stage of hypertension depend on how it is measured: it is vital that correct technique is used (see page 82) so that the appropriate criteria are accurately applied (**Table 9.2**).

Hypertension is caused by increased peripheral vascular resistance (primarily due to increased constriction in small arteries and arterioles), fluid retention or both. There are two forms:

- **Primary hypertension,** also called essential hypertension: this is hypertension of unknown cause, with multiple risk factors contributing to the elevated pressure
- **Secondary hypertension:** this is hypertension that occurs secondary to one of a number of conditions, including certain renal and endocrine disorders (see **Table 9.3**)

More than 90% of patients with hypertension have primary hypertension. However, it is largely asymptomatic and therefore many people are unaware of their disease and consequently do not present for treatment.

Epidemiology

Up to a third of the adult population in Europe and North America have hypertension. The rate in low- and middle-income countries is even higher; for example, some areas of Africa have a prevalence of >45%. Prevalence increases with age.

Stages of hypertension	
Stage	Criteria
1	Clinic BP ≥ 140/90 mmHg AND subsequent ABPM daytime average OR HBPM average ≥ 135/85 mmHg
2	Clinic BP ≥ 160/100 mmHg AND subsequent ABPM daytime average OR HBPM average ≥ 150/95 mmHg
3 (severe)	Clinic systolic BP ≥ 180 mmHg OR clinic diastolic BP ≥ 110 mmHg
Accelerated	Same as stage 3 hypertension but with signs of grade 3 or 4 retinopathy
BP, blood pressure; ABPM, ambulatory blood pressure monitoring; HBPM, home blood pressure monitoring.	

Table 9.2 The stages of hypertension. The precise boundaries differ depending on the methods used and guideline followed. Repeat high readings are needed to establish a diagnosis of hypertension, as outlined in **Figure 9.2**.

> **Up to a fifth of patients are unaware that they have hypertension,** and up to half of patients with known hypertension are receiving inadequate treatment.

Secondary hypertension: causes		
Cause	Examples	Investigations
Renal disease	Renal parenchymal disease	Urinalysis, eGFR, renal US scan
	Renovascular disease	CT or MRI angiography
Endocrine disease	Hyperaldosteronism (Conn's syndrome)	Electrolytes (low potassium, high normal sodium), aldosterone, renin, CT scan (adrenal adenoma)
	Cushing's syndrome	Urinary cortisol, dexamethasone suppression test, CT scan (adrenal adenoma)
	Phaeochromocytoma	Urinary catecholamines and metanephrines, CT scan
Use of certain drugs	Steroids (corticosteroids, oral contraceptive pill), non-steroidal anti-inflammatory drugs	None
Cardiovascular	Coarctation of the aorta	Echocardiogram, CT scan
Miscellaneous	Pregnancy	None
	Obstructive sleep apnoea	Sleep studies

Table 9.3 Causes of secondary hypertension

Aetiology

Primary hypertension accounts for 95% of cases. It is by definition idiopathic, but there are a number of recognised risk factors. Some of these are not modifiable, for example ethnic origin. However 'lifestyle' risk factors are susceptible to modification to reduce the risk of developing hypertension or to help with treatment:

■ high salt intake (>6g/day)
■ obesity
■ physical inactivity
■ alcohol
■ poor diet
■ smoking

A wide range of conditions cause secondary hypertension; they are listed in **Table 9.3.**

Clinical features

Most patients are asymptomatic. Their hypertension is detected during:

■ health screening
■ consultation for another problem or
■ routine blood pressure monitoring in certain groups of patents (e.g. patients with renal disease)

Contrary to popular belief, hypertension rarely causes visual problems or headache, except in severe cases (e.g. accelerated hypertension; see page 279).

History and examination focuses on relevant lifestyle factors and possible end-organ damage (**Table 9.4**). Some causes of secondary hypertension also have characteristic clinical features. Secondary causes should also be considered if hypertension:

■ occurs at a young age (<40 years) or
■ is unusually severe or
■ is resistant to treatment

Diagnostic approach

Each new diagnosis of hypertension requires institution of significant and often lifelong pharmacological treatment and lifestyle modification. Therefore it is essential to understand that hypertension cannot be diagnosed from a single blood pressure reading, because this can be artificially or temporarily raised by factors unrelated to hypertensive disease.

It is important that the correct technique is followed when measuring blood pressure (see Chapter 2, page 82); if not seriously misleading results can be obtained. If a reading of >140/90mmHg is obtained, measurement is repeated during the same consultation. If the second reading differs significantly from the first, measurement is repeated again.

Hypertension: end-organ damage		
Organ	Features	Investigation(s)
Heart	Left ventricular hypertrophy Ischaemic heart disease	12-lead electrocardiogram
Eyes	Hypertensive retinopathy (see Figure 9.1) ■ Grade 1: silver wiring ■ Grade 2: arteriovenous nipping ■ Grade 3: haemorrhages and cotton wool spots ■ Grade 4: optic disc oedema, hard exudates	Fundoscopy
Kidneys	Renal impairment Proteinuria (mild)	Urinalysis Urea and electrolytes US scan
Brain	Stroke Vascular dementia	CT scan MRI scan

Table 9.4 Target end organ damage caused by hypertension. Eye changes are common, but do not usually cause serious problems with vision. Similarly mild degrees of left ventricular hypertrophy are common, usually cause no harm, and improve with treatment

The lower of the latter two readings is documented as the blood pressure.

> **In the presence of an irregular pulse, for example in atrial fibrillation, automated blood pressure devices often give inaccurate results.** Under these circumstances, a manual blood pressure reading with direct auscultation is carried out.

To establish the diagnosis of hypertension, recordings obtained by using a device for ambulatory blood pressure monitoring (ABPM) or home blood pressure monitoring should be used, if possible. ABPM recordings correlate more closely with the risk of target organ damage and the overall risk of cardiovascular disease, and home blood pressure readings are more accurate because of the lack of a 'white coat' effect (higher blood pressure due to anxiety in a clinical setting). When ABPM or home monitoring is used, an average waking blood pressure ≥ 130/85 mmHg is considered diagnostic of hypertension.

With blood pressure correctly measured according to the guidelines above, the approach to diagnosis and staging of primary hypertension is shown in **Figure 9.2**.

Assessment of cardiovascular risk

Because the main aim of treatment is to prevent atherosclerosis and cardiovascular disease, hypertension must be managed in the context of an estimate of the patient's cardiovascular risk. This is usually expressed as the risk of a cardiovascular disease event occurring in the next 10 years. It is calculated using an online risk calculator or reference table; these tools are based on massive population data sets and are region-specific, e.g. pan-European. Risk scores are not accurately predictive for the individual patient but do help in communicating risk in easily understood terms, especially for patients who are symptom-free, but have raised blood pressure. In this way, risk scores can motivate concordance to lifestyle changes and treatment.

Investigations

Investigations are primarily directed towards the detection of end-organ damage (**Table 9.4**). A reasonable minimum set of investigations is:

■ fundoscopy to assess for retinopathy
■ urinalysis for haematuria and proteinuria
■ 12-lead electrocardiography to assess for left ventricular hypertrophy, or evidence of ischaemic heart disease
■ blood tests to assess for renal function, and for measurement of glucose and lipid levels

These investigations also enable formal estimation of cardiovascular risk.

Specialist referral is usually indicated if secondary hypertension is suspected; investigations in secondary hypertension are shown in **Table 9.3**.

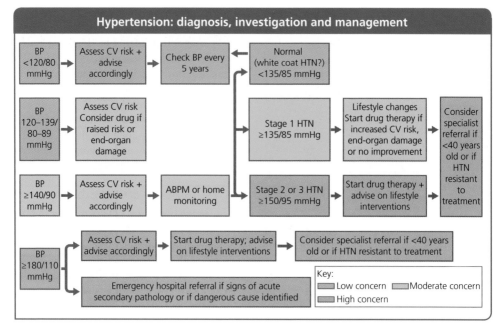

Figure 9.2 Diagnosis, investigation and management of hypertension. ABPM, ambulatory blood pressure monitoring; BP, blood pressure; CV, cardiovascular; HTN, hypertension.

Management

All patients must receive lifestyle advice (**Table 9.5**). The most beneficial recommendations with respect to blood pressure reduction are:

- weight loss; a 10 kg reduction decreases both systolic and diastolic blood pressure by 5–10 mmHg
- moderation of alcohol intake

Patient education is a vital element of management because of the asymptomatic nature of hypertension

Patients with stage 1 hypertension (see **Table 9.2**) and low cardiovascular risk (< 20% at 10 years) and with no evidence of end organ damage are treated initially with lifestyle measures alone. If these measures do not reduce blood pressure below the diagnostic thresholds for hypertension then drug therapy is indicated. Lifestyle measures may also be tried initially for patients with stage 2 hypertension, but drug therapy is usually

Management of hypertension: lifestyle modifications

Lifestyle modification	Recommendation
Decrease dietary salt intake	< 6 g/day
Lose weight (if overweight or obese)	Body mass index < 25 kg/m²
Increase physical activity	> 30 min/day
Decrease alcohol intake	Men: < 2 units/day
	Women: < 1 unit/day
Improve diet	Increase fruit and vegetable intake
	Decrease saturated fat intake
Stop smoking	Specialist smoking cessation services, nicotine replacement therapy

Table 9.5 Lifestyle modifications for the management of hypertension

required. Drugs are started immediately if the patient has severe hypertension, i.e. stage 3 (see **Table 9.2**).

Choice of antihypertensive drug depends on the patient's age and ethnicity

(**Figure 9.3**). The target is a blood pressure of < 140/90 mmHg (< 130/80 mmHg in patients with diabetes); it is often difficult to reach these targets.

> **Patients requiring antihypertensive therapy are warned that it is unusual to obtain adequate control with just one drug; usually two or three are needed.** As with all chronic conditions, patient education is a vital part of management, particularly in hypertension, because patients are usually asymptomatic.

Causes of secondary hypertension are managed appropriately. If the patient remains hypertensive, anti-hypertensive treatment is as described for primary hypertension.

Prognosis

This depends on the extent of end-organ damage. Effective control of blood pressure reduces the incidence of stroke and ischaemic heart disease and prolongs survival. Blood pressure is also generally the most important modifiable factor in slowing the rate of progression of chronic kidney disease (see page 166); by delaying the need for renal replacement therapy, good control is therefore of potentially great economic benefit in the population as a whole.

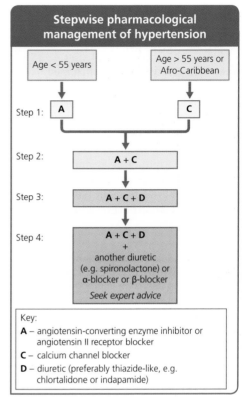

Figure 9.3 Stepwise pharmacological management of hypertension as per current guidelines. The patient is started on a step 1 drug and, if control is not achieved within a certain time, progresses through the stepped choices until blood pressure is adequately controlled.

Accelerated hypertension

Accelerated hypertension is the rapid development of severe hypertension (> 180/110 mmHg) with grade 3 or 4 hypertensive retinopathy. It can occur with hypertension of any cause, but underlying renal disease is common.

Clinical features

Patients are often asymptomatic. However, a minority have evidence of acute end organ damage such as breathlessness (as a result of left ventricular failure) and visual or neurological disturbance.

Investigations will often show evidence of renal impairment (e.g. raised creatinine concentration) and a minority of patient will have a microangiopathic blood film, with the presence of schistocytes as a consequence of damage to the microcirculation (see Figure 6.9).

> **Accelerated hypertension is occasionally referred to as 'malignant' hypertension, especially if optic disc oedema is present.** However, this term is best avoided because patients associate the word 'malignant' with cancer.

Management

Patients require admission and urgent treatment if:

- blood pressure is severely increased (≥ 220/120 mmHg)
- there is life-threatening organ damage (**Table 9.6**)

For patients in the latter group, treatment is with intravenous agents (sodium nitroprusside, glyceryl trinitrate or labetalol) in a high-dependency setting. The aim is to lower blood pressure over 2–6 h to about 160/100 mmHg, but with a reduction not exceeding 25% of the initial value.

> A key principle of management of accelerated hypertension is to avoid a rapid, steep reduction in blood pressure, which may cause further damage to organs that have lost their capacity to autoregulate blood flow, e.g. the brain and kidney.

If the situation is less urgent oral therapy is used instead, which is possible as an outpatient provided they are closely monitored.

- pre-existing antihypertensive medication is restarted or increased, as appropriate
- if there was no pre-existing antihypertensive therapy, the calcium-channel blocker nifedipine (sustained or modified release) is usually used initially, with other agents added as required

Renal complications

A minority of patients have renal impairment at initial presentation with accelerated hypertension. As blood pressure is lowered, it is not unusual for renal function to deteriorate, sometimes to the point at which renal replacement therapy is required. This deterioration may be caused by damage to the microcirculation combined with loss of autoregulation.

By the time of presentation, a minority of patients have experienced an excessive pressure–induced loss of sodium via the kidney (natriuresis) and are at risk of developing hypovolaemia, which may then contribute a prerenal element to the kidney injury. If this is the case, for example if the patient develops a significant postural drop in blood pressure during treatment (a fall of at least 20 mmHg in systolic or 10 mmHg in diastolic on standing), intravenous crystalloids are indicated.

Prognosis

Accelerated hypertension is one of the few conditions in which renal function can recover over a period of months (or 1–2 years), even if the patient requires dialysis initially.

Accelerated hypertension: life-threatening organ damage		
Complication	Mechanism	Clinical features
Pulmonary oedema	Raised systemic vascular resistance causes acute left ventricular failure with pulmonary congestion	Breathlessness; may be exacerbated when lying flat (orthopnoea)
Acute coronary syndromes	Increased afterload (systemic vascular resistance) increases myocardial oxygen demands	Chest pain, arrhythmias, heart failure
Aortic dissection	Raised pressure causes blood to dissect between layers of the aorta	'Tearing' chest pain radiating to the back; blood pressure may differ in each arm if base of relevant artery is affected
Hypertensive encephalopathy	Direct damage to small blood vessels in the brain, loss of cerebral autoregulation, intracranial hemorrhage	Confusion, seizures, focal signs, coma
Pre-eclampsia or eclampsia (pregnancy-specific)	Unknown; may be due to problems with placental perfusion	None for pre-eclampsia Eclampsia as for hypertensive encephalopathy

Table 9.6 Life-threatening organ damage in accelerated hypertension

It is sometimes unclear whether a patient with accelerated hypertension and renal impairment has an underlying primary renal disease predisposing to hypertension or has renal impairment secondary to the very high blood pressure. Once blood pressure has been controlled, it may be necessary to obtain a renal biopsy to resolve this question. The changes due to accelerated hypertension are seen in the arterioles. They consist of a thickened smooth muscle layer and a thickened duplicated basement membrane resulting in an 'onion-skinning' appearance with a narrowed lumen.

Renovascular disease

Renovascular disease is very common. It is caused by:

- atheroma (by far the most common cause), the deposition of fatty immune cells in the renal arteries, or
- fibromuscular dysplasia (much rarer), a non-atheromatous condition caused by thickening of the walls of the arteries.

Both may cause stenosis (narrowing) of the renal arteries, but atheroma is usually accompanied by atherosclerosis causing disease elsewhere, including peripheral vascular disease, cerebrovascular disease or ischaemic heart disease.

In either type of renovascular disease, the kidneys are critically dependent on the tone (i.e. diameter) of the efferent arteriole to maintain intraglomerular pressure and therefore glomerular filtration. This depends heavily on levels of angiotensin II (see page 18). This dependency on the efferent arteriole occurs because of the reduced perfusion pressure in the glomerulus due to the upstream stenosis. Therefore a sudden or exaggerated decrease in renal function after starting an angiotensin-converting enzyme inhibitor or angiotensin II receptor blocker may indicate renovascular disease.

Although a rare finding, renal artery stenosis may be accompanied by a bruit. This is best heard by listening with the stethoscope in the epigastric regions on the anterior abdomen.

Atheromatous renovascular disease

Atheromatous renovascular disease is a frequent finding in the population at risk of atheroma. The principle risk factors are increasing age, male gender, smoking, hypertension and diabetes. As a cause of renovascular disease it is far more common than fibromuscular dysplasia.

The pathology is the same as that in the vast majority of ischaemic heart disease, cerebrovascular disease and peripheral vascular disease: atheroma formation. This takes place in the main renal artery and the immediate large branch vessels.

Clinical features and investigations

The usual presentation is with renal impairment and hypertension in a patient with risk factors for, or actual evidence of, atheromatous disease in other territories (heart, brain, and periphery, usually the legs). Proteinuria and haematuria are typically absent. An US scan may show asymmetrical kidneys, particularly if there is macroscopic disease causing renal artery stenosis.

Atheromatous embolism

In a small subset of patients with atheromatous disease, the plaques proximal to the kidney can rupture; these are usually in the aorta upstream of the origin of the renal arteries, but sometimes in the main renal artery itself. The rupture may occur spontaneously or secondary to instrumentation of the arterial tree, for example during angiography. The resulting shower of atheromatous material produces the syndrome of cholesterol embolisation. This may be clinically obvious, with purplish discoloration of the feet, often with preserved pulses (so-called 'trash foot'; **Figure 9.4).**

Renovascular disease is often a diagnosis of exclusion. In the typical patient with risk factors for atheroma, renal impairment, hypertension, absence of proteinuria or haematuria, and with or without an US scan that shows small or asymmetrical kidneys, further investigations are not indicated. However, evidence for myeloma should be sought by electrophoresis of serum proteins, looking for a paraprotein and testing the urine for Bence Jones proteins (free immunoglobulin light chains, which are not detected by dipstick analysis)

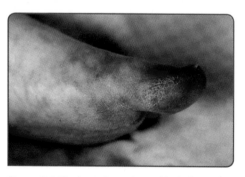

Figure 9.4 The foot of a patient with cholesterol emboli. The mottled discoloration over the middle portion is known as livedo reticularis, and together with the purple toe, is typical of this condition.

In the kidney, the material lodges in small blood vessels and incites a surrounding inflammatory response. Investigations show a deterioration of renal function over subsequent days and weeks, sometimes accompanied by consumption of complement components and eosinophilia. Renal biopsy shows characteristically shaped clefts in the lumen of small arteries where cholesterol within atheromatous emboli has dissolved during processing of the biopsied material. The outlook for recovery of renal function is poor.

Management

Management of atheromatous renovascular disease is with blood pressure control and risk factor modification (see page 278). There is little evidence that treating atheromatous stenosis directly with angioplasty, stenting or both makes any difference to the natural history of the disease; therefore it is unusual to proceed to angiography, which will not influence management and carries risk.

Fibromuscular dysplasia

Fibromuscular dysplasia is a rare cause of renal artery stenosis. There is non-atherosclerotic thickening of the wall of the renal artery, usually affecting the media layer of the artery. In most patients, the stenosis is unilateral. The aetiology is unknown, but there may be a genetic predisposition. It characteristically occurs in women in their thirties.

Fibromuscular dysplasia is suggested by the presence of a renal artery bruit. If suspected, angiography is carried out and typically shows a beaded appearance (**Figure 9.5).**

Unlike atheromatous disease, this condition responds to angioplasty: balloon dilatation of the narrowed artery, with or without the use of a stent to maintain the dilatation. If this is successful, the patient may be able to stop or reduce antihypertensive medication.

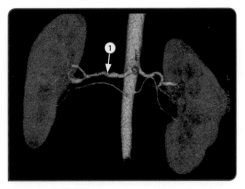

Figure 9.5 Three-dimensional reconstruction from a CT angiogram of a patient with fibromuscular dysplasia affecting the right renal artery (1), showing the characteristic beaded appearance. The left renal artery is normal. Courtesy of Dr Uday Patel.

Hypertension in special cases

There are two situations in which the general principles of management of hypertension require modification.

Hypertension in pregnancy

Hypertension in the setting of pregnancy may be chronic, i.e. pre-existing hypertension of any cause, or may arise specifically in pregnancy. The latter is termed gestational hypertension and usually arises after 20 weeks' gestation. There are two types:

- gestational hypertension in the absence of proteinuria
- pre-eclampsia in the presence of proteinuria

Both chronic and gestational hypertension also predispose to the development of pre-eclampsia as an additional complication.

> **Pregnancy in a patient with renal impairment carries significant risks for both fetus and mother.** The incidence of miscarriage increases steeply as eGFR decreases. For the mother, there is often an irreversible decline in glomerular filtration rate. Expert counselling and shared renal–obstetric care is required.

Management

Management of hypertension in pregnancy is complicated by:

- need to avoid under-perfusion of the placenta
- the more limited range of suitable drugs, (e.g. both angiotensin-converting enzyme inhibitors and angiotensin II receptor blockers can cause fetal abnormalities, and should be avoided).

As a result, the target for blood pressure is < 150/100 mmHg, with acute treatment only if blood pressure is > 150–160/100–110 mmHg. **Table 9.7** lists drugs that are safe to use in pregnancy.

Hypertension in diabetes

Diabetes, especially type 2 diabetes, is a common cause of chronic kidney disease (see page 160). Good glycaemic control and good control of blood pressure are two vital aspects of management that can help prevent or delay the development of diabetic nephropathy.

Antihypertensives used in pregnancy	
Oral	Intravenous
α-Methyldopa	Labetalol
Labetalol	Hydralazine
Nifedipine (long-acting preparation)	

Table 9.7 Antihypertensive agents safe for use in pregnancy

Management

Blood pressure is regularly assessed in all diabetic patients. Because of the importance of good blood pressure control in diabetes guidelines suggest the lower target of <130/80 mmHg in type 2 diabetes with kidney (microalbuminuria is the earliest manifestation), eye or cerebrovascular damage. In type 1 diabetes the target is <135/85 mmHg unless there is albuminuria or features of the metabolic syndrome, in which case it is <130/80 mmHg. Achieving these targets nearly always requires multiple drug therapy.

An angiotensin-converting enzyme inhibitor or an angiotensin II receptor blocker should be a component of the regime because these agents are particularly effective at lowering intraglomerular pressure via their vasodilatory effects on the efferent arteriole. Intraglomerular pressure is the main driver for the hyperfiltration that occurs early in the natural history of diabetic nephropathy, and which is thought to then cause further damage to the glomerulus.

Answers to starter questions

1. Angiotensin-converting enzyme inhibitors (ACEIs) comprise one of the most effective and widely-used classes of antihypertensive drug. Their initial development was prompted by the observation that peptides in the venom of *Bothrops jararaca* had ACEI activity. Although these peptides were not active taken orally, research on them led to captopril, the first clinically useful ACEI.

2. The pulse pressure is determined by the elasticity of the arterial tree distal to the heart. With elastic arteries, part of the energy in the expelled stroke volume of blood is absorbed by dilation of the artery, buffering the rise in blood pressure. During diastole, elastic recoil of the arteries boosts diastolic pressure. The net effect is a reduced pulse pressure. With age, and particularly with CKD, elasticity is lost, leading to a widening of pulse pressure. It is likely that this stiffening makes a significant contribution to the markedly increased cardiovascular mortality seen in CKD.

3. Atheromatous renovascular disease (e.g. renal artery stenosis) is a common contributor to hypertension in the older population. Much less commonly, fibromuscular dysplasia may cause hypertension in younger patients. In either case, the decreased renal perfusion causes an increase in renin production by the kidney, leading to hypertension, and the narrowing of the renal artery may produce an audible bruit, best heard either side of the midline in the epigastric region.

4. Hypertension associated with episodic symptoms such as sweating, pallor, and panic attacks is a classical presentation of phaeochromocytoma. Although these catecholamine-secreting tumours are a rare cause of hypertension, it is important not to miss the diagnosis: they are cured by surgery, and untreated may result in life-threatening hypertensive crises.

5. There are at least two reasons for visual disturbance in a patient with hypertension. With its fine and delicate arteries, the retina is an 'end' organ for hypertensive damage; hypertensive retinopathy. In severe cases, this may include a large retinal haemorrhage that may interfere with vision. The other situation arises secondary to accelerated hypertension (> 180/110 mmHg with grade 3 or 4 hypertensive retinopathy) where cerebral autoregulation of blood flow is impaired, and a decrease in blood pressure can cause cerebral underperfusion. The occipital lobes, which contain the visual cortex, are particularly vulnerable. This is why blood pressure should not be reduced too rapidly in treating accelerated hypertension.

Chapter 10
Tubulointerstitial disease

Starter questions

Answers to the following questions are on page 295.

1. A patient presents with heavy proteinuria, oedema, and hypoalbuminaemia (i.e. the nephrotic syndrome; see page 176). A renal biopsy shows apparently normal glomeruli and an interstitial nephritis. What should the patient be specifically asked about?
2. Why might a patient with disease affecting the tubulointerstitial compartment of the kidney pass large amounts of urine?
3. Why might a patient with a chronic manic-depressive illness be referred to a nephrologist?
4. What does the M in MRSA stand for? Why is it no longer used?
5. How may imaging be helpful in a patient admitted with a suspected upper urinary tract infection?

Introduction

Tubulointerstitial diseases affect the proximal and distal convoluted tubules, loop of Henle, collecting duct and the surrounding supporting tissues (see page 9).

Tubulointerstitial disease includes both hereditary (see Chapter 11) and acquired diseases (this chapter); the latter being either acute or chronic. Both types result in one of, or several of, various clinical syndromes caused by disturbance of normal tubular function. The acute conditions are usually reversible, but the chronic diseases are a significant cause of end-stage renal failure (10–20% of cases).

The level of damage to the tubulointerstitial compartment is the key determinant of prognosis in renal disease, even if the primary disease affects the glomerulus. The extent of interstitial fibrosis and tubular atrophy found on renal biopsy is often a more accurate predictor of the likelihood of progressive chronic kidney disease than glomerular changes (Chapters 5 and 6).

Case 12 Excessive passage of urine

Presentation

Rosemary Wilkins, aged 54 years, presents to her general practitioner (GP) with increasing tiredness. She has also been passing more urine than usual, particularly at night, for several months.

Initial interpretation

Tiredness is a common and non-specific symptom with multiple mental and physical causes. However, the history of polyuria (the passage of large amounts of urine, usually accompanied by increased urinary frequency) suggests conditions such as diabetes and kidney disease. She should be asked about any history of renal disease (e.g. frequent urinary tract infections as a child) and whether there is a family history of diabetes. The examination will include measuring blood pressure, examining the fundi for any evidence of hypertensive or diabetic retinopathy, and testing her urine.

Further history

Mrs Wilkins is well known to the practice, where she has received treatment for bipolar disorder for the past 20 years. Her symptoms have been controlled by lithium therapy for the last 10 years under psychiatric supervision. She has had no other problems with her health and has no family history of diabetes or other significant disease.

Examination

Her mental state is normal. No abnormal features are found on physical examination, including fundoscopy. Mrs Wilkins' blood pressure is 145/86 mmHg. Dipstick urinalysis gives a positive result (+) for proteinuria only.

Interpretation of findings

The absence of glycosuria shown by dipstick urinalysis makes diabetes unlikely to be the cause of her polyuria. Increased blood pressure is a very common finding in people of Mrs Wilkins' age. Although the pressure is not particularly high, hypertension together with proteinuria means that significant kidney disease must be considered and investigated for.

The history of long-term lithium use together with polyuria suggest lithium nephropathy is a possibility. This complication develops in 20–30% of patients on long-term lithium treatment and manifests with varying degrees of failure to produce a concentrated urine and chronic kidney disease. Mrs Wilkins' renal function must therefore be estimated using relevant blood and urine tests.

Investigations

Blood and urine tests are ordered to estimate her glomerular filtration rate (from serum creatinine concentration), quantify her proteinuria (using urinary albumin:creatinine ratio) and check her glycosylated haemoglobin for evidence of diabetes (**Table 10.1**). Additionally, a search through Mrs Wilkins' records shows that 2 years ago her creatinine concentration was at the upper limit of normal, which suggests significant renal impairment at that time. Because serum creatinine concentration is inversely related to glomerular filtration rate, by the time serum creatinine is at the upper limit of normal the patient will typically have lost about a third of their renal function.

Case 12 continued

One of the most useful – and cheapest – 'investigations' in nephrology is a look at previous estimations of renal function. Obtaining information about the timescale of a deterioration in renal function is often key to formulating a working diagnosis and plan of investigation.

Diagnosis

Mrs Wilkins' current and previous creatinine levels show that her renal function has worsened significantly, having probably been abnormal 2 years ago. Her normal glycosylated haemoglobin levels rule out diabetes as a cause.

The clinical picture suggests lithium nephropathy because of the combination of probable chronic kidney disease and polyuria in a patient who has been on this drug for a number of years. The slight increase in urinary protein excretion is also consistent with this diagnosis. She should be referred to a nephrologist to confirm the diagnosis; stopping her lithium will have significant implications for her mental state.

Mrs Wilkins is seen in the local nephrology clinic where her history, examination and initial investigations are reviewed. A renal ultrasound is arranged and shows two normal-sized kidneys. A subsequent renal biopsy shows tubular atrophy, interstitial fibrosis and a sparse infiltrate of chronic inflammatory cells. These biopsy appearances are found in a range of chronic conditions, but are also consistent with lithium nephropathy, which has no specific features.

The exact causal relationship between lithium and the changes found at biopsy is unclear. However, the evidence for lithium nephropathy is sufficiently strong that Mrs Wilkins is switched to another drug to treat her bipolar disorder and her renal function stabilises.

Rosemary Wilkins' blood test results

Test	Result	Normal range or target
Urine albumin:creatinine ratio	9.7 mg/mmol	< 3 mg/mmol
Serum creatinine	193 µmol/L	50–110 µmol/L
Serum albumin	36 g/L	35–50 g/L
Haemoglobin A1c	39 mmol/mol	< 48 mmol/mol

Table 10.1 Blood test results for Rosemary Wilkins

Tubular syndromes

Several hereditary and acquired syndromes affect specific parts, and therefore functions, of the renal tubule (Figure 10.1). This is then reflected in their varying clinical presentations. They are accompanied by some degree of proteinuria, usually less than 1–2 g/day; larger amounts suggest concomitant glomerular disease.

The most common syndrome found in clinical practice is difficulty producing concentrated urine, i.e. a degree of nephrogenic diabetes insipidus. The other syndromes below are much rarer, but a single underlying pathology, depending upon how many segments of the tubule are affected, may exhibit features of more than one of these tubular syndromes.

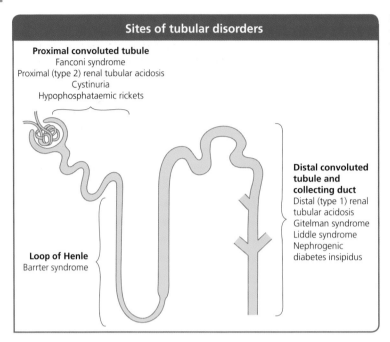

Sites of tubular disorders

Proximal convoluted tubule
Fanconi syndrome
Proximal (type 2) renal tubular acidosis
Cystinuria
Hypophosphataemic rickets

Distal convoluted tubule and collecting duct
Distal (type 1) renal tubular acidosis
Gitelman syndrome
Liddle syndrome
Nephrogenic diabetes insipidus

Loop of Henle
Barrter syndrome

Figure 10.1 Sites of tubular disorders in the renal tubule.

Problems in renal sodium, potassium and water transport

Any cause of tubulointerstitial disease, particularly if it is chronic (see page 291), tends to cause sodium wasting and an acquired nephrogenic diabetes insipidus. This is because the renal tubule normally reabsorbs 99% of the glomerular filtrate, so even mild tubular problems result in significant losses.

Several hereditary syndromes cause derangements in the renal tubular transport of sodium, potassium and water (see page 19):

- Bartter's and Gitelman's syndromes (causes excessive loss of electrolytes)
- Liddle's syndrome (causes retention of sodium)
- nephrogenic diabetes insipidus (causes an inability to concentrate the urine)

> **Patients with tubulointerstitial diseases tend to waste excessive amounts of sodium and water** (at least in the early stages), whereas patients with diseases affecting their glomeruli tend to have sodium and water retention.

Fanconi's syndrome

Fanconi's syndrome is caused by disease processes that predominantly affect the proximal tubule. This is the main site for reabsorption of glucose, amino acids, phosphate, bicarbonate, sodium, potassium and water; consequently, all these substances appear in excess in the urine. Patients are affected by:

- acidosis
- growth failure (in children)
- rickets or osteomalacia (the effect of phosphate loss is exacerbated by failure of production of active form of vitamin D; see page 41)
- hypokalaemia
- polyuria, polydipsia and hypovolaemia

Aetiology

The syndrome may be caused by a number of hereditary defects (see Chapter 11) or acquired causes including:

- myeloma (or other monoclonal gammopathies)
- the use of certain drugs (e.g. tenofovir, used in the treatment of HIV infection)
- heavy metal poisoning

Many of these conditions also result in chronic kidney disease (CKD; see Chapter 4).

Management

Treatment is directed at the underlying cause. Replacement therapy (bicarbonate, vitamin D, potassium) may also be needed.

Renal tubular acidosis

The exchange of ions and other molecules throughout the length of the renal tubule regulates acid–base balance. Therefore diseases at various sites may be accompanied by acidosis. In fact, any cause of low glomerular filtration rate in advanced CKD can cause acidosis due to a failure to excrete the acid products of metabolism.

There are two main types of renal tubular acidosis: type 1 and type 2 (**Table 10.2**).

Pathogenesis and clinical features

Decreases in plasma bicarbonate concentration are accompanied by increases in chloride concentration to maintain electroneutrality. Therefore renal tubular acidosis results in a hyperchloraemic acidosis with a normal anion gap (see page 259). Renal acidosis is usually associated with hyperkalaemia, but the effect on plasma potassium concentration is variable. Type 1, for example, occasionally presents with hypokalaemia, but this is unusual.

Management

Any underlying condition (**Table 10.2**) is treated. The acidosis is treated with oral sodium bicarbonate.

Hyporeninaemic hypoaldosteronism, sometimes called renal tubular acidosis type 4, is most commonly seen in diabetic nephropathy. The main clinical consequence is hyperkalaemia, which makes management with angiotensin-converting enzyme inhibitors or angiotensin II receptor blockers difficult because these agents favour retention of potassium via their block of aldosterone release. Dietary control of potassium is helpful, together with treatment with oral sodium bicarbonate.

Renal tubular acidosis types 1 and 2		
	Type 1	Type 2
Site affected	Distal renal tubule	Proximal renal tubule
Causes	Genetic, nephrocalcinosis, autoimmune diseases, use of certain drugs	Genetic, causes of Fanconi's syndrome, use of certain drugs
Features	Minor loss of bicarbonate (< 100 mmol/day) Urine pH > 5.5 Failure to thrive (in children) Osteomalacia (in adults)	Large loss of bicarbonate Urine pH < 5.5 Osteomalacia Nephrocalcinosis and renal calculi
Treatment	Small amounts of bicarbonate are sufficient	Difficult: large doses of bicarbonate required

Table 10.2 Comparison of renal tubular acidosis types 1 and 2

Acute tubulointerstitial disorders

Acute disorders affecting the tubulointerstitial compartment present with acute kidney injury (AKI), a clinical picture resembling rapidly progressive glomerulonephritis, or both (see page 179). Occasionally they also have features of a tubular syndrome (see page 287).

Acute tubular necrosis is a very common finding in acute kidney injury (see Chapter 3). Acute tubulointerstitial nephritis is a rarer condition, but important to recognise because it can be given specific treatment.

Acute tubulointerstitial nephritis

Acute tubulointerstitial nephritis is an acute inflammatory disorder characterised by inflammatory infiltrates (e.g. lymphocytes, macrophages, oedema, occasionally eosinophils) affecting both tubules (tubulitis) and the interstitium.

The disorder is found in up to 10% of patients with intrarenal AKI.

Aetiology

Various drugs, infections and systemic diseases can cause acute tubulointerstitial nephritis (**Table 10.3**). In some cases an aberrant immune response is implicated, for example drug hypersensitivity, but in others the detailed pathogenic mechanisms are unknown. Up to a third of cases have no obvious precipitant.

Pathogenesis

Whatever the cause, the inflammatory cells attack and disrupt the normal function of the tubules. The accompanying oedema increases intrarenal pressure and further impedes normal filtration.

Clinical features and investigations

The condition presents with deteriorating renal function over days or weeks. There may be a history of a relevant precipitating factor or associated systemic disease, and other manifestations of hypersensitivity in the form of a rash or arthralgia. Proteinuria is usually moderate (protein: creatinine ratio < 70). Eosinophilia, eosinophiluria or both may be present depending on the cause, but a renal biopsy is required for definitive diagnosis.

Management

Any precipitating factor is treated and potentially causative drugs stopped. If the condition fails to improve or if there is no obvious cause to address then corticosteroids are

Acute tubulointerstitial nephritis		
Causes	Examples	Comments
Drugs	Antibiotics (rifampicin), non-steroidal anti-inflammatory drugs, omeprazole Many other drugs have been implicated	In some cases, an immune response to the drug is detected
Infections	HIV, hantavirus, leptospirosis and many others	Some cases represent direct involvement, others a hypersensitivity reaction
Autoimmune diseases	Systemic lupus erythematosus, Sjögren's syndrome	Probably immune complex-mediated
Miscellaneous	Sarcoid Tubulointerstitial nephritis with uveitis syndrome Transplant rejection	Sarcoid produces a granulomatous interstitial nephritis

Table 10.3 Causes of acute tubulointerstitial nephritis

indicated. Supportive management is the same as for other causes of AKI (see page 150).

If a cause can be identified and treated or if the condition responds to corticosteroids then the prognosis is usually good. In other cases, it eventually results in chronic kidney disease (CKD) or end-stage renal failure.

Acute tubular necrosis

Acute tubular necrosis is a loose term used to describe the acute tubular injury found in AKI (see page 139), particularly when this is caused by ischaemic or toxic insults, or both.

The term is used loosely because a biopsy is not usually carried out so the detailed pathology is unknown. Even if a biopsy is examined, the tubules are usually not necrotic.

There is swelling of the tubular cells depending on the severity of the acute insult. This, combined with detachment of cells in cases of actual necrosis, causes tubular obstruction. Recovery requires regeneration of tubular cells, characterised by the appearance of dilated tubules with flattened epithelium containing mitotic figures.

Other aspects of the history and management of acute tubular necrosis are covered in Chapter 3.

Chronic tubulointerstitial nephritis

Chronic tubulointerstitial (or interstitial) nephritis is caused by chronic damage to the tubulointerstitial compartment; it may or may not be inflammatory in nature.

Tubular atrophy and interstitial fibrosis, the end results of damage to the tubulointerstitial compartment, are a common consequence of many forms of chronic glomerulonephritis: as glomeruli sclerose and become obsolescent their associated tubule atrophies. A similar histological picture, with varying degrees of chronic inflammatory infiltrate, is produced by a wide range of other insults (**Table 10.4**), which together account for 10% of cases of CKD.

Aetiology

A variety of toxic, immunological and physical factors cause damage to the tubulointerstitial compartment (**Table 10.4**).

Pathogenesis

The exact pathogenesis depends on the underlying cause, but always involves the production of various pro-inflammatory and pro-fibrogenic cytokines by tubular and interstitial cells, which drives the proliferation of fibroblasts and generation of interstitial fibrosis.

Clinical features

The clinical features are the same as those of CKD (see page 162), with or without a tubular syndrome (see page 287).

Investigations

Specific investigations are performed to confirm any underlying precipitants suggested

Chronic tubulointerstitial nephritis: causes		
Causes	Examples	Comments
Use of certain drugs	Phenacetin (analgesic nephropathy)	Now rarely seen
	Lithium	All patients on long-term lithium need renal monitoring
	Mesalazine	May have an acute presentation
Autoimmune diseases	Systemic lupus erythematosus, Sjögren's syndrome	Rare; glomerular involvement is usual
Toxins	Heavy metals (lead, mercury)	Rare
	Plant-derived toxins (herbs used in traditional Chinese medicine, Balkan endemic nephropathy)	Probably both caused by contamination with *Aristolochia* alkaloids
Miscellaneous	Radiation-induced nephritis	History of radiotherapy
	Post-reflux or obstructive nephropathy	

Table 10.4 Causes of chronic tubulointerstitial nephritis

by the patient's history. Ultrasound (US) imaging often shows small kidneys, in which case a renal biopsy is not usually carried out because it carries a higher risk than with normal-sized kidneys and the information gained is unlikely to affect management.

Management

Any specific causes are addressed, for example any toxins or causative drugs are withdrawn and autoimmune conditions treated with immunosuppression. Otherwise, management is the same as for CKD (see page 166). If an underlying cause can be treated then renal function may stabilise, but in many cases the patient will progress to end-stage renal failure.

Tubulointerstitial infections

Tubulointerstitial infections are infections of the renal substance; they are either acute or chronic. Lower urinary tract infections are a very common problem, particularly in women where the shorter urethra means infections can ascend to the bladder more easily. They are usually managed in primary care, but recurrent, complicated or chronic infections of the lower urinary tract are referred to an urologist, urogynaecologist or a nephrologist.

Lower urinary tract infections are the most common precursor to an ascending infection involving the renal substance: acute pyelonephritis.

Pyelonephritis

Pyelonephritis is an acute inflammation of the renal substance caused by an infection. The severity of its symptoms varies from mild loin pain and pyrexia, to a life-threatening illness if accompanied by septicaemia.

Aetiology and clinical features

Pyelonephritis is caused by lower urinary tract infections that ascend to the kidney. *Escherichia coli* is the most common causative organism (70–90% of cases); other causes include *Staphylococcus saprophyticus*, *Enterococcus* and *Proteus*.

Patients present with severe loin pain, systemic upset and pyrexia. If the patient is hypotensive, or has other systemic signs of sepsis, they will require hospital admission.

Diagnostic approach

A diagnosis is made with a typical history, pyrexia and loin tenderness on examination, and the results of urine and blood cultures showing a typical organism. If suggested by the history, e.g. a history of renal colic, US scans and CT urograms are used to detect complicating features such as renal calculi or obstruction.

Management

Treatment is with antibiotics targeted at the causative organism. They are given intravenously with fluids if the patient is admitted to hospital. Recovery is usually complete, but there may be residual scarring of the renal substance, particularly if the acute infection was complicated by abscess formation.

> **Ascending infections, usually with Gram-negative bacilli, can produce a renal corticomedullary abscess.** On the other hand a renal cortical abscess is produced by haematogenous spread. *Staphylococcus aureus* is then the causative organism in most cases.

An infected, obstructed collecting system is an emergency. Without prompt management the kidney will be destroyed and reduced to a bag of pus (a pyonephrosis). In addition to antibiotics, treatment usually requires percutaneous drainage with insertion of a nephrostomy tube under radiological guidance.

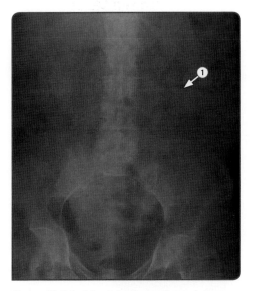

Figure 10.2 A plain abdominal radiograph from a patient with emphysematous pyelonephritis. Gas is visible outlining the collecting system of the left kidney ①.

A rare variant which also requires prompt drainage is emphysematous pyelonephritis. It is caused by gas-producing organisms (**Figure 10.2**) and typically occurs in patients with diabetes.

Renal tuberculosis

Renal tuberculosis is a chronic infection of the kidneys with *Mycobacterium tuberculosis*. It occurs following seeding from a primary infection, usually in the lungs. It is rare, but is sometimes found in residents of endemic regions (e.g. South Asia) or immigrants from these areas.

Patients present with sterile pyuria. They may also have disease in other organ systems (e.g. the lower urogenital tract) or systemic symptoms of infection (e.g. pyrexia, night sweats and weight loss).

Imaging (e.g. a CT urogram) shows calcification of the kidney and strictures of the collecting system or ureters. A prolonged urine culture is required to identify the causative microorganism. Treatment is with standard antituberculous chemotherapy.

Xanthogranulomatous pyelonephritis

Xanthogranulomatous pyelonephritis is a rare form of chronic bacterial infection that occurs as a complication of infected renal stones. The kidney is largely replaced by a chronic inflammatory mass which mimics a renal tumour.

The name comes from the yellowish appearance of the mass (Greek: xanthos, 'yellow'); the colour of lipid-laden macrophages. Treatment requires nephrectomy.

Malacoplakia

Malakoplakia is caused by an abnormal response by macrophages to a chronic infection, usually with *E. coli*. It presents as inflammatory plaques involving any part of the urinary system, but other tissues may also be involved. Histopathology shows characteristic Michaelis–Guttmann bodies.

Papillary necrosis

In papillary necrosis the renal papillae become necrotic. They are then either sloughed into the collecting system or remain in situ and calcify. Papillary necrosis is caused by toxic, ischaemic or infective insults.

Aetiology

Papillary necrosis is a rare condition with the following causes:

- complication of sickle cell disease
- complication of diabetes

- severe pyelonephritis
- urinary tract obstruction
- excessive analgesic intake

Clinical features and investigations

If a papilla is sloughed, its passage down the ureter produces symptoms similar to renal colic caused by a calculus or clot. Similarly, it can cause obstruction. Patients also have an inability to concentrate urine, leading to polyuria, nocturia and polydipsia.

Investigations show sterile pyuria, haematuria, CKD and hypertension. Imaging of the kidneys shows cortical irregularities, distorted calyces (**Figure 10.3**) and papillary calcification. The calcification is best visualised with CT; US is valuable if obstruction is suspected.

Management

Any underlying condition is treated. An obstruction requires urological and radiological intervention. Salt and water depletion is avoided in patients with a concentrating defect.

> **Remember to always consider over-the-counter preparations and ask the patient specifically about them.** Patients may not see these as typical drugs and do not always mention them when asked about their medication history.

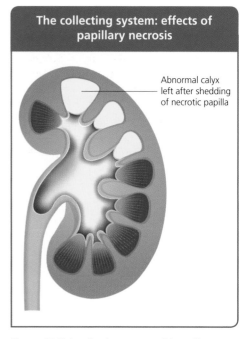

The collecting system: effects of papillary necrosis

Abnormal calyx left after shedding of necrotic papilla

Figure 10.3 A collecting system with papillary necrosis affecting the upper calyces. There is an abnormal space which represents the gap left by the shed necrotic papilla.

Answers to starter questions

1. Has he or she taken any painkillers recently? Nephrotic range proteinuria is very unusual in interstitial nephritis. However, the combination of interstitial nephritis and minimal change nephropathy, the latter responsible for the heavy proteinuria, is almost pathognomonic of non-steroidal anti-inflammatory drug (NSAID) use, as these agents can cause both of these renal lesions.

2. It is worth recalling that with a glomerular filtration rate of 100 mL/min, the glomeruli are producing 100 x 60 x 24 mL (i.e. 144 L) of filtrate per day. Obviously, the vast majority of this is reabsorbed by the renal tubules or else fatal dehydration would occur very quickly. However, even a moderate disturbance of tubular function by tubulointerstitial disease may interfere with this reabsorption, resulting in dangerously large volumes of urine.

3. Lithium, often used in manic-depressive illness, may cause an acute renal problem with nephrogenic diabetes insipidus with or without acute kidney injury, and has been implicated in chronic tubulointerstitial nephritis. An alternative mood stabilizer may be tried, but unfortunately, some patients appear dependant on lithium.

4. MRSA stands for methicillin (or meticillin)-resistant *Staphylococcus aureus*. Methicillin was one of the first penicillins to be developed with significant activity against *Staphylococcus*. Unfortunately, it caused an interstitial nephritis in a high proportion of patients (10-20% if treated for more than 10 days). For this and other reasons it has been superseded by drugs such as flucloxacillin and is no longer used clinically.

5. Plain abdominal X-ray, renal ultrasound and CT of the kidneys, ureters and bladder (KUB) is indicated in patients with suspected upper urinary tract infection. Acute pyelonephritis may show radiological features including calculi (in the kidney or ureter), hydronephrosis and gas in the urinary collecting system (i.e. the calyces, ureters and bladder) that suggest a more complicated case requiring urgent urological and/or radiological intervention.

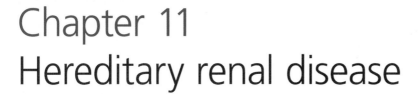

Chapter 11
Hereditary renal disease

Starter questions

Answers to the following questions are on page 306.

1. Why is it important to ask a patient with newly diagnosed autosomal dominant polycystic kidney disease (ADPKD) about a family history of stroke?
2. Why should a man presenting with haematuria and renal impairment, with a family history of other affected male members, be asked about their eyesight and hearing?
3. When might a patient with polyuria and polydipsia be treated with diuretics to reduce urine volume?

Introduction

Inherited renal disease accounts for about 10% of cases of end-stage renal failure and causes biochemical abnormalities in individuals with less severe renal disease. Disease is either localised to the kidney, i.e. primary inherited kidney disease, or a systemic disease that involves the kidney.

Inherited renal disease is usually due to a single gene mutation. All components of the kidney can be affected by one or more of these mutations. The commonest inherited renal disease is autosomal dominant polycystic kidney disease (ADPKD), in which multiple cysts develop gradually from the renal tubules and lead to renal failure.

Presentations reflect the function of the genes or cells involved. For example:

- glomerular basement membrane defects lead to haematuria, proteinuria and chronic kidney disease (e.g. Alport's syndrome)
- podocyte defects cause nephrotic syndrome and progressive renal impairment (e.g. congenital focal segmental glomerulosclerosis)
- tubule defects lead to electrolyte derangements (e.g. Bartter's and Gitelman's syndromes)
- tumour suppressor gene defects lead to tumour syndromes

Close collaboration with clinical geneticists is needed for detailed molecular diagnosis, which may be relevant to prognosis, and for genetic counseling of families.

Case 13 Flank pain

Presentation

Philip Porter, aged 35 years, presents to his general practitioner (GP) with right-sided flank pain. This started suddenly the previous day and is moderately severe, although perhaps improving a little. He also noted that his urine was blood-stained at the time, but this is now clearing.

Initial interpretation

Flank pain has many causes, including renal colic, cholecystitis and a musculoskeletal origin.

Patients often worry that the pain may be coming from the kidney, but this is unusual unless renal calculi are responsible. A musculoskeletal origin, for example pain due to degenerative spinal disease, is a much commoner cause. However, in this case the presence of haematuria, even though it is now resolving, suggests a urinary tract source.

Further history

Philip is worried that the pain may be caused by kidney trouble, because his father died in his sixties from renal failure. The GP takes a further family history and discovers that a paternal uncle died in his thirties from an intracranial haemorrhage. Philip is married, but does not have any children.

Examination

Philip's blood pressure is 155/95 mmHg. On abdominal examination, the GP can feel masses in both flanks, which are bimanually palpable (ballotable).

Interpretation of findings

The family history of renal disease and the finding of probable enlarged kidneys make the diagnosis of ADPKD very likely.

However, this diagnosis needs to be confirmed because it has implications for other members of the family, especially if Philip has children in the future.

Philip's hypertension (blood pressure >140/90 mmHg) is probably secondary to his renal disease, because the distortion of the renal substance produced by the growth of the cysts will have interfered with the blood supply, triggering increased renin release. ADPKD is associated with an increased incidence of intracranial berry aneurysms, so it could well account for his uncle's death.

Investigations

The GP arranges blood tests to determine renal function, as well as an abdominal ultrasound scan. Blood test results show a reduced eGFR of 42 mL/min/1.73 m^2 (Table 11.1). Ultrasound shows two enlarged kidneys with multiple cysts; a few cysts are also visible in the liver.

> **Pain in polycystic kidneys is fairly common, and is usually the result of haemorrhage in a cyst.** It may be accompanied by visible haematuria. Usually nothing more than reassurance and simple analgesia are needed. More rarely, infection of a cyst produces pain with pyrexia and systemic upset; a prolonged course of antibiotics is usually needed in such cases.

Diagnosis

The diagnosis of ADPKD is confirmed by findings on the ultrasound. Although multiple simple cysts, i.e. sporadic cysts not due to ADPKD, sometimes cause diagnostic confusion, simple cysts are not associated with enlarged kidneys or with cysts in the liver. Philip is referred to a nephrologist for further follow-up and management.

Case 13 *continued*

Philip Porter's blood test results		
Test	Result	Normal range or target
Urine albumin:creatinine ratio (mg/mmol)	2	< 3
eGFR (mL/min/1.73 m^2)	42	> 60
Serum albumin (g/L)	44	35–50
Haemoglobin A1c (mmol/mol)	27	< 48

Table 11.1 Blood test results for Philip Porter

Philip requires annual reviews to check his blood pressure control and monitor the progression of renal impairment. He is reassured that progression is likely to be slow and predictable, and that there will be plenty of time to plan for renal replacement therapy in the future. The implications for any future children, each of which will have a 50% chance of inheriting the condition, are discussed with him. Because of his family history of intracranial haemorrhage, a magnetic resonance angiogram is organised to screen for berry aneurysms. It is normal.

Cystic kidney disease

Cystic kidney disease is characterised by the development of fluid-filled spaces of various sizes within the renal substance. Autosomal dominant polycystic kidney disease is the most common form and accounts for 5–10% cases of end-stage renal failure. The recessive form, autosomal recessive polycystic kidney disease (ARPKD), is rarely seen in adults because it has a high mortality rate in children. A number of other conditions previously termed 'medullary cystic kidney disease' are better termed autosomal dominant tubulointerstitial kidney disease. This is a more accurate description because they are not always characterised by obvious cysts (see page 304).

- In about 85% of patients there is a mutation in the *PKD1* gene, encoding polycystin-1, on chromosome 16
- In 15% there is a mutation in the *PKD2* gene, encoding polycystin-2, on chromosome 4

The products of PKD1 and PKD2 form a heterodimer, i.e. a protein comprising two different polypeptide chains, on the surface of tubular cells, explaining the similar phenotype in all patients. However, patients with defects in polycystin-2 tend to have a slower progression to renal failure.

A substantial proportion of patients with ADPKD do not have an obvious family history. In 10% of these patients the disease is due to a new mutation. In the other 90% the disease has not been recognised in previous generations.

Autosomal dominant polycystic kidney disease

This is the most common form of inherited cystic disease seen in adults; it is extremely rare in childhood because cysts only develop from the late teens onwards.

Aetiology

The global prevalence of ADPKD is about 1 in 1000.

Although only about 10% of tubules develop cysts, the growth of these gradually compresses and damages the remaining normal renal tissue (**Figure 11.1**).

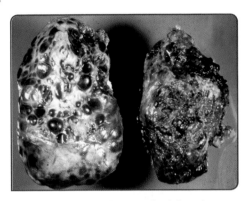

Figure 11.1 Polycystic kidneys after bilateral nephrectomy. Each kidney is largely made up of cysts, with little remaining normal renal tissue.

Clinical features

The main feature of ADPKD is progressive renal impairment leading to end-stage renal failure, usually after the age of 40 years. Other features include cystic haemorrhage or infection, and an increased incidence of hypertension. Rarely, the kidneys are so large that nutritional status is affected. There is also a raised risk of malignancy.

Cysts also commonly occur in the liver and, more rarely, in the pancreas. These are usually asymptomatic, but massive hepatomegaly occasionally develops, particularly in women.

The most significant extrarenal manifestation is an increased incidence of intracranial berry aneurysms. These are found in 10–20% of patients. If present, they confer an increased risk of intracranial, usually subarachnoid, haemorrhage.

Investigations

The most helpful investigation to confirm the diagnosis of ADPKD is renal ultrasound: it is cheap, non-invasive, readily available, and gives good visualisation of the cysts. Other imaging modalities, such as CT scans, can be used. Cysts appear on ultrasound as multiple, echo-free spaces within the kidneys, which are enlarged as a result.

Screening for intracranial aneurysms with magnetic resonance angiography (MRA) is recommended in patients with any family history of intracranial bleeds. Whether a detected aneurysm is treated depends on its characteristics. Prophylactic endovascular coiling is carried out for large accessible aneurysms. Small aneurysms are monitored by repeat MRA every few years.

Management

Management is as for other causes of progressive kidney disease (see page 166); there is no direct treatment for the defect. Good control of blood pressure, although probably having only a minor effect on the rate of progression of renal impairment, is beneficial for general cardiovascular health.

Tolvaptan, an antidiuretic hormone (ADH) antagonist, can slow the progression of renal impairment in ADPKD. However, with the predictable consequences of inducing polyuria, nocturia, thirst and polydipsia, it is unclear how much of a role this drug will have in management.

Prognosis

The progression to end-stage renal failure is not inevitable; by the age of 70 years, about 75% of patients have reached this stage. When end-stage renal failure does occur, it is usually slow and predictable, which allows planning for any of the usual options for end-stage management.

Renal screening

It is recommended that potentially affected family members over the age of 18 years are offered screening with renal ultrasound. Diagnostic criteria have been published that relate age, number of cysts detected on imaging and probability of having inherited the condition.

Screening apparently unaffected individuals for polycystic kidney disease, as with screening for other genetic diseases, is a complex issue that needs to be carefully discussed with the patient. There will be implications, for example, for life insurance and for the patient's children.

Other inherited cystic disease

Autosomal recessive polycystic kidney disease is much rarer than ADPKD; it affects 1 in 10,000–40,000 live births. It is caused by a mutation in the *PKHD1* gene on chromosome 6, which encodes fibrocystin.

In contrast to the autosomal dominant form, ARPKD often presents with renal complications early in life; mortality is up to 70–80% for very early presentations (within weeks or months of birth). Increasingly it is being recognised that children may survive to or present in adult life, when hepatic complications secondary to fibrosis are a significant feature.

Inherited glomerular disease

With the exception of some of the collagen chain defects, inherited glomerular disease is relatively rare. They present with combinations of haematuria and proteinuria, and with progressive renal impairment in many patients. The most common conditions are summarised in **Table 11.2.**

Collagen chain defects

These are defects of the collagen chains that are components of the glomerular basement membrane.

X-linked Alport's syndrome

X-linked Alport's syndrome has a global prevalence of 1 in 10,000–50,000. Renal involvement manifests as haematuria and progressive renal impairment, leading to end-stage renal failure in the late teenage years to early adulthood. Other features are hearing and ocular involvement, namely high-tone deafness and lenticonus (an anterior bulging of the lens), respectively. Depending on the degree of random inactivation (lyonisation) of the

Inherited glomerular diseases			
Category	Genes*	Diseases	Pattern of inheritance
Collagen chain defects	COL4A5	X-linked Alport's syndrome	X-linked
	CO4A3, COL4A4	Autosomal recessive Alport's syndrome	Autosomal recessive
	COL4A3	Benign familiar haematuria, also known as thin basement membrane disease	Autosomal dominant
Congenital nephrotic syndrome and focal segmental glomerulosclerosis	NPHS1	Nephrin deficiency: Finnish-type congenital nephrotic syndrome	Autosomal recessive
	NPHS2	Podocin deficiency	Autosomal recessive
	WT1	A transcription factor deficiency: Denys–Drash syndrome	Autosomal dominant
Systemic diseases with significant glomerular involvement	GLA	α-Galactosidase A deficiency: Fabry's disease	X-linked
	Various, including APOA1, which encodes apolipoprotein A-I	Familial amyloidoses (all autosomal dominant)	Autosomal dominant

*The genes are not comprehensive lists; in many cases of these diseases, mutations of other genes are known to produce a similar phenotype.

Table 11.2 Inherited glomerular diseases

normal X chromosome in the kidneys, female patients may be affected to a variable degree, but generally much less severely than male patients (end-stage renal failure, for example, is extremely rare in female patients).

Other collagen chain defects

More common than X-linked Alport's syndrome are other defects of collagen, including heterozygous carriers of autosomal recessive Alport's syndrome. These conditions present with intermittent or persistent non-visible haematuria, which may be familial in 30–50% of cases (benign familial haematuria).

Renal biopsy is usually not indicated, but if carried out shows diffuse thinning of the glomerular basement membrane (thin membrane disease). The prognosis is excellent because one normal gene is present; if patients develop renal impairment, this is usually caused by a separate disease.

Congenital nephrotic syndrome and focal segmental glomerular sclerosis

A number of congenital nephrotic syndromes lead to focal segmental glomerulosclerosis. As listed in **Table 11.2** several different gene defects, many coding for components of the glomerular filtration apparatus, manifest with proteinuria in the nephrotic range (>3 g/day) in childhood. In some patients this occurs from birth. The proteinuria usually results in the development of focal segmental glomerulosclerosis and renal failure. Treatment is supportive and the same as for other causes of end-stage renal failure. Renal transplantation is associated with a very low risk of recurrence, except in the case of *NPHS1* mutations, in which antibodies to nephrin may develop in up to 25% of cases.

The high prevalence (at least 10–30%) of genetic causes in cases of childhood focal segmental glomerulosclerosis means that screening for known mutations is probably worthwhile in this group. A precise genetic diagnosis will inform prognosis and genetic counseling. Screening is not currently indicated in adult practice, but the rapid improvements in the cost and speed of DNA sequencing may make this possible in the future.

Systemic disease with glomerular involvement

Fabry's disease

Fabry's disease is rare, affecting only 1 in 40,000 live births, but it is thought to be underdiagnosed in the male population with end-stage renal failure. It produces a characteristic rash (angiokeratoma corporis diffusum: small red papules, usually around the thighs, groin and lower abdomen), but this is not always obvious. Pain resulting from nerve involvement, defects in sweating, corneal clouding and cardiac complications may also suggest the diagnosis.

Amyloidosis

Many different abnormal proteins may deposit in various tissues, including the kidney, as amyloid. This produces amyloidosis, which usually presents with proteinuria and progressive renal impairment. It can be difficult to distinguish these rare hereditary types from the commoner acquired AA and AL amyloidosis (see page 204); referral to a specialist centre may be indicated. The National Amyloidosis Centre at University College London is the only UK centre specialising in amyloidosis.

Inherited tubulointerstitial disease

Inherited tubulointerstitial diseases are rare. They present with one or a combination of the tubular syndromes discusssed in Chapter 10, renal impairment or stone formation (**Table 11.3**).

Disorders of renal tubular sodium transport

Genetic defects that affect the Na$^+$–K$^+$–2Cl$^-$ cotransporter in the ascending limb of the loop of Henle (see page 23) cause Bartter's syndrome, whereas defects of the Na$^+$–Cl$^-$ cotransporter in the distal tubule (see page 23) cause Gitelman's syndrome. These are rare conditions, with variable ages of presentation. In general, Bartter's syndrome presents in the first few years of life, whereas Gitelman's syndrome does not present until early adult life.

Clinical features

The effects of Bartter's syndrome and Gitelman's syndrome mimic those of loop

Category	Gene(s)*	Disease(s)	Pattern of inheritance
Disorders of renal tubular sodium handling	SLC12A1	Deficiency of Na$^+$–K$^+$–2Cl$^-$ cotransporter: Bartter's syndrome	Autosomal recessive
	SLC12A3	Deficiency of Na$^+$–Cl$^-$ cotransporter: Gitelman's syndrome	Autosomal recessive
	SCNN1G	Gain-of-function sodium channel: Liddle's syndrome	Autosomal dominant
Disorders of acid–base balance (see Chapters 8 and 10)	SLC4A4	Deficiency of bicarbonate cotransporter: proximal renal tubular acidosis	Autosomal recessive
	SLC4A1	Deficiency of anion transport protein: distal renal tubular acidosis	Autosomal dominant
Autosomal dominant tubulointerstitial kidney disease	UMOD, REN and MUC1	Medullary cystic kidney disease and familial juvenile hyperuricaemic nephropathy	All autosomal dominant
Disorders of water handling	AVPR2	Deficiency of ADH receptor: nephrogenic diabetes insipidus	X-linked
Renal stone disease	SLC3A1 and SLC7A9	Deficiency of dibasic amino acid transporter: cystinuria	Variable inheritance
	CLCN5	Deficiency of Cl$^-$–H$^+$ exchanger: Dent's disease	X-linked

Inherited tubulointerstitial diseases

ADH, antidiuretic hormone.
*The genes listed are not comprehensive; in many cases of these diseases, mutations of other genes are known to produce a similar phenotype.

Table 11.3 Inherited tubulointerstitial diseases

diuretics and thiazide diuretics, respectively, and lead to loss of sodium. The resulting decrease in the volume of body fluid (i.e. volume contraction) causes secondary hyperaldosteronism, which leads to hypokalaemia and metabolic alkalosis; however, blood pressure is usually normal.

Urinary calcium excretion differentiates between the two syndromes because, again mimicking the effects of the two classes of diuretics, urinary calcium is normal or high in Bartter's syndrome but reduced in Gitelman's syndrome. Bartter's syndrome is also associated with defective urine-concentrating ability, resulting in polyuria and polydipsia.

Management

These syndromes are managed by electrolyte replacement (potassium and magnesium) and the use of potassium-sparing diuretics. Fluid replacement is usually required for Bartter's syndrome, and non-steroidal anti-inflammatory drugs may also be useful because the condition is associated with excessive prostaglandin synthesis, which exacerbates the metabolic features.

> **Because Bartter's and Gitelman's syndromes mimic the effects of diuretics, surreptitious abuse of diuretics is a key other cause of the metabolic disturbances associated with these conditions.** Another cause is electrolyte loss due to excessive vomiting, e.g. in bulimia nervosa.

Liddle's syndrome

Liddle's syndrome is caused by a gain-of-function mutation (the mutant protein is overactive) in the amiloride-sensitive sodium channels of the distal tubule and collecting duct. In contrast to Bartter's and Gitelman's syndromes, this leads to excessive reabsorption rather than loss of sodium, and a clinical picture of hypertension and hypokalaemia that mimics mineralocorticoid excess. It is treated by blocking the sodium channel with amiloride or triamterene.

Autosomal dominant tubulointerstitial kidney disease

This is the umbrella term for a group of disorders previously known by names such as medullary cystic kidney disease and familial juvenile hyperuricaemic nephropathy. They present with slowly progressive renal impairment (end-stage renal failure in middle age), minimal proteinuria or haematuria, and tubulointerstitial fibrosis on renal biopsy.

Nephrogenic diabetes insipidus

Nephrogenic diabetes insipidus is caused by mutations of the genes encoding the ADH receptor (X-linked) or the water channel protein aquaporin 2 (autosomal dominant or recessive). These produce a clinical picture of polyuria and polydipsia. This is similar to the clinical picture for central diabetes insipidus, which is caused by failure to produce ADH.

The two conditions are distinguished by the failure of diabetes insipidus with a nephrogenic cause to respond to administration of the ADH analogue desmopressin. Paradoxically, treatment with thiazide diuretics helps reduce urine volumes in nephrogenic diabetes insipidus, probably in part because the volume contraction that they cause promotes proximal tubular reabsorption of sodium and water.

Cystinuria

Cystinuria is the most common inherited renal stone disease, with an incidence of 1 in 10,000 live births. In cystinuria, mutations affect the proteins responsible for renal reabsorption of the dibasic amino acids cystine, ornithine, arginine and lysine, but only cystine is of sufficiently low solubility to form renal stones.

Inheritance is usually autosomal recessive. However, heterozygous individuals can have increased urine concentrations of cystine, in some cases sufficient to lead to stone formation. In this situation, the disease is behaving more like an autosomal dominant condition with variable penetrance.

Clinical features

Diagnosis is by visualisation of the characteristic hexagonal cystine crystals on urine microscopy and quantification of the relevant amino acids in the urine. The complications of cystinuria are those associated with any cause of renal stone (see page 309):

- renal colic
- infections
- obstruction
- in severe cases, chronic kidney disease progressing to end-stage renal failure

Management

Cystinuria is managed by increasing fluid intake and alkalinising the urine. If these measures are ineffective, chelating agents that bind to cystine and increase its solubility are used e.g. D-penicillamine.

Inherited tumour syndromes

Tuberous sclerosis and Von Hippel–Lindau disease are caused by mutations of autosomal dominant tumour suppressor genes. These mutations 'take the brakes off' cell cycle checkpoints, thereby allowing unregulated cell division, the mechanism underlying many cancers. For the disease to manifest, there must be a 'second hit' mutation of the remaining normal allele in somatic cells. This can lead to tumour development in various parts of the body.

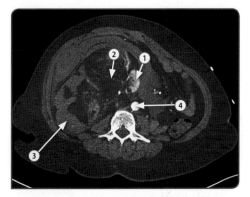

Figure 11.2 Contrast-enhanced CT scan showing acute bleeding ① into a massive angiomyolipoma ② in a patient with tuberous sclerosis. The angiomyolipoma is of low attenuation because of its high fat content. The patient had undergone emergency left nephrectomy to treat life-threatening bleeding into an angiomyolipoma on that side. ③, normal renal tissue ④, contrast in abdominal aorta.

Tuberous sclerosis

Tuberous sclerosis is caused by mutations in either the *TSC1* or *TSC2* gene. It affects 1 in 5000–10,000 live births. Benign hamartomas develop in a number of organs, most obviously the skin, eye and brain. These may be associated with severe problems manifesting in early childhood, such as seizures, developmental delay and behavioural difficulties.

In 60–80% of patients, angiomyolipomas develop in the kidney. These are benign tumours with vascular, adipose and smooth muscle components. Small tumours are asymptomatic, but larger ones may cause potentially life-threatening bleeding (**Figure 11.2**). Management of larger tumours with either surgery or radiology-guided embolization, while sparing normal renal tissue, can be difficult. The drug everolimus, which targets the underlying cellular dysregulation, has shown considerable promise in reversing the growth of these tumours.

Von Hippel–Lindau disease

Von Hippel–Lindau disease is caused by mutations affecting the *VHL* gene and affects 1 in 36,000 live births. The most serious extrarenal features are retinal angiomas, haemangioblastomas of the central nervous system and phaeochromocytomas.

In the kidney, the condition eventually leads to the development of renal carcinoma in at least 50% of patients. Regular screening with imaging of the kidneys is recommended.

Answers to starter questions

1. ADPKD is associated with an increased incidence of intracranial aneurysms (found in 10–20% of cases of ADPKD versus 1–5% in the general population). Patients therefore have a raised risk of aneurysmal rupture leading to intracranial haemorrhage. Screening for such aneurysms is advised if there is any family history of stroke or subarachnoid haemorrhage, which might be due to aneurysmal rupture.

2. Alport's syndrome is one of the more common inherited diseases that affect the glomerulus. It presents with haematuria and renal impairment. In most patients it is X-linked and due to a mutation of the gene coding for a collagen chain found in the glomerular basement membrane. The same collagen chain is also present in the eye and ear, so patients will often have lenticonus, an anterior bulging of the lens, and high tone hearing loss.

3. Thiazide diuretics have surprisingly been shown to reduce urine volumes in nephrogenic diabetes insipidus. The mechanism is not completely understood, but appears to involve increased sodium and water reabsorption in the proximal tubule, which is a regulatory response to the volume contraction caused by the diuretics. This decreases the volume of tubular fluid delivered to the distal nephron, where the defect in water reabsorption in this condition occurs.

Chapter 12
Urological nephrology

Starter questions

Answers to the following questions are on page 316.

1. Why should a patient with recurrent renal stones be advised against eating large amounts of rhubarb?
2. Why might a patient with a chronic partial obstruction of the urinary tract pass excessive amounts of urine?
3. What advice should be given to a woman known to have renal scarring who is pregnant with her first child?
4. Why should a patient presenting with a raised haemoglobin concentration (i.e. polycythaemia) be asked whether they have noticed any blood in their urine?

Introduction

Urology is the surgical speciality that deals with disorders of the urogenital tract. It encompasses urodynamics, oncology, stone disease, reconstruction, paediatric urology and andrology. The conditions it deals with are common, and account for up to a third of all surgical hospital admissions.

Joint management by urologists and nephrologists is needed when urological conditions have a significant impact on renal function and when medical management is appropriate, for example in certain cases of renal stone disease and retroperitoneal fibrosis.

Very few urological conditions are immediately life-threatening on presentation, but they often severely affect patients' quality of life. Therefore early diagnosis and management are essential. This is particularly true of malignant conditions: urinary tract tumours are common, e.g. bladder cancer is the seventh commonest cancer in the UK.

Case 14 Severe loin pain

Presentation

John Wilkinson, a 45-year-old butcher, presents to the emergency department. He is accompanied by his son. He awoke this morning with severe left-sided loin pain. The pain comes and goes in waves and is the worst he has ever experienced, making him feel sweaty and nauseous. It radiates down into his left groin, and makes him try to move around for relief.

Initial interpretation

Pain is an extremely common symptom and must be carefully categorised to develop a list of possible causes (see **Table 2.2**). John's presentation is typical of renal colic, i.e. acute-onset episodic pain in the flank radiating to the groin.

Colic is pain that comes and goes in waves and makes the patient move around. In contrast, the pain of peritonism, i.e. inflammation of the lining of the abdominal cavity (the peritoneum), tends to be constant and makes the patient lie still.

The distribution of the pain reflects the dermatomes that share the innervation of the renal tract (see Figure 2.2).

Further history

John recalls a similar but much less severe episode 2 years ago after a 2-week summer holiday in Spain. After that episode, he also remembers passing some grit in his urine. He is otherwise well, with no other significant past medical history.

Examination

Examination shows a man in obvious discomfort with left loin tenderness. He is sweaty but observations are otherwise normal.

Interpretation of findings

This clinical picture strongly suggests renal stone disease: the nature of the pain points to a ureteric origin, and the previous history suggests that this is caused by a stone. Similar pain can be produced by the passage down the ureter of blood clots or sloughed renal papillae (see page 293). However, the history of grit in the urine after a holiday in a hot country suggests that renal calculi are much more likely. In hotter climates, urine concentration tends to increase, thereby increasing the likelihood of calculi forming n the urinary tract.

John is referred to the urology team at the local hospital for investigation and management.

Investigations

After arrival in the emergency department, John provides a fresh urine sample. Dipstick urinalysis gives a ++ result for blood, confirming the likelihood of pathology in the renal tract. The urinalysis does not show any evidence of an associated infection, which would be indicated by the presence of nitrite and white blood cells. CT of the kidneys, ureters and bladder shows a 0.5-cm renal calculus at the left ureterovesical junction. Given that John has a history of renal calculi, blood and urine samples are sent to screen for metabolic conditions such as hypercalcaemia. The results are all normal except for a urine test result indicating excessive calcium excretion, i.e. hypercalciuria (**Table 12.1**).

> Renal calculi tend to lodge at the narrowest points of the urinary tract: the pelviureteric junction, pelvic brim and ureterovesical junction.

Case 14 continued

John Wilkinson's blood and urine test results		
Test	Result	Normal range
Dipstick urine	Blood ++	Negative
Serum calcium	2.43 mmol/L	2.2–2.7 mmol/L
Urine calcium excretion	7.3 mmol/24 h	1.2–6.2 mmol/24 h

Table 12.1 Blood and urine test results for John Wilkinson

Diagnosis

The diagnosis is a renal calculus as visualised on CT, secondary to idiopathic hypercalciuria, as detected by the urine test. John is advised about maintaining good fluid intake and reducing the amount of salt in his diet (which reduces calcium excretion), because these are essential steps to prevent recurrence.

John is treated with analgesia and intravenous fluids. He passes the stone spontaneously within a day while still an inpatient. He is discharged with arrangements for follow up in the urology stone clinic.

Renal stone disease

In renal stone disease, a discrete stone (calculus) or stones (calculi) form in the collecting system of urinary tract. It is one of the more common disorders affecting the urinary tract, occurring in up to 5% of women and 10% of men at some point in their lives.

Nephrocalcinosis is the formation of more diffuse calcification involving the renal cortex and medulla. It is seen in renal tubular acidosis or systemic conditions causing hypercalcaemia.

Aetiology

Renal stones form when substances exceed their solubility threshold in urine. Therefore any factor that leads to increased urine concentration, such as low fluid intake, living in a hot climate or both, predisposes to stone formation.

Stones of different composition have different causes (**Table 12.2**). The commonest type of stone (80% of cases) contains calcium combined with oxalate, phosphate or both; most of these stones are the result of idiopathic hypercalciuria, the excretion of an excessive concentration of calcium in the urine that is not associated with hypercalcaemia.

Clinical features

Small stones, or stones retained within a calyx, may be asymptomatic. Passage of larger stones down the ureter causes renal colic: severe colicky pain radiating from loin to groin; haematuria (visible or invisible) is frequent. Complicating infection may cause pyrexia and systemic upset.

Investigations

Initial investigations are carried out to identify the stone through imaging studies. Urine and blood tests are done to identify a cause.

Imaging

CT is used to visualise the stone unless radiation dosage is a concern, in which case ultrasound is used (e.g. in women who are or might be pregnant).

On CT scan, renal stones appear as discrete areas of increased density within the renal tract (**Figure 12.1**). They are usually round unless they occupy a significant portion of the pelvicalyceal system ('stag horn' calculi).

Renal stones: types and causes		
Type of stone	Frequency (% of stones)	Causes
Calcium containing	80	Any cause of hypercalcaemia, especially primary hyperparathyroidism
		Hypercalciuria (without hypercalcaemia)
		Hyperoxaluria: increased intake of oxalate (rhubarb, spinach, chocolate), enteric hyperoxaluria or primary hyperoxaluria
		Hypocitraturia: distal renal tubule disorder (citrate binds calcium)
Uric acid	10	Idiopathic
		Hyperuricaemia: in association with gout, high cell turnover or tumour lysis
		Hyperuricosuria (without hyperuricosaemia): high urate intake or proximal renal tubule disorder
		Acid urine
Magnesium ammonium phosphate (struvite), usually with calcium	3	Infection with urease-producing bacteria (e.g. *Proteus*)
Cystine	2	Cystinuria (see page 304)
Other	1–3	Hereditary: xanthinuria or Dent's disease
		Use of certain drugs (e.g. indinavir, ritonavir)

Table 12.2 Types of renal stone and their causes

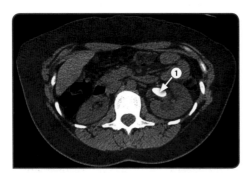

Figure 12.1 Transverse CT scan showing a renal calculus ① in the left kidney.

On US, they appear as areas of increased echogenicity, usually with a posterior acoustic shadow, where there is a relative lack of penetration by the ultrasound beam due to reflection by the calculus.

Blood and urine tests

Urine is examined for blood and signs of infection, i.e. nitrites and white cells on dipstick testing. If the latter are present, urine should be sent for microbiological analysis.

Particularly if stones are recurrent, further analysis of blood and urine is directed towards identification of one of the underlying metabolic causes (see **Table 12.2**). If the stone is available, then laboratory analysis of its chemical composition will help identify any underlying cause.

> **Calcium and, to a lesser extent, cystine stones are radiopaque and visible on plain radiographs.** Uric acid stones are radiolucent on plain films but visible on CT. Stones composed of indinavir, an antiretroviral drug, are radiolucent even on CT.

Management

Management of renal stone disease includes pain relief, usually with non-steroidal anti-inflammatory drugs, and fluids, which need to be intravenous if the patient is nauseated. Most stones pass spontaneously. However, if this does not occur, stones may be removed by various approaches, including endoscopic surgery, percutaneous nephrolithotomy, extracorporeal shockwave lithotripsy or open surgery.

Ensuring ample fluid intake is the primary way to prevent formation of further stones. Depending on the exact cause, more specific long-term medical management may be necessary, as described in **Table 12.3**.

> **An infected, obstructed renal tract is a medical emergency.** In addition to antibiotics to treat the infection, urgent urological intervention, radiological intervention or both are required to relieve the obstruction.

Prognosis

Renal stones often recur but rarely result in serious permanent damage. However, the following may lead to significant loss of renal tissue, and in extreme cases end-stage renal disease:

- multiple stones, especially if caused by a metabolic disorder such as cystinuria

Renal stone disease: medical management	
Type of stone	Management
Calcium containing	Treat any cause of hypercalcaemia
	Decrease salt intake to decrease calcium excretion
	For idiopathic hypercalciuria:
	■ thiazide diuretics to decrease calcium excretion
	■ potassium citrate (citrate binds calcium)
Uric acid	Allopurinol
	Potassium citrate to alkalinise the urine
Cystine	D-penicillamine
Infection associated	Appropriate antibiotics

Table 12.3 Medical management of renal stone disease

- large stones, for example staghorn calculi involving two or more calyces, particularly if associated with infection

Obstructive uropathy

The urinary tract can become obstructed at any level from the pelviureteric junction in the kidney down to the urethra. Acute bilateral obstruction or obstruction of a single functioning kidney are key differential diagnoses in acute kidney injury (see Chapter 3). In this situation, prompt recognition and relief of the obstruction are vital parts of management.

Aetiology

The causes of obstructive uropathy are:

- intralumenal, for example stones
- within the wall of the urinary tract, e.g. strictures
- the result of external compression, e.g. fibrosis or tumours

The most common causes are bladder outflow obstruction secondary to prostatic disease in men and renal calculi.

Clinical features

Chronic obstruction, particularly if unilateral, is often asymptomatic. In advanced disease, the symptoms are those of chronic kidney disease (see page 162), accompanied by any features of the underlying cause.

> **In obstruction, the volume of urine produced may be misleading.** Chronic partial obstruction damages the renal tubules, effectively inducing a state of nephrogenic diabetes insipidus. As a result the patient somewhat paradoxically may have polyuria and polydipsia.

Investigations

Investigations are directed towards identifying the site and cause of the obstruction.

Therefore imaging is a key investigation; US (**Figure 12.2**), CT or both are used. There is sometimes uncertainty as to whether an identified dilated portion of the urinary tract represents a functionally significant obstruction; nuclear medicine scanning may be helpful in these circumstances, because it gives dynamic information concerning the flow of urine and thus identifies significant obstruction.

Management

Functionally significant obstructions need to be relieved as soon as possible after identification. The chosen method depends upon the obstruction, for example:

- bladder outflow obstruction due to prostatic disease is relieved with a urethral catheter in the short term; a subsequent operation is needed.
- Higher levels of obstruction, for example due to retroperitoneal disease, require insertion of tubes under radiological guidance through the skin of the flanks directly into the collecting system of the kidney (nephrostomies).
- Medical management has a significant role in the relief of obstruction in retroperitoneal fibrosis (see below).

With relief of the obstruction, patients may experience a post-obstructive diuresis. This is partly the result of an osmotic diuresis as

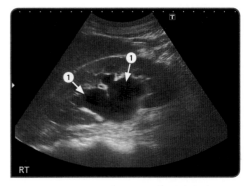

Figure 12.2 US image of an obstructed kidney, showing a dilated pelvicalyceal system ①. This is sometimes referred to as the 'Mickey Mouse' sign.

previously retained low-molecular-weight compounds are cleared, and partly a consequence of the tubular damage, which produces salt and water wasting. Post-obstructive diuresis, which can persist for days and sometimes weeks, must be treated with appropriate fluid replacement to avoid the development of a prerenal component to the renal injury.

Prognosis

Depending on the length and degree of the obstruction, there may be permanent damage to one or both kidneys in the form of tubulointerstitial fibrosis. As with most causes of chronic kidney disease, this may progress to end-stage renal disease (see page 168).

Retroperitoneal fibrosis

Retroperitoneal fibrosis is characterised by inflammation and fibrosis in the retroperitoneal compartment. It has an annual incidence of 1 in 200,000–500,000 of the population, but is being increasingly recognised. The pathology usually occurs around the aorta (periaortitis) but may extend along the pelvic vessels. The ureters are commonly involved in the inflammatory mass, leading to obstruction.

The condition is seen in middle to old age. It is more common in men than in women.

Aetiology

The causes of retroperitoneal fibrosis are:

- Idiopathic or immunoglobulin G4 (IgG4) related disease
- Pathology linked to underlying aortic atheroma and/or aortic aneurysm (see below)
- Drugs (e.g. methysergide and hydralazine)
- Neoplasia (e.g. retroperitoneal lymphoma and sarcoma)
- Infection

It used to be thought that fibrosis associated with underlying aortic disease was caused by an immune response to the lipid components of atheroma. However, it is now thought that both this and 'idiopathic' retroperitoneal fibrosis are probably types of immunoglobulin G4-related disease. In IgG4 disease there is chronic inflammation with a lymphoplasmacytic infiltrate rich in IgG4-positive plasma cells and fibrosis in one or more types of tissue. The cause is unclear but may include an autoimmune component.

Clinical features and investigations

As well as symptoms related to obstruction and renal failure, patients may experience systemic upset, with malaise, tiredness and weight loss. There may be a normochromic normocytic anaemia and, characteristically, increased measures of inflammatory markers such as erythrocyte sedimentation rate and C-reactive protein levels.

Computerised tomography is the best imaging modality for investigation of retroperitoneal fibrosis (**Figure 12.3**). Biopsy may be required if there is uncertainty about the diagnosis, for example if malignancy or infection is suspected.

Management

If there is an identifiable underlying cause this is treated. First-line medical treatment for idiopathic IgG4-related retroperitoneal fibrosis is with glucocorticoids (usually prednisolone). Other immunosuppressants, such

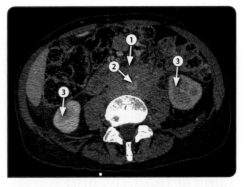

Figure 12.3 CT scan in a patient with retroperitoneal fibrosis, showing an inflammatory and fibrotic mass surrounding the aorta ①. Aorta enhanced by contrast ②. Lower pole of kidneys ③ enhanced by contrast. The dilated pelvicalyceal systems of the kidneys are out of the plane of this cross-sectional image.

as azathioprine and mycophenolate mofetil, may be introduced later as steroid-sparing agents or if there is insufficient response to prednisolone.

Response to treatment is monitored by the effect on inflammatory markers and improvement in renal function. If there are problems with medical management, for example lack of response or intolerable side effects, then the following are considered:

- stenting of the ureters
- ureterolysis, i.e. freeing the ureters from the fibrous tissue and wrapping in omentum to prevent recurrence

The outlook is usually good. However, prognosis depends on the extent of obstructive damage.

Reflux nephropathy

Reflux nephropathy is also known as 'chronic pyelonephritis'. It describes a pattern of renal cortical scarring that in many cases is associated with vesicoureteric reflux of urine and urinary infections, usually in infancy or early childhood. Vesicoureteric reflux is found in up to 10% of the population and is a common cause of chronic kidney disease and end-stage renal disease, particularly in children.

Aetiology

Secondary vesicoureteric reflux occurs in the setting of bladder outflow obstruction as a result of, for example, posterior urethral valves (a developmental abnormality which results in an obstructing membrane in the posterior urethra in men). Primary reflux is caused by an incompetent vesicoureteric junction, reflecting delayed development of the junction's valvular function. It is found predominantly in women.

There is a familial basis for the primary disease, with reflux occurring in up to a third of siblings or children of affected individuals. Scarring of the renal cortex probably requires the combination of vesicoureteric reflux and intrarenal reflux of infected urine, and happens early in life.

Clinical features and investigations

Reflux is associated with urinary tract infections in infancy. This may be because the failure to fully void all urine favours the multiplication of bacteria. The extent to which such infections should be investigated is controversial, as is whether investigations should focus on detection of renal scarring (with ultrasound or dimercaptosuccinic acid scan; **Figure 12.4**) or reflux (some form of micturating cystogram).

If not associated with infections then reflux nephropathy is usually asymptomatic and detected only during investigations for chronic kidney disease, proteinuria or hypertension. Patients may go on to develop end-stage renal disease (see page 168).

> **Renal scars are commonly identified incidentally during renal imaging.** If not associated with renal impairment, hypertension or proteinuria, they are unlikely to be of long-term significance.

Management and prognosis

If the condition is detected in infancy, perhaps as the result of screening of a relative of an affected individual, prophylactic antibiotics may be given for the first few years of life, addressing the role of infection in causing scarring. Surgical treatment is reserved for:

- patients who have problems with antibiotics, such as side effects or poor compliance
- patients who have more severe degrees of reflux

Surgical treatment employs minimally invasive measures to narrow the vesicoureteric junction. Less commonly, ureteric reimplantation may be considered. Surgery is usually required if reflux is secondary to obstruction.

Prognosis depends on the extent of renal scarring and the degree of chronic kidney disease.

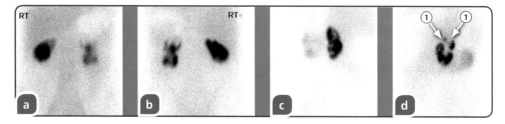

Figure 12.4 DMSA nuclear medicine scan showing renal scarring. ① Scarring (lack of uptake of tracer) has particularly affected the upper pole of the left kidney. Panels show gamma camera images acquired from (a) anterior, (b) posterior, (c) right posterior oblique and (d) left posterior oblique views.

Urinary tract tumours

The most common types of malignant tumour affecting the urinary tract are those arising from the urothelium, i.e. transitional cell carcinoma, and from the renal substance itself, i.e. renal carcinoma.

Haematuria

Both transitional cell carcinoma and renal carcinoma commonly present with haematuria , often visible, which is why this symptom must be thoroughly investigated, particularly in at-risk groups such as older patients and smokers.

Haematuria may also be due to glomerular disease, and it is important to distinguish this 'nephrological' cause from haematuria due to 'urological' diseases (renal calculi, tumours). Coexisting proteinuria suggests referral initially to a nephrologist, and visible haematuria to a urologist, but there is often cross-referral between the specialities during investigation of haematuria.

Benign tumours

The commonest type of benign tumour is an angiomyolipoma. Angiomyolipomas are usually an incidental finding, and when small usually require no further action. Multiple or large angiomyolipomas may occur in tuberous sclerosis (see page 305); large tumours are at risk of bleeding and may require resection or embolisation.

> **Treatment for any form of renal neoplasia usually requires loss of normal renal tissue.** If this risks precipitating end-stage renal disease, detailed discussion with the patient and planning for renal replacement therapy are vital.

Transitional cell carcinoma

Transitional cell carcinoma is common, with bladder cancer accounting for about 1 in 30 new cancers. It behaves as a superficial tumour, easily treated with local therapy, or as an invasive metastatic disease. It may occur anywhere from the tips of the renal papillae down to the proximal urethra, but the bladder is the commonest site. It is multi-centric in 30–40% of cases. Haematuria is the usual presentation, but depending on the site there may also be obstructive features.

Management

Treatment is surgical resection. For early non-invasive tumours this is via a cystoscopic approach. Other tumours may require more radical surgery.

Supplemental medical treatment with intravesical chemotherapy or bacillus Calmette–Guérin vaccine is used to control local disease, particularly if it is multicentric.

> **It is not known how the bacillus Calmette–Guérin (BCG) vaccine controls transitional cell carcinomas.** As a derivative of *Mycobacterium bovis* it probably activates immune cells that then attack cancer cells. Flu-like symptoms with its use are common, but systemic infections are rare.

Renal carcinoma

Renal carcinoma is common, accounting for just under 2% of all cancers. Presentation with haematuria is common, but these tumours are also often incidental findings on imaging carried out for other reasons.

Patients may also present with systemic upset, i.e. malaise, pyrexia and weight loss, or with a paraneoplastic syndrome resulting from production of excess hormones, for example:

- polycythaemia as a consequence of excess production of erythropoietin
- hypercalcaemia resulting from excess parathyroid hormone-related protein

Management

Treatment is with surgical resection. If anatomically feasible, this is of only part of the kidney, i.e. partial nephrectomy. In other cases total nephrectomy is required. Alternatively, for patients who are not fit enough for major surgery, treatment is with various forms of radiologically guided ablation. Conservative management may be appropriate for smaller tumours in older patients.

Answers to starter questions

1. Calcium oxalate is a common constituent of renal stones. Although most oxalate is a product of metabolism, there is a contribution to urinary excretion from oxalate rich foods such as rhubarb, spinach and chocolate.

2. Chronic obstruction damages the renal tubules via the effect of back pressure. This impairs their ability to produce a concentrated urine; in effect, a state of nephrogenic diabetes insipidus. As a result, and somewhat deceptively, chronic obstruction may be associated with polyuria and polydipsia.

3. Renal scarring is often secondary to reflux of infected urine in infancy, even in the absence of a clear history. There is often an inherited component, with the condition occurring in up to a third of first degree relatives. Screening of the newborn, with a view to antibiotic prophylaxis if reflux is identified, should be discussed with the mother.

4. An underlying renal cancer may be causing both the visible haematuria and the polycythaemia, the former by direct bleeding from the tumour and the latter via production of excess erythropoietin.

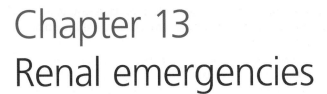

Chapter 13
Renal emergencies

Introduction

Medical emergencies associated with the renal system are common and therefore often present to other medical and surgical specialties. The most frequently encountered are pulmonary oedema secondary to fluid overload, electrolyte disturbances, sepsis originating in the urinary tract and renal colic.

Patients on renal replacement therapy are particularly at risk, primarily due to their difficulties controlling fluid and electrolyte balance. Dialysis patients, particularly those on haemodialysis with little residual urine output, are very prone to fluid overload and hyperkalaemia. Dialysis patients are also at risk of sepsis associated with their access, i.e. intravenous or intraperitoneal catheters. Renal transplant patients are immunosuppressed and therefore have an increased risk of infection, sometimes from unusual organisms (opportunistic infections).

As with any emergency, the approach to management is structured to ensure rapid treatment of the most life-threatening features.

Case 15 Breathlessness

Presentation

Joyce Withers, who is 65 years old, presents to the emergency department with breathlessness. She is unable to lie flat because of this, but she is more comfortable sitting up and denies chest pain. Her pulse rate is 110 beats/min; blood pressure, 175/95 mmHg; oxygen saturation 88% on room air; and respiratory rate, 24 breaths/min. She is apyrexial.

Initial interpretation

Breathlessness is a common symptom in patients presenting to hospital, but it has many varied causes including pulmonary oedema, pneumonia, acute asthma,

Case 15 *continued*

exacerbation of chronic obstructive pulmonary disease and pulmonary embolus. The initial history and examination is directed towards the respiratory and cardiovascular systems because they are where pathology is most likely to be located. In view of Mrs Withers' low oxygen saturation, oxygen therapy is started via a non-rebreathing mask and titrated to achieve 94–98% saturation.

Further history and examination

Mrs Withers has felt tired for the past couple of weeks but has otherwise been reasonably well. She has no fever but is coughing up small amounts of white frothy sputum. She required a coronary artery bypass graft for ischaemic heart disease 3 years ago and she had a transient ischaemic attack 6 months ago.

On examination, there is ankle and sacral oedema, and her jugular venous pressure is raised at 6 cm above the sternal angle. On auscultation of the chest, widespread fine inspiratory crepitations are audible in the mid and lower zones.

Working diagnosis and investigations

Mrs Withers' examination findings suggest fluid overload: there is peripheral oedema (ankle and sacral) and the white frothy sputum together with the fine crepitations in the chest are consistent with pulmonary oedema. Along with this evidence of increased fluid in the interstitial compartment, the raised jugular venous pressure is also consistent with a raised intravascular volume. The non-purulent sputum and absence of pyrexia are evidence against an infective component. Several investigations are ordered:

■ A chest X-ray to confirm the pulmonary oedema

■ Urea and electrolytes to determine renal function: a deterioration might be contributing to the fluid overload
■ Electrocardiography: a further ischaemic cardiac event could have caused acute left ventricular dysfunction, which might to contributing to Mrs Withers' symptoms

Mrs Withers' radiograph shows bilateral perihilar infiltration and pleural effusions, which is consistent with pulmonary oedema (**Figure 13.1**). Her blood test results are: urea 45 mmol/L and creatinine, 750 µmol/L (3 months previously they had been 6 mmol/L and 120 µmol/L, respectively). Her ECG is unremarkable.

Immediate intervention

Mrs Withers has features of acute pulmonary oedema (breathlessness worsened by lying flat, crepitations on auscultation, bilateral perihilar infiltration and pleural effusions on X-ray) in the context of an acute kidney injury (significant deterioration in renal function over a short time). The low oxygen saturation on admission indicates that the pulmonary oedema is

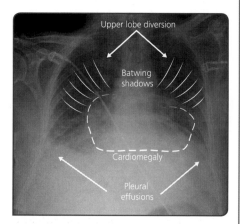

Figure 13.1 Chest radiograph showing features of pulmonary oedema: upper lobe venous diversion, batwing opacities (a pattern of perihilar shadowing) and bilateral pleural effusions.

Case 15 *continued*

sufficient to affect oxygen uptake, putting Mrs Withers at risk of hypoxic complications, particularly of the brain and heart.

Mrs Withers is initially started on intravenous furosemide to promote a diuresis and relieve the fluid overload, and an infusion of glyceryl trinitrate to cause vasodilation which will decrease the load on the heart by reducing preload and afterload. The combined aim of these treatments is to reduce the raised left ventricular end diastolic pressure, which is the cause of her pulmonary oedema. However, after 2 hours her condition appears to be getting worse and the senior doctor in charge of her management decides to insert a temporary central venous catheter and arrange for urgent haemodialysis on the renal unit.

Acute kidney injury

Acute kidney injury is characterised by a sudden increase in creatinine levels resulting from a decrease in glomerular filtration rate (see Chapter 3) and is frequently encountered in the emergency setting. It affects patients with many different conditions, but the principles underlying its emergency investigation and management are the same in all cases.

Fluid management

The fluid status of all patients with acute kidney injury is assessed regularly to guide fluid management (at least daily, but up to once or twice an hour in an emergency situation). Heart rate, blood pressure, jugular venous pressure, capillary refill time and level of consciousness are all recorded so that changes over time can be observed. If the patient has signs of volume depletion, intravenous fluid boluses are given (250–500 mL of crystalloid, e.g. 0.9% sodium chloride) until volume is restored.

Senior review should be sought if the patient remains oliguric despite having received > 2 L of fluid.

- If the patient is euvolaemic, maintenance fluids are given (estimated urine output + 500 mL per day)
- If they are hypervolaemic, diuretics are started and an infusion of glyceryl trinitrate considered

Urgent haemodialysis is required if the patient fails to respond to these measures.

Monitoring

A urinary catheter is inserted to collect urine to monitor the volume produced. However, it risks introducing infection and should only be used if accurately measuring urine output is very important and cannot be determined any other way. Urea, creatinine, electrolytes and bicarbonate concentrations are measured at least once a day because they can change quickly. In addition to routine observations, the patient's weight is recorded daily and an accurate record of fluid intake and output is kept. Because recording this accurately is very difficult changes in weight are the best way to monitor changes in fluid balance on a day-to-day basis.

Investigations

The following investigations are urgently carried out to investigate the cause of acute kidney injury:

- Dipstick urinalysis, followed by a protein: creatinine ratio for more accurate quantification if proteinuria is present
- Ultrasound of the renal tract within 24 h to exclude obstruction, unless an alternative cause of acute kidney injury is clear

- More specialised tests are indicated as required:

  - liver function tests (in suspected hepatorenal syndrome)
  - C-reactive protein test (for sepsis)
  - bone profile (to exclude hypercalcaemia, e.g. due to myeloma)
  - creatine kinase test (for rhabdomyolysis)
  - platelets, blood film, lactate dehydrogenase test, bilirubin test, reticulocyte count (for haemolytic–uraemic syndrome or thrombotic thrombocytopenic purpura)
  - urine and blood for paraprotein (myeloma)
  - blood for decreased immunoglobulins (myeloma)

Emergency management

In addition to fluid management, emergency management of acute kidney injury requires the following:

- Treatment of sepsis
- Cessation of nephrotoxic drugs:
  - non-steroidal anti-inflammatory drugs
  - angiotensin-converting enzyme (ACE) inhibitors
  - angiotensin II receptor blockers
  - potassium-sparing diuretics (risk of hyperkalaemia)
  - metformin (risk of lactic acidosis)
- Stop diuretics, at least temporarily, in cases of hypovolaemia
- Review of drug doses; these may need to be altered
- Administration of a proton pump inhibitor for gastric protection
- Avoidance of intravenous radiographic contrast media (e.g. for contrast enhanced CT scan or coronary angiography). If its use is necessary, intravenous fluids are given to hydrate the patient before and after the procedure

Case 16 Bradycardia in a patient with chronic kidney disease

Presentation

Adam Jenkins, aged 38 years, has chronic kidney disease secondary to immunoglobulin A nephropathy and is well known to the renal team. He is a difficult character with poor adherence to his dietary limitations. He presents to the emergency department complaining of feeling generally unwell after a weekend away with friends.

His observations are: heart rate 35 beats/min, blood pressure 113/76 mmHg, respiratory rate 16 breaths/min, oxygen saturation 98% on room air and temperature 36.5°C.

Initial interpretation

Poor adherence to dietary recommendations can lead to various problems for patients with chronic kidney disease. Too much salt results in poorly-controlled blood pressure, too much fluid results in fluid overload and pulmonary oedema, and too much potassium leads to hyperkalaemia.

Further history and examination

Adam admits to drinking excessive amounts of fruit juice over the weekend, and eating a large amount of chocolate. There are no notable findings on examination and in particular no evidence of fluid overload.

Investigations

Electrocardiography is carried out to assess heart rhythm in view of his bradycardia. Blood is taken to estimate urea and electrolyte concentrations and is sent to the laboratory for urgent analysis. Meanwhile, the ECG is found to be markedly abnormal, with tall, tented T waves, absent P waves, a prolonged PR interval and prolonged QRS complexes with abnormal morphology

Diagnosis

The ECG changes are consistent with hyperkalaemia. In the context of chronic kidney disease and Adam's history this should be treated immediately without waiting for the blood test results, because he is at imminent risk of cardiac arrest.

Immediate intervention

Intravenous access is established and 10 mL of 10% calcium gluconate at a rate of no more than 2 mL/min is started immediately. After this, an infusion of 10 units of soluble human insulin in 50 mL of 50% glucose over 15 min is started.

Adam's potassium concentration is rechecked after the infusion and further treatment given if necessary. If Adam fails to respond to medical management, dialysis will be needed to ensure that his potassium levels are brought within a safe range.

The use of ion exchange resins such as calcium resonium is no longer recommended. They were previously used for the management of hyperkalaemia, but evidence for their effectiveness is lacking and they could be harmful.

Acute severe hyperkalaemia

Acute severe hyperkalaemia most commonly occurs in cases of:

- acute kidney injury secondary to the use of drugs such as ACE inhibitors, angiotensin II receptor blockers and potassium-sparing diuretics
- tissue injury, for example from rhabdomyolysis or surgery

Immediate action is required if any of the following are present:

- potassium concentration > 6.5 mmol/L
- characteristic symptoms associated with hyperkalaemia, for example weakness
- ECG changes: tall, tented T waves, absent P waves, a prolonged PR interval and bizarre QRS complexes (see Figure 7.2)

Initial management consists of:

- 10 mL of 10% calcium gluconate or calcium carbonate intravenously at a rate of no more than 2 mL/min, followed by:
- 10–20 units of soluble human insulin in 50 mL of 50% glucose over 15 min

If severe acidosis is present without fluid overload, intravenous sodium bicarbonate is also given. However, this is avoided in patients with hypocalcaemia (because the increase in pH further reduces levels of ionised calcium), and in patients with type 2 respiratory failure (because this will be exacerbated by the CO_2 load produced as the bicarbonate buffers the excess acid). Salbutamol nebulisers are given to increase cellular uptake of potassium, but care is needed because they can cause tachycardia.

Case 17 Acute loin to groin pain

Presentation

Derek Sykes, who is 45 years old, presents to the emergency department with sudden onset pain in his left side. The pain is severe, comes and goes in waves, and moves down towards his groin. He has also been vomiting and is unable to keep any fluids or medications down.

Initial interpretation

Acute onset of pain in the flank and radiating to the groin, i.e. renal colic, is the classic symptom of renal stones. This tends to affect men in their twenties to forties. Because Derek is vomiting and unable to keep down any food or drink, he is at risk of becoming dehydrated.

Further history and examination

Derek had a similar episode of pain a few years ago, but it was not as severe as this one and resolved with the use of analgesics provided by his general practitioner. He has no other medical problems.

On examination, he has tachycardia but his blood pressure is normal and he is afebrile. His left flank is tender and he is unable to lie still for long. There are no current signs of fluid depletion.

Working diagnosis and investigations

The symptoms of severe unilateral flank pain in a middle-aged man, with a similar episode in the past, suggest renal stones. Derek's tachycardia is being caused by the pain.

Blood tests and dipstick urinalysis are carried out as soon as possible to exclude a urinary infection.

Immediate intervention

Because Derek is unable to maintain any oral intake, intravenous access is urgently established. He is started on intravenous fluids to ensure that he remains hydrated.

Analgesia is given as soon as possible: intramuscular diclofenac is usually the first-line treatment, but he will require subcutaneous or intravenous morphine if this is ineffective. Because he is vomiting, an intravenous antiemetic such as metoclopramide should be considered because opiates are likely to exacerbate this symptom. While fluids and analgesia are being dealt with, imaging, usually in the form of a CT in the next few hours, is performed to confirm the diagnosis.

Renal stones

Renal stones have a lifetime prevalence of approximately 15% in men and 10% in women. Although many cases are asymptomatic, acute renal colic requires emergency management because the pain is severe and necessitates rapid relief. Occasionally there is an accompanying infection and if this is not treated urgently the associated kidney is at risk. Key differential diagnoses include non-renal and renal causes (**Table 13.1**).

Differential diagnoses for renal stones	
Renal causes	Non-renal causes
Tumour	Appendicitis
Pyelonephritis	Diverticulitis
Retroperitoneal fibrosis	Ectopic pregnancy
Ureteric stricture	Acute salpingitis
Papillary necrosis	Rupture or torsion of an ovarian cyst
Clot colic	Abdominal aortic aneurysm

Table 13.1 Differential diagnoses for renal stones

Immediate intervention

Immediate intervention consists of intravenous access, fluid resuscitation and analgesia. Patients with volume depletion because of poor oral intake and vomiting are given intravenous fluids.

Pain is usually the most prominent symptom, so effective analgesia is vital. Intramuscular diclofenac is usually effective, but intravenous or subcutaneous morphine may also be required. Antiemetics are also considered: the patient may have nausea and vomiting because of the severe pain or as a complication of opiate use.

Further management of renal stones depends on their size and the patient's symptoms (see page 310).

Investigations

A plain CT of the kidneys is carried out to visualise the stone and exclude ureteric obstruction. Urinary tract infections must be excluded based on the history, basic observations and the results of blood tests (white cell count and C-reactive protein concentration), dipstick urinalysis and urine microscopy, culture and sensitivity.

The presence of an infected, obstructed system is a urological emergency that requires the administration of antibiotics and urgent decompression with a nephrostomy.

Hospital admission

Renal stones are usually managed at home. However, patients are admitted to hospital if they:

- have shock, fever or other signs of systemic infection
- are at increased risk of loss of renal function, for example if they have a single kidney, chronic kidney disease or bilateral obstructing stones, or have had a renal transplant
- are unresponsive to analgesia and antiemetics within 1 h, or have severe or recurrent pain
- are vomiting or dehydrated, and therefore require intravenous fluids
- are pregnant
- are unable to cope alone at home

Hospital admission is also warranted in cases of diagnostic uncertainty, for example for patients:

- at risk of ectopic pregnancy
- in whom leaking abdominal aortic aneurysm cannot be excluded

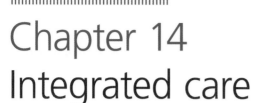

Chapter 14
Integrated care

Starter questions

Answers to the following questions are on page 332.

1. When should general practitioners refer patients with renal dysfunction to secondary care?
2. How is the decision to start a patient on dialysis made?
3. When is the right time to discuss advanced care planning with patients approaching the end of their life?

Introduction

For the majority of patients, stable renal disease is managed in the community by their general practitioner (GP), or is managed jointly between primary and secondary care. Common renal disorders for which this is the case include chronic kidney disease (CKD), renal stones, hypertension and proteinuria.

GPs are usually the first point of contact for patients with renal disorders. They have the responsibility for recognising CKD early on, despite the frequently non-specific nature of its presenting symptoms. This early recognition and prompt initiation of treatment are central to preventing or slowing its progression. GPs must also be alert to renal disease that requires referral to secondary care.

Many patients never need to visit a specialist renal physician in secondary care. However, for those who do, good communication between consultants and GPs is vital to ensure that optimal care is provided. Renal medicine is a multidisciplinary specialty requiring close teamwork (see **Table 14.1**).

Case 18 Starting on dialysis

Presentation

Ipsita Kaur, aged 44 years, has diabetic nephropathy secondary to type 1 diabetes. Over the past year, she has been seen every 3 months in a clinic for patients with advanced CKD. She presents to Dr Butler, a nephrologist, for her appointment and reports feeling increasingly tired and short of breath over the past month. Six months ago, Ipsita had surgery to create an arteriovenous fistula in preparation for starting haemodialysis (Figure 2.39) having decided that she would prefer haemodialysis over peritoneal dialysis. She is waiting for a transplant, but has not found a suitable donor.

Initial interpretation

Ipsita's tiredness and shortness of breath are relatively non-specific symptoms. However, she is known to have progressive CKD and this is the most likely cause for the worsening of her symptoms. However, it is important to keep an open mind: patients with CKD are also at risk of other pathologies that cause similar problems, such as cardiovascular disease.

Further history

Ipsita has been attending the advanced kidney care clinic for the past year, because of her deteriorating renal function. She has met with various members of the multidisciplinary team (Table 14.1). She has discussed her preferences for dialysis with Dr Butler and Sue, the specialist nurse, and has decided to opt for haemodialysis. She does not like the idea of connecting herself to a peritoneal dialysis machine.

She explains that she is concerned that her current symptoms are reducing her ability to work. She wonders whether she may feel better if she starts dialysis.

Examination

Jugular venous pressure is elevated, but Ipsita's heart sounds are normal. Bibasal crackles are audible on auscultation of her chest. Her abdomen is soft and

The renal multidisciplinary team	
Job	Role
Consultant nephrologist	Coordinates patients' specialist medical treatment
General practitioner	Coordinates patients' medical care in the community
Specialist nurse	Provides specialist care for patients with chronic kidney disease, including those who will soon require dialysis, haemodialysis patients, peritoneal dialysis patients and renal transplant patients
Renal dietician	Gives specialist advice on dietary matters specific to renal patients, such as low-phosphate and low-potassium diets, low-salt diets and adequate calorie intake
Physiotherapist	Helps patients improve their mobility, and helps rehabilitate patients after hospital admissions
Occupational therapist	Helps patients participate as fully as possible in activities of daily living
Psychologist	Provides specialist psychological support for renal patients, for example to help them cope with living with a chronic disease

Table 14.1 The renal multidisciplinary team

Case 18 *continued*

non-tender, and there is a palpable thrill and an audible bruit on palpation and auscultation of her fistula.

Interpretation of findings

Ipsita has symptoms consistent with chronic uraemia: tiredness and shortness of breath. She also has signs consistent with fluid overload: raised JVP and bilateral crackles. She is likely to be at the point at which dialysis should be started: although none of her symptoms and signs are absolute indications, they are having a significant impact on her life and will only get worse.

The palpable thrill and audible bruit over her fistula suggest that it is functioning well.

Investigations

Blood tests are arranged to confirm that Ipsita's symptoms and signs are associated with a worsening of her CKD (**Table 14.2**). These show that her eGFR has dropped to 7 mL/min/1.73 m²; it was 12 mL/min/1.73 m² 3 months ago.

Ipsita Kaur's blood test results

Test	Result	Normal range
Sodium	145 mmol/L	135–146 mmol/L
Potassium	5.8 mmol/L	3.5–5.0 mmol/L
Urea	42.8 mmol/L	2.5–6.7 mmol/L
Creatinine	568 µmol/L	79–118 µmol/L
eGFR	7 mL/min/1.73 m	80–125 mL/min/1.73 m²

Table 14.2 Blood test results for Ipsita Kaur

Diagnosis

Ipsita has end-stage renal failure, as confirmed by her eGFR of 7 mL/min/1.73 m². She is symptomatic, with fluid overload and uraemia.

Dialysis should start as soon as possible; it will improve her symptoms and prevent the need for emergency admission to hospital to treat fluid overload or hyperkalaemia. Her condition is stable and her potassium concentration is at a safe level, so she can begin dialysis as an outpatient within the next few days.

When to refer to a nephrologist

In general, patients should be referred to a nephrologist if they have a significant decrease in GFR, proteinuria, hypertension that is difficult to control, are suspected to have an underlying significant renal disease or have any of the other indications listed in **Table 14.3**.

These clinical situations do not, in general, require urgent referral. However, if a systemic disease such as vasculitis is suspected, e.g. the patient has deteriorating renal function, blood and protein in the urine, and systemic upset, then this is a medical emergency. In cases where there is doubt, the local renal unit should be consulted for advice on the appropriate timescale for referral.

Indications for referral to a nephrologist
■ GFR < 30mL, with or without diabetes
■ ACR ≥70 mg/mmol, unless known to be caused by diabetes and already appropriately treated
■ ACR ≥30 mg/mmol, together with haematuria
■ Sustained decrease in GFR of ≥25% or sustained decrease in GFR of ≥15 mL within 12 months
■ Hypertension that remains poorly controlled despite use of at least 4 antihypertensive drugs at therapeutic doses
■ Known or suspected rare or genetic causes of CKD
■ Suspected renal artery stenosis
GFR, glomerular filtration rate; ACR, albumin/creatinine ratio; CKD, chronic kidney disease.

Table 14.3 Indications for referral to a nephrologist

Chronic kidney disease

Chronic kidney disease is a lifelong condition that requires long-term management and follow-up. Although only a small proportion of patients progress to end-stage renal failure, treatment prevents or delays progression and decreases the risk of associated complications such as cardiovascular disease.

Screening

Because earlier stages of CKD are asymptomatic, patients in at-risk populations are offered testing in primary care to enable earlier detection. This involves taking blood for measurement of urea and creatinine concentrations and eGFR and urine dipstick testing for blood and protein. Delayed detection results in increased morbidity and mortality and higher risk of cardiovascular complications.

Chapter 4 lists the predisposing risk factors that are regarded as criteria for screening (see Table 4.6). Many are common in the elderly population, e.g. diabetes, hypertension and cardiovascular disease.

Preventing CKD in patients with cardiovascular disease and diabetes

The pathophysiological processes in cardiovascular disease and diabetes damage the kidneys and greatly raise an individual's risk of renal deterioration and development of CKD (see page 158). This risk can be reduced by paying particular attention to tight control of blood pressure and tight glycaemic control in diabetes. There is substantial evidence that this slows or prevents development and progression of CKD. Along with appropriate pharmacotherapy, lifestyle changes and frequent monitoring are required for tight control. These require patient involvement and are most effectively achieved as a partnership between patient, primary care and, when appropriate, secondary care.

Psychosocial health

The World Health Organization defines health as 'a state of complete physical, mental and social well-being and not merely the absence of disease or infirmity'. In the context of CKD, complete physical health is not achievable, but good psychosocial health must be an aim. Educating the patient, involving them in management and encouraging them to take responsibility for aspects of their treatment are the best ways to approach the mental and social aspects.

Mild depression is common in patients with CKD, particularly when coming to terms with the diagnosis. This is an urgent issue if the prospect of end-stage renal failure is being discussed. Other members of the multidisciplinary team, such as psychologists and nurses, have a particular role to play in providing support to patients with depression or those having difficulty accepting a new diagnosis or disease progression.

Advanced chronic kidney disease

Patients with advanced CKD (stage 5 or progressive stage 4), are seen regularly by their renal physician to allow education around renal replacement therapy and explanation of the options, e.g. haemodialysis, peritoneal dialysis, transplantation and conservative care, and discussion of the patient's preferences.

Planning the patient's pathway through the various options available (**Figure 14.1**) is the responsibility of the renal multidisciplinary team. However, the general practitioner continues to be involved: there are many simple health problems which can be resolved by a convenient visit to the local surgery, rather than a more involved trip to the renal unit. This is especially the case if the patient has chosen a conservative care pathway: care under these circumstances is based largely at home or in a hospice, and the general practitioner is best placed to coordinate this.

Palliative care

A need for palliative care arises in two situations in renal medicine:

■ patients choosing a conservative care pathway for end-stage renal failure

■ patients who are withdrawing from dialysis

In both situations early involvement of and shared care with the hospital or community palliative care team is helpful.

In patients who have capacity, decisions of this gravity should be made after thorough discussion of the options, an explanation of the consequences of not starting or withdrawing from dialysis, and, ultimately, where the patient would wish to die. Patients can be reassured that death from uraemia is not painful; usually a progressively comatose state develops or there is sudden death from hyperkalaemia. More distressing symptoms, such as breathlessness, are best managed by the palliative care team, whether at home, in a hospice or in hospital.

> **A common question from patients and relatives, particularly when withdrawing from dialysis, is how long it will take to die.** This is extremely variable and partly depends on whether there is any residual renal function. If the patient is anuric, then survival for more than a week or so would be very unusual. If there is a significant urine output, then survival can be much longer and difficult to predict.

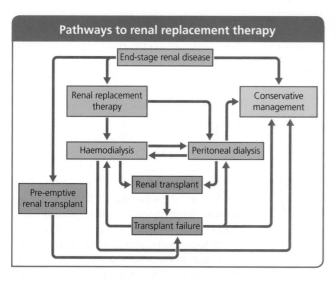

Pathways to renal replacement therapy

Figure 14.1 Pathways to renal replacement therapy.

Renal disease in the elderly

Ageing results in a number of structural and functional changes in the kidneys (**Table 14.5**) and is associated with a decline in renal function. For example, after the age of 30 years eGFR declines by about 8 mL/min/1.73 m^2 per decade. It is unclear whether the age-related decline in renal function is a consequence of the effects of comorbidities or reflects physiological age-related decline. However, changes in renal function are accentuated by comorbidities that have increased incidence in the elderly, such as hypertension, diabetes, heart failure, atherosclerosis and urinary outflow obstruction.

> **Aggressive management of hypertension may be inappropriate in an elderly patient.** The risk of falls or worsening of cognitive function (particularly if the patient already has a degree of memory impairment) associated with hypotensive episodes may outweigh the treatment benefits.

Primary care management

Many elderly patients with CKD present asymptomatically, and the majority never progress to end-stage disease. Most of these patients are safely treated in primary care.

As with younger patients with CKD, management is focused on preventing the adverse effects of renal disease by controlling hypertension and diabetes, if present. However, it requires a more individualised approach that takes into account each patient's comorbidities, functional status, life expectancy and health priorities.

Renal replacement therapy

Although many elderly patients with CKD die before needing renal replacement therapy, some reach the stage at which it is considered. There is no age limit to dialysis, and an increasing number of elderly people are on either peritoneal dialysis or haemodialysis. However, on a population basis there is little robust evidence to show that dialysis prolongs life if started after the age of 70 years. This is because the increasing co-morbidities seen with age independently limit life and increase the complications of dialysis. The question of whether any relief of uraemic symptoms outweighs the

Renal changes associated with ageing		
Type of changes	Renal change	Effect
Structural	Decreased renal mass	Decreased GFR
	Decreased renal cortex size	Decreased GFR
	Loss of glomeruli	Decreased GFR
	Increased glomerular sclerosis	Decreased GFR
	Tubulointerstitial fibrosis and scarring	Impaired ability to maintain water and sodium balance
	Loss of tubular mass	Impaired ability to maintain water and sodium balance
Functional	Decreased renal blood flow	Decreased GFR
	Increased renal vascular resistance	Contributes to decreased renal blood flow
	Decreased tubular function	Diminished capacity to produce both a concentrated and a dilute urine
	Impaired sodium handling	Failure to maintain constant volume and composition of extracellular fluid, especially in acute illness

Table 14.5 Structural and functional changes in the kidney associated with ageing. GFR, glomerular filtration rate

burden of dialysis is difficult and requires discussion and decision making on an individual basis.

Similarly, there is no upper age limit to transplantation. However, it is generally accepted that the expected life expectancy of the patient should be ≥ 5 years for transplantation to be a viable option. Transplantation may be appropriate for some elderly patients, but for others the risks of a major operation and the need

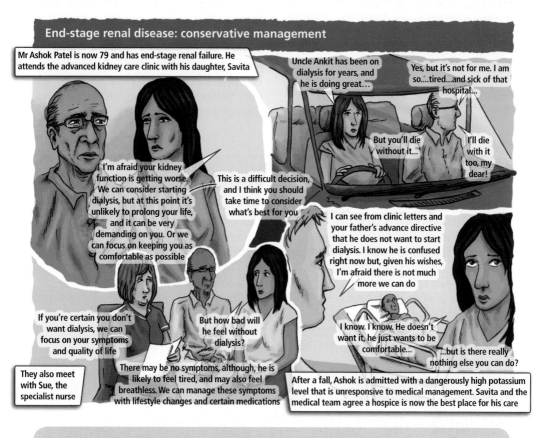

End-stage renal disease: conservative management

Mr Ashok Patel is now 79 and has end-stage renal failure. He attends the advanced kidney care clinic with his daughter, Savita

Uncle Ankit has been on dialysis for years, and he is doing great...

Yes, but it's not for me. I am so....tired...and sick of that hospital...

But you'll die without it...

I'll die with it too, my dear!

I'm afraid your kidney function is getting worse. We can consider starting dialysis, but at this point it's unlikely to prolong your life, and it can be very demanding on you. Or we can focus on keeping you as comfortable as possible

This is a difficult decision, and I think you should take time to consider what's best for you

I can see from clinic letters and your father's advance directive that he does not want to start dialysis. I know he is confused right now but, given his wishes, I'm afraid there is not much more we can do

If you're certain you don't want dialysis, we can focus on your symptoms and quality of life

But how bad will he feel without dialysis?

I know. I know. He doesn't want it, he just wants to be comfortable...

...but is there really nothing else you can do?

They also meet with Sue, the specialist nurse

There may be no symptoms, although, he is likely to feel tired, and may also feel breathless. We can manage these symptoms with lifestyle changes and certain medications

After a fall, Ashok is admitted with a dangerously high potassium level that is unresponsive to medical management. Savita and the medical team agree a hospice is now the best place for his care

Graeme Harrison, an 83-year-old man, visits his GP complaining of increasing tiredness. He has had hypertension for 15 years and type 2 diabetes for 10 years. Six years ago he had a coronary artery bypass graft, following which he has had a degree of left ventricular failure. His wife, who has come with him, says that he is becoming more forgetful. His current medications are ramipril, furosemide, metformin and amlodipine. In addition to tiredness, he is getting up 3–4 times per night to pass reasonable volumes of urine. There is nothing to find on examination.

Investigations show his haemoglobin is 84 g/L and his eGFR 13 mL/min/1.73 m². When he was last seen 5 years ago his eGFR was 34 mL/min /1.73 m². He is referred to his local renal unit, where further investigations are unremarkable apart from a renal ultrasound showing small kidneys.

The renal team explain to Mr Harrison that he has near end-stage renal failure, which will not improve. Given his age and comorbidities, it is unlikely that dialysis will prolong his life. Mr Harrison considers this information and talks it over with his wife and GP, and decides that dialysis is not for him. The GP adjusts his drug regime (stops metformin, starts glicazide) and the renal unit arranges for intravenous iron. With this, his haemoglobin improves to 100 g/L and he feels less tired. Eleven months later, he develops worsening left ventricular failure with increasing breathlessness. The community palliative care team are involved and successfully relieve his dyspnoea. He dies peacefully at home 6 days later.

for lifelong immunosuppression outweigh the benefits.

Conservative care

Surgery is riskier in older patients in terms of both morbidity and mortality. However, surgery to create a fistula for haemodialysis can be avoided, because a temporary or long-term intravenous line can be used instead.

Some patients may choose conservative care, which focuses on symptom control and quality of life. Common reasons are wanting to avoid the use of dialysis lines, surgery to site catheters for peritoneal dialysis or to create fistulae, and the inconvenience of frequent visits to hospital for dialysis.

Some patients who choose conservative can live as long as those who opt for dialysis. It is common for other conditions, such as cardiovascular events, to cause death before progressive renal failure produces symptoms and serious metabolic derangements (e.g. severe hyperkalaemia) that need managing. If it does, palliative care as outlined in the previous section is indicated.

Answers to starter questions

1. Patients with renal dysfunction should be referred to secondary care when they have progressive dysfunction, or conditions that put them at increased risk of such progression. These include diabetes, hypertension, cardiovascular disease, structural renal tract abnormalities, multisystem diseases with potential for renal involvement, family history of CKD stage 5 or hereditary renal disease or presence of haematuria or proteinuria. General practitioners do not need to refer stable, mild (stages 1–3) CKD patients without any complicating features.

2. The decision to commence dialysis is based upon laboratory parameters and symptomatology. It involves discussion between the nephrologist, patient and family (or other carers if involved), and rests ultimately on the patient's decision. Some patients are relatively asymptomatic but develop resistant hyperkalaemia or metabolic acidosis, resulting in the need to commence dialysis. Conversely, other patients have reasonable blood parameters but troublesome symptoms such as fatigue, anorexia and nausea that will likely improve with dialysis.

3. Decisions regarding care for patients nearing or at the end of their lives must take their preferences into account, as well as their general health. There is usually no ideal time to discuss advanced care plans, but a series of discussions may be needed. Patients and their families often need time to consider and discuss these questions. The role of the doctor is to provide information concerning the possible choices and their consequences, and to facilitate referral to other relevant services, such as palliative care.

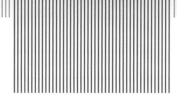

Chapter 15
Self-assessment

SBA questions

Acute kidney injury

1. A 78-year-old woman is admitted to hospital with dysuria and fevers for the past 48 h. Her medical history reveals hypertension and type 2 diabetes. Her temperature is 38.5°C, her heart rate is 107 bpm, her respiratory rate is 22 breaths/min, her blood pressure is 98/50 mmHg and her oxygen saturation is 94% on room air. Her blood tests show a urea concentration of 24.6 mmol/L and a creatinine concentration of 243 µmol/L.
What is the single most likely underlying kidney pathology?

A Acute glomerulonephritis
B Acute interstitial nephritis
C Acute tubular injury
D Focal segmental glomerulosclerosis
E Renal vein thrombosis

2. A 42-year-old man with alcoholism is found collapsed at home, having last been seen by a neighbor 2 days before. In hospital, he is confused and drowsy. His temperature is 35°C, his heart rate is 102 bpm, his respiratory rate is 20 breaths/min, his blood pressure is 115/63 mmHg and his oxygen saturation is 92% on room air. His blood tests show a urea concentration of 18.9 mmol/L and a creatinine concentration of 189 µmol/L. A bladder catheter is introduced in the emergency department, and dark urine is removed.
Which single blood test is most likely to confirm the cause of his AKI?

A Alkaline phosphatase
B Bilirubin
C Corrected calcium

D C-reactive protein
E Creatine kinase

3. A 36-year-old woman with bipolar disorder took a lithium overdose 7 h ago. She is vomiting and tremulous and complains of muscular cramps. Her blood tests show a urea concentration of 18.3 mmol/L and a creatinine concentration of 169 µmol/L. Her blood lithium concentration is significantly increased (3.4 mmol/L; therapeutic range 0.4-1).
What is the single most effective treatment?

A Activated charcoal
B Gastric lavage
C Haemodialysis
D IV 0.9% sodium chloride
E Quinine sulphate

4. A 65-year-old woman had a right hemicolectomy for colon cancer 3 days ago. She has a bladder catheter, and her urine output has decreased significantly over the past 12 h. Her temperature is 36.8°C, her heart rate is 98 bpm, her respiratory rate is 24 breaths/min, her blood pressure is 103/67 mmHg and her oxygen saturation is 98% on 2 L/min of oxygen via nasal cannula. Her blood tests show a urea concentration of 9.8 mmol/L, a creatinine concentration of 134 µmol/L, a haemoglobin concentration of 91 g/L and a C-reactive protein concentration of 145 mg/L. On examination, her capillary refill time is 3 s and her mucous membranes are dry.
What is the single most appropriate next action?

A IV 5% glucose 250 mL over 30 min
B IV 0.9% sodium chloride 250 mL over 30 min

C IV 0.9% sodium chloride 1 L over 8 h
D IV benzylpenicillin and gentamicin
E Transfuse 1 unit of packed red blood cells over 2 h

5. A previously well 73-year-old woman has a 6-month history of weight loss, back pain and fatigue. Her blood test results are haemoglobin, 98 g/L; white cell count, 3.8 × 10⁹/L; erythrocyte sedimentation rate, 99 mm/h; urea concentration, 12.5 mmol/L; creatinine concentration, 178 µmol/L; and corrected calcium concentration, 3.1 mmol/L.
Which single investigation would be most useful in confirming the underlying diagnosis?

A CT of the chest, abdomen and pelvis
B MRI of the whole spine
C Renal biopsy
D Urine Bence Jones protein
E US of the renal tract

6. A 32-year-old man has a 3-day history of fever, abdominal pain, vomiting and bloody diarrhoea. His medical history is non-significant. At home, he has been taking paracetamol and ibuprofen for his abdominal pain but is on no regular medications. In the emergency department, blood tests show haemoglobin, 9.2 g/L; white cell count, 5.4 × 10⁹/L; platelets, 75 × 10⁹/L; urea concentration, 43.2 mmol/L; and creatinine concentration, 595 µmol/L. Blood film shows fragmented red blood cells (schistocytes).
What is the single most likely cause of his acute kidney injury (AKI)?

A Acute tubular injury secondary to sepsis
B Analgesic nephropathy
C Haemolytic–uraemic syndrome
D Non-steroidal anti-inflammatory drug (NSAID) nephrotoxicity
E Volume depletion

Chronic kidney disease

1. A 58-year-old man with diet-controlled type 2 diabetes presents to his general practitioner (GP) for a routine review. Dipstick testing of his urine shows proteinuria +, and his blood pressure is 135/87 mmHg. His recent blood tests show a urea concentration of 10.6 mmol/L, a creatinine concentration of 191 µmol/L and a haemoglobin A1c value, 55 mmol/mol.
What is the single most appropriate next management step?

A Regular exercise and dietary modification
B Start bisoprolol

C Start insulin
D Start metformin
E Start ramipril

2. A 72-year-old woman with chronic kidney disease (CKD) attends the emergency department with a 48-h history of severe pain and swelling affecting her ankle. Her temperature is 37.3°C, her heart rate is 91 bpm, her respiratory rate is 18 breaths/min, her oxygen saturation is 99% on room air and her blood pressure is 148/89 mmHg. On examination, the left ankle is erythematous, swollen and warm to touch.
What is the single most likely diagnosis?

A Gout
B Pseudogout
C Renal osteodystrophy
D Rheumatoid arthritis
E Septic arthritis

3. A 43-year-old man with end-stage renal disease (ESRD) and on haemodialysis is seen in the nephrology clinic. He is generally well, and his observations are within normal limits. Recent blood tests show haemoglobin, 82 g/L; mean corpuscular volume, 85 fL; and ferritin, 50 µg/L.
What is the single most appropriate next step?

A Blood transfusion
B Erythropoiesis-stimulating agent
C IV iron
D Oral iron supplements
E Repeat blood tests in 3 months

4. A 59-year-old man with CKD is reviewed in the nephrology clinic. He describes low energy levels but feels otherwise well. Routine blood tests show sodium, 141 mmol/L; potassium, 4.7 mmol/L; urea, 10.9 mmol/L; creatinine, 189 µmol/L; corrected calcium, 2.18 mmol/L; phosphate, 1.3 mmol/L; and parathyroid hormone (PTH), 55 pg/mL.
What is the single most appropriate next step in managing this patient's abnormal bone profile?

A Admit for IV calcium replacement
B Repeat blood tests in 3 months
C Start alfacalcidol
D Start haemodialysis
E Start phosphate binder

5. A 46-year-old woman on peritoneal dialysis presents to her local renal unit complaining of cloudy peritoneal fluid and mild abdominal pain. She is otherwise well. Her heart rate is 97 bpm, her respiratory rate is 18 breaths/min, her oxygen saturation is 99% on room air, her blood pressure is 143/87 mmHg and her temperature is 37.5°C.

What is the single most important next investigation?

A Blood cultures
B Chest radiograph
C CT of the abdomen
D Peritoneal fluid microscopy, culture and sensitivity
E Plain abdominal radiograph

6. A 35-year-old woman is referred to the nephrology clinic by her GP after blood tests taken for persistent fatigue showed a urea concentration of 15.4 mmol/L and a creatinine concentration of 259 µmol/L. Her medical history includes asthma and urinary tract infections in childhood. She takes the combined oral contraceptive pill but no other medications. Her blood pressure is 146/77 mmHg, and other observations are within normal limits; however, her body mass index (BMI) is 30 kg/m². What is the single most likely cause of her renal impairment?

A Combined oral contraceptive pill use
B Hypertension
C Post-streptococcal glomerulonephritis
D Prediabetes
E Vesicoureteric reflux

7. A 67-year-old man visits his GP for a routine review. He has a past medical history of hypertension and type 2 diabetes and reports a recent sore throat. He takes amlodipine and metformin. Blood tests taken before the appointment show sodium, 143 mmol/L; potassium, 4.1 mmol/L; urea, 7.6 mmol/L; creatinine, 129 µmol/L; and haemoglobin A1c value, 69 mmol/mol. A urine dipstick test shows proteinuria ++. What is the single most likely cause of his renal impairment?

A Diabetic nephropathy
B Hypertensive nephropathy
C Immunoglobulin (Ig) A nephropathy
D Metformin-induced nephropathy
E Post-streptococcal glomerulonephritis

Primary glomerular disease

1. An 8-year-old boy develops swelling of his ankles, and swelling around his eyes in the mornings. His parents have noticed these changes over the past 3–4 days. He had an upper respiratory tract infection, with a sore throat and pyrexia for 1–2 days, a week ago, but has otherwise been well. Examination shows pitting oedema of his lower legs to mid-shins. Dipstick testing of his urine shows ++++ protein but no blood.

What is the single most likely cause of his proteinuria?

A Focal segmental glomerulosclerosis
B IgA nephropathy
C Membranous nephropathy
D Minimal change nephropathy
E Post-infectious glomerulonephritis

2. A 55-year-old man has had progressive swelling of his legs over the past 3 weeks. Examination shows pitting oedema to his knees. His blood pressure is 154/95 mmHg. Investigations show a urine albumin:creatinine ratio of 270 mg/mmol, a serum albumin concentration of 28 g/L and a creatinine concentration of 84 µmol/L. A renal biopsy gives a diagnosis of membranous nephropathy. His oedema is controlled with furosemide. What would be the single most appropriate agent to add to his treatment?

A Angiotensin converting enzyme (ACE) inhibitor (e.g. ramipril)
B Calcineurin inhibitor (e.g. tacrolimus)
C Corticosteroid (e.g. prednisolone)
D Oral anticoagulant (e.g. warfarin)
E Ponticelli regimen (corticosteroids plus alkylating agent such as cyclophosphamide)

3. A 68-year-old man has a cough, which he has had for a few weeks; he has noticed some blood in his sputum for the past few days. He has a 35-pack-year history of smoking. Examination reveals ankle oedema and some wheezes in his right upper chest. Investigations show +++ proteinuria, an albumin concentration of 24 g/L and a creatinine concentration of 93 µmol/L. A chest radiograph shows a mass in the right upper zone. What is the single most likely cause of his proteinuria?

A Focal segmental glomerulosclerosis
B Goodpasture's disease
C IgA nephropathy
D Membranous nephropathy
E Minimal change nephropathy

4. A 45-year-old woman is found to have +++ proteinuria at a life insurance examination; she also has a BMI of 32 kg/m². Her blood pressure is 138/86 mmHg. Further investigations show that her serum creatinine concentration is 213 µmol/L (which gives a calculated glomerular filtration rate, GFR, of 24 mL/min), and that she has two normal-sized kidneys on renal US. She proceeds to renal biopsy, which gives a diagnosis of focal segmental glomerulosclerosis. After her biopsy, she is seen in the nephrology outpatient clinic to talk about this diagnosis.

What single aspect of the patient's condition will it be most important to discuss with her?

A Good control of blood pressure will be important if it becomes increased

B Immunosuppression may help some patients

C Progression to ESRD is almost inevitable

D She should try to lose weight

E There is no clear cause known for focal segmental glomerulosclerosis

5. A 23-year-old white woman comes to her GP with visible haematuria. She has had a moderately severe sore throat for the preceding 3 days and has felt generally unwell. She has been off work, but felt it necessary to come to the surgery only when she noted blood in her urine this morning. There is no significant past medical history, and she is not on medication. Direct questioning reveals vague joint pains for the previous few weeks. Her blood pressure is 148/94 mmHg. Dipstick testing of her urine shows ++ protein and +++ blood. Blood tests show a creatinine concentration of 124 µmol/L. What is the single most likely diagnosis?

A IgA nephropathy

B Minimal change nephropathy

C Post-infectious glomerulonephritis

D Systemic lupus erythematosus

E Urinary tract infection

6. A 45-year-old man comes to his GP feeling more tired than usual. There is no significant past medical history. Examination is normal; his blood pressure is 155/90 mmHg. Dipstick testing of his urine shows proteinuria ++ and haematuria ++. Investigations show a creatinine concentration of 282 µmol/L and a haemoglobin concentration of 113 g/L. Renal US shows small kidneys (8.2 cm and 8.4 cm in length) with increased echogenicity.
What is the single most likely underlying renal diagnosis?

A Hypertensive renal disease

B IgA nephropathy

C Membranous nephropathy

D Minimal change nephropathy

E Small vessel vasculitis

7. An 18-year-old woman has had swelling around her eyes and a decrease in her urine output over the past 2 days. Two weeks ago, she was treated for a severe sore throat, which a throat swab done at the time showed to be caused by *Streptococcus pyogenes*. On examination, she has periorbital and ankle oedema, and her blood pressure is 156/98 mmHg. Dipstick testing of her urine shows proteinuria ++ and

haematuria +++. Initial blood tests show a creatinine concentration of 147 µmol/L. What single further investigation will be most helpful in confirming the diagnosis?

A Anti-double-stranded DNA antibody

B Anti-glomerular basement membrane antibody

C Antineutrophil cytoplasmic antibody (ANCA)

D C-reactive protein

E Complement profile

8. A 35-year-old man has been feeling more tired than usual for the past few weeks. He has also noticed that his ankles occasionally swell, but that his face appears thinner; his friends have asked him whether he has lost weight. Examination shows some ankle oedema and a blood pressure of 148/94 mmHg; his cheeks have a rather sunken appearance. A urine dipstick test shows proteinuria ++ and haematuria +. Blood tests show a creatinine concentration of 138 µmol/L, an albumin concentration of 31 g/L and complement component C4 and C3 concentrations of 0.35 g/L and 0.1 g/L, respectively. What is the single most likely diagnosis?

A Infective endocarditis

B Post-infectious glomerulonephritis

C Systemic lupus erythematosus

D Type 2 mesangiocapillary glomerulonephritis

E Type 2 (essential) cryoglobulinaemia

Secondary glomerular disease

1. A 62-year-old man has been feeling generally unwell and tired for the last few weeks. Over the past week, he has noticed a rash developing on his legs. Yesterday, he started to cough up small amounts of blood. On examination, there is a palpable purpuric rash on his legs. Urinalysis shows ++ proteinuria and +++ haematuria. Investigations show a haemoglobin concentration of 93 g/L and a creatinine concentration of 249 µmol/L. A blood test 3 months ago showed a creatinine concentration of 84 µmol/L. What further single blood test is most likely to help with the diagnosis?

A Anti-double-stranded DNA antibody

B Anti-glomerular basement membrane antibody

C Anti-neutrophil cytoplasm antibody (ANCA)

D Complement profile

E Eosinophil count

2. A 24-year-old woman has had intermittent fever and joint pains for the past 3–4 weeks. She has now come to see her GP because she has noticed some lumps in her neck, shortness of breath, and pain on the left side of her chest when she coughs or takes a deep breath. Examination shows some splinter haemorrhages on her fingernails, enlarged lymph nodes in her neck, and poor air entry with stony dullness to percussion at the left lung base. Urinalysis shows +++ proteinuria and ++ haematuria. A chest radiograph confirms a left pleural effusion.

What single investigation would be most likely to help with the diagnosis?

A Anti-double-stranded DNA antibody
B Blood cultures
C Complement profile
D Lymph node biopsy
E Pleural fluid aspiration and analysis

3. A 32-year-old woman is being treated for anti-glomerular basement membrane disease with regular dialysis, plasma exchange and immunosuppression with prednisolone and cyclophosphamide. One week into treatment, she becomes breathless and coughs up a small amount of blood. On examination, she is apyrexial; there are inspiratory crackles at both lung bases. A chest radiograph shows ill-defined shadowing in both lower zones.

What is the single most likely explanation for the chest radiograph appearances?

A Bilateral pleural effusions
B Hospital-acquired pneumonia
C Pulmonary embolism
D Pulmonary haemorrhage
E Pulmonary oedema

4. A 75-year-old man has a 2-week history of worsening back pain. He gets up at night three or four times to pass urine, and has had some difficulty in passing urine for the past year. On examination, he is euvolaemic; his bladder is just palpable. Rectal examination reveals an enlarged smooth prostate. Investigations show a haemoglobin concentration of 95 g/L, a creatinine concentration of 388 µmol/L and a corrected calcium concentration of 3.1 mmol/L. Urinalysis shows ++ proteinuria. Renal ultrasound (US) shows a moderately enlarged bladder, which empties incompletely, and normal-sized kidneys with no pelvicalyceal dilation.

What is the single most likely diagnosis?

A Carcinoma of the prostate
B Membranous nephropathy

C Myeloma
D Obstructive uropathy
E Primary hyperparathyroidism

5. A 35-year-old man is found to have ++ proteinuria and ++ haematuria at a routine check-up. He has a history of regular sex with other men, but no other significant past medical history. Examination is unremarkable apart from a blood pressure of 154/94 mmHg. Initial investigations show a creatinine concentration of 138 µmol/L, C3 concentration of 0.65 g/L, C4 concentration of 0.01 g/L and a rheumatoid factor concentration of 260 IU/mL.

What single further blood test is most likely to help with diagnosing the underlying cause?

A Anti-double-stranded DNA antibody
B Anti-streptolysin O titre
C Hepatitis B surface antigen
D Hepatitis C antibody
E HIV antigen and antibody screen

6. A 54-year-old man has recently been diagnosed with type 2 diabetes mellitus. He has no other notable past medical history and is not on medication. On examination, his BMI is 28.4 kg/m² and his blood pressure is 145/90 mmHg. Investigations show a creatinine concentration of 76 µmol/L and a haemoglobin A1c value of 52 mmol/mol. Urinalysis shows an albumin:creatinine ratio of 6.7 mg/mmol.

In addition to lifestyle (including dietary) advice, what is the single next best step in management?

A Arrange renal biopsy
B Start amlodipine
C Start insulin
D Start metformin
E Start ramipril

7. A 61-year-old woman received a diagnosis of type 2 diabetes 2 years ago; management has been with diet and ramipril 5 mg a day. At regular review, there is no evidence of diabetic retinopathy. Her blood pressure is 129/78 mmHg. Investigations show a creatinine concentration of 161 µmol/L (a year ago, this was 72 µmol/L) and a haemoglobin A1c value of 47 mmol/mol. Urinalysis shows ++ proteinuria and ++ haematuria.

What is the single next best step in management?

A Add metformin to improve glycaemic control
B Arrange a renal US scan in preparation for renal biopsy
C Create arteriovenous fistula in preparation for haemodialysis

D Evaluate family and friends for a potential kidney donor

E Increase ramipril to improve blood pressure control

8. An 18-year-old man has had profuse diarrhoea, associated with some abdominal pain and intermittent fever, for the last 6 days; he has noticed blood in his stool for the past day. Ten days ago he had eaten an undercooked hamburger. On examination, he looks unwell but is euvolaemic. There is diffuse abdominal tenderness. His blood pressure is 155/100 mmHg. Investigations show haemoglobin, 96 g/L, and platelets, 110 × 10⁹/L. A blood film shows fragmented red blood cells. He has a creatinine concentration of 187 µmol/L.
What is the single most likely diagnosis?

A Accelerated hypertension
B Haemolytic–uraemic syndrome
C Post-infectious glomerulonephritis
D Prerenal AKI
E Thrombotic thrombocytopenic purpura

Electrolyte disorders

1. A 66-year-old man presents to his GP for a routine medication review. He has a history of hypertension and takes amlodipine and bendroflumethiazide. He is feeling well, and his blood pressure is 137/74 mmHg. Blood tests taken before the appointment show sodium concentration, 129 mmol/L; potassium concentration, 4.5 mmol/L; urea concentration, 4.6 mmol/L; and creatinine concentration, 74 µmol/L.
What is the single most appropriate next step in managing this patient's hyponatraemia?

A Admit to hospital for IV fluids
B Repeat blood tests in 2 weeks
C Send paired urine and serum osmolalities
D Stop amlodipine
E Stop bendroflumethiazide

2. A 93-year-old woman from a nursing home attends the emergency department with poor oral intake for the past 5 days. On arrival, she is drowsy and observations show a heart rate of 96 bpm, a respiratory rate of 16 breaths/min, oxygen saturation of 97% on room air, a blood pressure of 110/75 mmHg and a temperature of 35.9°C. On examination, she has cool peripheries, her capillary refill time is 2 s, her jugular venous pressure is not visible and she has dry mucous membranes. Examination is otherwise unremarkable. Blood tests show sodium concentration, 156 mmol/L; potassium concentration, 3.4 mmol/L; urea concentration, 10.4 mmol/L; creatinine concentration, 159 µmol/L; haemoglobin concentration,

112 g/L; white cell count, 11.4 × 10⁹/L; neutrophils, 7.1 × 10⁹/L; and platelets 465 × 10⁹/L.
What is the single most appropriate initial treatment for her hypernatraemia?

A Enteral water via nasogastric tube
B IV 5% glucose infusion
C IV 0.18% saline
D IV alternating bags of 5% glucose plus 0.18% sodium chloride and 0.9% sodium chloride
E IV boluses of colloid

3. An 18-year-old woman attends the emergency department with acute severe asthma and receives emergency treatment with salbutamol and ipratropium nebulisers, IV hydrocortisone, IV magnesium and IV 0.9% sodium chloride. Her symptoms improve, and she is admitted to the respiratory ward for observation. Blood tests taken after her initial treatment show sodium concentration, 143 mmol/L; potassium concentration, 2.6 mmol/L; urea concentration, 4.2 mmol/L; creatinine concentration, 56 µmol/L; haemoglobin, 129 g/L; white cell count, 4.5 × 10⁹/L; and platelets, 179 × 10⁹/L.
What is the single most likely cause of her hypokalaemia?

A Administration of 0.9% sodium chloride
B Administration of ipratropium nebulisers
C Administration of IV hydrocortisone
D Administration of IV magnesium
E Administration of salbutamol nebulisers

4. A 69-year-old man is on the vascular ward 4 days after amputation of his right foot for severe peripheral vascular disease. He has become unwell, with a temperature of 38.5°C, blood pressure of 85/50 mmHg, heart rate of 110 bpm, respiratory rate of 22 breaths/min and oxygen saturation of 93% on 3 L/min oxygen. A fluid bolus is given, and his blood pressure improves. Arterial blood gases show pH, 7.28; partial pressure of oxygen (Po_2), 12 kPa; partial pressure of carbon dioxide (Pco_2), 5 kPa; base excess, -7 mEq/L; bicarbonate (HCO_3^-), 18 mmol/L; and potassium concentration, 6.9 mmol/L. Electrocardiography (ECG) shows prominent T waves in the chest leads.
What is the single most appropriate next step?

A Insulin and glucose infusion
B IV calcium gluconate
C IV sodium bicarbonate
D Salbutamol nebulisers
E Start broad-spectrum antibiotics

5. A 75-year-old woman with multiple myeloma presents to the emergency department, feeling unwell with abdominal pain and nausea. Her heart rate is 95 bpm, her respiratory rate is 18 breaths/min, her oxygen saturation is 97% on

room air, her blood pressure is 112/76 mmHg and her temperature is 36.4°C. Blood tests show haemoglobin, 94 g/L; white cell count, 12×10^9/L; neutrophils, 8.2×10^9/L; platelets, 345×10^9/L; sodium concentration, 144 mmol/L; potassium concentration, 4.2 mmol/L; urea concentration, 9.2 mmol/L; creatinine concentration, 132 µmol/L; and corrected calcium concentration, 2.98 mmol/L.

What is the single most appropriate initial action?

A Cinacalcet
B Haemodialysis
C IV 0.9% sodium chloride
D IV furosemide
E IV pamidronate

6. A 55-year-old man with an ileostomy following a total colectomy for ulcerative colitis attends the emergency department, complaining of palpitations. He also reports increased output through his stoma for the past few days. He appears unwell and is moved to the resuscitation area, where the cardiac monitor shows runs of non-sustained ventricular tachycardia. What is the most likely cause of his arrhythmia?

A Hyperkalaemia
B Hypomagnesaemia
C Hyponatraemia
D Ischaemic heart disease
E Valvular heart disease

7. A 42-year-old woman with a history of alcoholism presents to the emergency department after being found collapsed at home. On arrival, she is alert but appears confused. Her heart rate is 138 bpm, her blood pressure is 98/52 mmHg, her respiratory rate is 16 breaths/min, her oxygen saturation is 97% on room air and her temperature is 36.1°C. ECG shows atrial fibrillation. Blood tests show sodium concentration, 134 mmol/L; potassium concentration, 3.1 mmol/L; urea concentration, 4.3 mmol/L; creatinine concentration, 43 µmol/L; corrected calcium concentration, 2.1 mmol/L; magnesium concentration, 0.28 mmol/L; and phosphate concentration, 0.7 mmol/L.

What is the single most appropriate next step in her management?

A Direct current cardioversion
B IV magnesium replacement
C IV metoprolol
D Oral digoxin
E Oral magnesium replacement

8. A 56-year-old woman with stage 4 CKD attends the renal clinic for a routine review. She takes Calcichew (calcium carbonate),

omeprazole, ramipril and amlodipine. Recent blood tests show sodium concentration, 142 mmol/L; potassium concentration, 4.6 mmol/L; urea concentration, 16.2 mmol/L; creatinine concentration, 179 µmol/L; corrected calcium concentration, 2.09 mmol/L; phosphate concentration, 2.1 mmol/L; and PTH concentration, 110 ng/L.

What is the single most appropriate next step in the management of her electrolyte abnormality?

A Admit for IV calcium gluconate infusion
B Increase Calcichew dose
C Increase dietary calcium intake
D Start alfacalcidol
E Start haemodialysis

9. A 44-year-old woman presents to her GP with a 2-month history of fatigue, generalised joint pain and intermittent nausea. She has been taking regular multivitamins. A physical examination is unremarkable. Blood tests show haemoglobin concentration, 125 g/L; white cell count, 5.5×10^9/L; neutrophils, 3.1×10^9/L; platelets, 213×10^9/L; sodium concentration, 138 mmol/L; potassium concentration, 4.1 mmol/L; urea concentration, 4.5 mmol/L; creatinine concentration, 73 µmol/L; corrected calcium concentration, 2.65 mmol/L; and PTH concentration, 7.3 pmol/L.

What is the single most likely cause of her hypercalcaemia?

A Multiple myeloma
B Primary hyperparathyroidism
C Sarcoidosis
D Thyrotoxicosis
E Vitamin D excess

10. A 31-year-old man recently started chemotherapy for a high-grade non-Hodgkin's lymphoma. Three days into treatment, he becomes unwell with abdominal pain, palpitations, dysuria and lethargy. Blood tests show sodium concentration, 132 mmol/L; potassium concentration, 5.9 mmol/L; urea concentration, 13.2 mmol/L; creatinine concentration, 156 µmol/L; corrected calcium concentration, 2.08 mmol/L; phosphate concentration, 2.6 mmol/L; and uric acid concentration, 550 µmol/L.

What is the single most likely cause of this patient's electrolyte derangement?

A Drug toxicity
B Haemolysis
C Rhabdomyolysis
D Tumour lysis syndrome
E Urinary tract infection

Acid–base balance

1. A 22-year-old man presents to the emergency department with abdominal pain and vomiting. He is drowsy and unable to give a history, but his girlfriend explains that for the past 2 weeks he has continuously felt thirsty and has been going to the toilet more frequently than normal. He has also had a cough for the past few days. On examination, he is cold and hypotensive (his blood pressure is 94/60 mmHg). He is tachypnoeic (respiratory rate, 30 breaths/min), but his chest is clear. His abdomen is soft but tender all over. Arterial blood gases on air show pH, 7.04; Po_2, 19.4 kPa; Pco_2, 3.1 kPa; HCO_3^-, 7 mmol/L; and base excess, -12 mEq/L; lactate concentration, 4 mmol/L; and glucose concentration, 35 mmol/L. Blood tests show sodium concentration, 129 mmol/L; potassium concentration, 4.6 mmol/L; urea concentration, 12.3 mmol/L; creatinine concentration, 126 µmol/L; corrected calcium concentration, 2.4 mmol/L; haemoglobin concentration, 134 g/L; white cell count, 14.1×10^9/L; platelets, 254×10^9/L; and C-reactive protein concentration, 19 mg/L. What it the single most likely cause of this patient's acid–base abnormality?

    A AKI
    B Ketosis
    C Methanol poisoning
    D Sepsis
    E Type 2 respiratory failure

2. A 78-year-old man with chronic obstructive pulmonary disease (COPD), type 2 diabetes and stage 4 CKD is seen on the medical assessment unit with a 2-week history of increasing shortness of breath and lethargy. He was last admitted 3 months ago with an exacerbation of COPD, for which he required non-invasive ventilation. He is normally able to walk to the shops and back but currently feels short of breath at rest. He has his usual cough, and his sputum is clear. His inhalers have not helped. He also reports he has had a bad back after a fall 6 weeks ago and has been taking over-the-counter analgesia. On examination, he appears unwell. His blood pressure is 160/55 mmHg and his heart rate is 110 bpm. His respiratory rate is 32 breaths/min with crackles at both bases. He has bilateral pitting oedema to the knees. Arterial blood gases on 2 L/min oxygen show pH, 7.21; Po_2, 9.2 kPa; Pco_2, 5.1 kPa; HCO_3^-, 13 mmol/L; base excess, –12 mEq/L; and lactate concentration, 1.9 mmol/L. What is the single most likely cause of his acid–base abnormality?

    A Acute infective exacerbation of COPD

    B Acute-on-chronic renal impairment
    C Bacterial pneumonia
    D Diabetic ketoacidosis
    E Drug overdose

3. A 68-year-old man with hypertension presents to the emergency department with a 3-day history of vomiting and diarrhoea. He has a history of gastrointestinal reflux, asthma and hypertension, and normally takes omeprazole and amlodipine and uses a beclomethasone inhaler. On examination, he is drowsy and has volume depletion. His heart rate is 113 bpm, his blood pressure is 109/78 mmHg, his respiratory rate is 20 breaths/min, his oxygen saturation is 97% on 4 L/min oxygen; and his temperature is 36.3°C. Arterial blood gases on 4 L/min oxygen show pH, 7.51; Po_2, 14.2 kPa; Pco_2, 5.9 kPa; HCO_3^-, 28 mmol/L; base excess, 4 mEq/L; and lactate concentration, 1.8 mmol/L. What is the single most likely cause of this patient's acid–base abnormality?

    A Amlodipine
    B Beclomethasone inhaler
    C Omeprazole
    D Persistent vomiting
    E Persistent diarrhoea

4. A 72-year-old man with a history of COPD and diabetes develops gangrene in his right big toe. A blood gas test on room air taken on admission shows pH, 7.28; Po_2, 8.9 kPa; Pco_2, 7.1 kPa; base excess, -6.2 mEq/L; HCO_3^-, 19 mmol/L; and lactate concentration, 1.9 mmol/L. What is the single most appropriate description of his acid–base balance?

    A Metabolic acidosis
    B Mixed metabolic and respiratory acidosis
    C Mixed metabolic and respiratory alkalosis
    D Respiratory acidosis
    E Respiratory alkalosis

5. A 19-year-old woman presents to the emergency department having taken an aspirin overdose. On arrival, she is alert but appears breathless and complains of nausea and feeling generally unwell. Observations show a heart rate of 98 bpm, a blood pressure of 113/68 mmHg, a respiratory rate of 28 breaths/min, oxygen saturation of 100% on 4 L/min oxygen and a temperature of 36.7°. A blood gas test on 4 L/min oxygen shows pH, 7.51; Po_2, 19.7 kPa; Pco_2, 3.1 kPa; base excess, 2.1 mEq/L; and HCO_3^-, 20.8 mmol/L. What is the single most appropriate description of her acid–base status?

    A Compensated metabolic alkalosis
    B Compensated respiratory alkalosis
    C Metabolic alkalosis

D Mixed respiratory and metabolic alkalosis
E Respiratory alkalosis

6. A 61-year-old woman has a severe kyphoscoliosis resulting from poliomyelitis as a child. She experiences frequent respiratory tract infections and requires non-invasive ventilation overnight. She is admitted to hospital with drowsiness and acute shortness of breath. Observations show a heart rate of 95 bpm, a blood pressure of 132/69 mmHg, a respiratory rate of 27 breaths/min, oxygen saturation 87% on 2 L/min oxygen and a temperature of 36.8°C. Arterial blood gases on 2 L/min oxygen show pH, 7.28; Po_2, 7.9 kPa; Pco_2, 8.4 kPa; base excess, 5.7 mEq/L; and HCO_3^-, 30.1 mmol/L.
What is the single most appropriate description of her acid–base balance?

A Metabolic acidosis with complete compensation
B Metabolic acidosis with partial compensation
C Mixed respiratory and metabolic acidosis
D Respiratory acidosis with complete compensation
E Respiratory acidosis with partial compensation

Hypertension

1. A 52-year-old man is found on routine screening to have hypertension (his ambulatory blood pressure monitoring daytime average is 160/102 mmHg). Examination is normal apart from grade 1 hypertensive retinopathy. Initial investigations show borderline left ventricular hypertrophy on ECG, and a potassium concentration of 3.2 mmol/L. His blood pressure is successfully controlled with adherence to lifestyle advice and maximal doses of an ACE inhibitor and a calcium channel blocker.
What single feature suggests a secondary cause of his hypertension?

A Age
B Borderline left ventricular hypertrophy
C Hypertensive retinopathy
D Need for two agents
E Low potassium concentration

2. A 57-year-old woman is found to be hypertensive on routine screening, with an average blood pressure of 155/90 mmHg. She has smoked five cigarettes a day for 30 years. Her diet contains a lot of processed foods; she drinks 15 units of alcohol per week. She walks 3–4 km two or three times a week. Her BMI is 32 kg/m².

Which single lifestyle change will contribute most to control of her hypertension?

A Decrease alcohol intake
B Decrease processed food intake
C Increase exercise
D Stop smoking
E Weight loss

3. A 63-year-old African–Caribbean man is found to have hypertension on routine screening. Examination and investigations show no evidence of target organ damage. Lifestyle advice does not produce adequate control of his blood pressure.
What would be the single best agent to start?

A Alpha blocker (e.g. doxazosin)
B ACE inhibitor (e.g. ramipril)
C Beta blocker (e.g. metoprolol)
D Calcium channel blocker (e.g. nifedipine)
E Diuretic (e.g. bendroflumethiazide)

4. A 78-year-old smoker is investigated for hypertension. Urinalysis is normal. His creatinine concentration is 149 µmol/L and renal US shows kidneys measuring 8.4 cm and 10.7 cm.
What is the single most likely cause of his renal impairment and hypertension?

A Atheromatous renovascular disease
B Chronic glomerulonephritis
C Chronic interstitial nephritis
D Myeloma
E Reflux nephropathy

5. A 74-year-old patient with type 2 diabetes mellitus is investigated for hypertension. Urinalysis is normal. His creatinine concentration is 127 µmol/L. Renal US shows two kidneys, 9 cm and 11 cm in length. He is started on ramipril 2.5 mg/day. The result of a repeat creatinine test 10 days later is 138 µmol/L.
What would be the single best next step in management?

A Recheck creatinine in a week's time
B Refer for renal angiography
C Stop the ramipril
D Switch to an angiotensin II receptor blocker (e.g. candesartan)
E Switch to a calcium channel blocker (e.g. nifedipine)

6. A 36-year-old man presents with a headache and blurred vision. His blood pressure is found to be 212/125 mmHg. Fundoscopy shows grade 4 hypertensive retinopathy. The patient is admitted, and a plan made to lower his blood pressure gradually over the next few hours to 160/100 mmHg.

What is the single most serious complication that might result from a too rapid reduction in his blood pressure?

A AKI
B Cerebral infarction
C Digital ischaemia
D Hepatic necrosis
E Left ventricular failure

7. A 26-year-old woman, 26 weeks into her first pregnancy, is found to be hypertensive on routine review. There is no ankle oedema, and no proteinuria on urinalysis.
If drug treatment is required, what is the single best agent to start?

A Bendroflumethiazide
B Candesartan
C Furosemide
D Methyldopa
E Ramipril

Tubulointerstitial disease

1. A 27-year-old man is receiving Truvada (combined emtricitabine and tenofovir) for the treatment of HIV infection. He develops a chest infection and is given a course of oral doxycycline. Routine testing of his urine at this time shows glycosuria. Subsequent blood tests show a fasting blood glucose concentration of 5.4 mmol/L (glycosuria reconfirmed at the time of this blood test) and a phosphate concentration of 0.65 mmol/L.
What is the most likely cause of this biochemical picture?

A Doxycycline
B Emtricitabine
C HIV-associated nephropathy
D Prediabetes
E Tenofovir

2. A 45-year-old woman with known stage 3 CKD presumed secondary to reflux nephropathy and scarring presents during the summer with mild postural dizziness and occasional nausea. Examination shows no peripheral oedema; blood pressure is 130/82 mmHg while seated and 115/75 mmHg while standing. Blood tests show that her eGFR has decreased from 45 to 38 mL/min.
What is the single next best step in management?

A Advise increased salt and water intake and review
B Arrange an echocardiogram
C Arrange short Synacthen test
D Prescribe fludrocortisone
E Refer for renal biopsy

3. A 64-year-old woman is treated for community-acquired pneumonia with amoxicillin (in the past she has felt nauseated with doxycycline). 12 days later, she feels increasingly unwell and develops a diffuse erythematous rash. Urinalysis shows blood +, protein +. Bloods tests show an eosinophil count of 3.2×10^9/mL and a creatinine concentration of 144 µmol/L.
What is the most likely cause of her renal impairment?

A Acute interstitial nephritis
B IgA nephropathy
C Prerenal AKI
D Post-infectious acute glomerulonephritis
E Small vessel vasculitis

4. A 33-year-old woman is reviewed because of recurrent lower urinary tract infections. She reports that her mother told her that she had urine infections frequently when she was a baby. Examination is normal apart from a blood pressure of 152/94 mmHg. Urinalysis shows proteinuria ++. Blood tests give an eGFR of 42 mL/min. A nuclear medicine renal scan is reported as showing upper pole scarring in both kidneys, probably as a result of reflux.
What is the single most important part of her subsequent management?

A Blood pressure control, ideally with an ACE inhibitor
B Long-term prophylactic antibiotics
C Reassure that renal function is likely to be stable
D Regular drinking of cranberry juice
E Reimplantation of her ureters

5. A 23-year-old woman is seen in the emergency department with a 2-day history of increasingly severe left loin pain. For the past 12 h, she has been experiencing intermittent pyrexia associated with chills and shaking. She also reports a burning pain on passing urine over this time. Examination shows an unwell woman with a temperature of 38.4°C and acute tenderness in the left loin. Urine and blood samples are taken for culture.
What single pathogen is most likely to be responsible for this clinical picture?

A *Candida albicans*
B *Enterococcus* species
C *Escherichia coli*
D *Proteus mirabilis*
E *Staphylococcus saprophyticus*

6. A 55-year-old man, originally from sub-Saharan Africa, is found to have pyuria on routine dip-stick testing. Subsequent urine culture shows no growth. Renal imaging is arranged and shows

calcification in both kidneys, with dilation of a few calyces.
What is the single most likely cause of these abnormalities?

A Primary hyperparathyroidism
B Reflux nephropathy
C Sarcoidosis
D Schistosomiasis
E Tuberculosis

7. A 22-year-old African–Caribbean man with sickle cell disease attends the emergency department with pyrexia and increasing right flank pain for the past 2 days. Urine and blood samples are sent for tests, and a renal US scan is ordered; this shows hydronephrosis of the right kidney.
What is the single most likely explanation for this US appearance?

A Pyelonephritis
B Retroperitoneal fibrosis
C Sloughed renal papilla
D Ureteric calculus
E Ureteric infarction

Hereditary renal disease

1. A 45-year-old woman with known autosomal dominant polycystic kidney disease presents with the sudden onset of right flank pain. She also sees some blood in her urine. She is otherwise well. On examination, she is apyrexial. There is tenderness in the right upper quadrant of the abdomen; both kidneys are palpable.
What is the single most likely cause of her pain?

A Bleed into a cyst
B Infected cyst
C Pyelonephritis
D Renal calculus
E Renal infarction

2. A 51-year-old man with autosomal dominant polycystic kidney disease is seen in the renal outpatient clinic. Review of his results shows that his eGFR has decreased from 45 to 35 mL/min over the past 3 years. He asks about the likely course of the condition in the future.
What is the single most accurate piece of information about his renal prognosis to give him at this stage?

A He is likely to reach ESRD in about 6–7 years
B He should talk to family and friends about a renal transplant in the next year or so
C His condition is likely to stabilise at this level of GFR

D It is impossible to give any useful information at this stage
E There is likely to be a rapid decline to ESRD over the next 1–2 years

3. A 23-year-old man is found to have blood and protein in his urine on routine dipstick testing. He has had some hearing difficulties since childhood. A maternal uncle is on haemodialysis.
What is the single most likely diagnosis?

A Alport's syndrome
B Autosomal dominant polycystic kidney disease
C Fabry's disease
D IgA nephropathy
E Reflux nephropathy

4. A 26-year old man with an unknown cause of renal failure has been on haemodialysis for the past 2 years. He is reviewed because he has developed a painful burning sensation in his feet. Examination shows some purplish papules scattered over his upper thighs.
What single investigation will help confirm the diagnosis?

A Renal biopsy for basement membrane morphology
B Sequencing of CLCN5 gene
C Sequencing of transthyretin gene
D Urine assay for dibasic amino acids
E White blood cell α-galactosidase activity

5. A 16-year-old girl collapses with marked weakness. She has been previously well but has always noted polyuria and polydipsia. There is no history of any medication, vomiting or diarrhoea. Investigations show a potassium concentration of 1.8 mmol/L. Urinary calcium excretion is normal.
What is the single most likely diagnosis?

A Bartter's syndrome
B Bulimia nervosa
C Diuretic abuse
D Gitelman's syndrome
E Purgative abuse

6. A 35-year-old man is reviewed following his second passage of a renal calculus. An US scan and a plain abdominal radiograph are normal. Microscopy of his urine shows hexagonal crystals.
What is the single best next step in management?

A Advise increased fluid intake
B Scan for parathyroid adenoma
C Start allopurinol
D Start D-penicillamine
E Start prophylactic trimethoprim

7. A 32-year-old woman collapses with the sudden onset of severe abdominal pain. On examination, she has shock, with a blood pressure of 90/50 mmHg and a pulse rate of 120 bpm. Small reddish bumps are noted around her nose and cheeks. An abdominal CT scan shows a large perinephric haematoma.
What is the single most likely source of the bleed from the kidney?

A Abscess
B Angiomyolipoma
C Arteriovenous malformation
D Renal calculus
E Renal carcinoma

Urological nephrology

1. A 56-year-old man has experienced multiple episodes of renal colic, with the passage of calcium-containing stones. Investigations have shown a high urinary calcium excretion. He has increased his fluid intake but has still experienced an episode of renal colic.
What single next step in management is most likely to be helpful?

A Increase fluid intake still further
B Low calcium diet
C Start allopurinol
D Start a loop diuretic
E Start a thiazide diuretic

2. A 72-year-old man is found on a routine blood test to have a creatinine concentration of 227 μmol/L. On questioning, he admits to some increased nocturia and frequency over the past year or so. Examination reveals a smooth swelling arising from the pelvis and extending halfway to the umbilicus.
What is the single most likely cause of this clinical picture?

A Benign prostatic hypertrophy
B Bladder cancer
C Cauda equina lesion
D Constipation
E Urethral stricture

3. A 65-year-old man presents with increasing tiredness and malaise over the previous few months. There is nothing to find on examination. Investigations show a haemoglobin concentration of 112 g/L, a creatinine concentration of 384 μmol/L and a C-reactive protein concentration of 112 mg/L. Renal US shows bilateral hydronephrosis; a subsequent abdominal CT scan shows a cuff of soft tissue encasing the lower aorta and involving the ureters.
What is the single best next step in management?

A Biopsy the soft tissue
B Insert bilateral nephrostomies
C Insert bilateral retrograde ureteric stents
D Laparotomy and ureterolysis (freeing of ureters)
E Start oral prednisolone

4. A 27-year-old woman with known reflux nephropathy (eGFR, 55 mL/min) is reviewed 12 weeks into her first pregnancy. Her mother has the same condition, but more advanced (stage 4 CKD). She asks whether any special measures are necessary in view of her renal history.
What single piece of advice will it be most important to give her?

A Consider ureteric reimplantation to reduce reflux during pregnancy
B Her baby should be screened for reflux soon after birth
C Reassure that her baby is unlikely to be affected by reflux
D Take antibiotic prophylaxis during her pregnancy
E Take plenty of fluids during her pregnancy

5. A 67-year-old man is seen following two episodes of visible haematuria. He has a 30-pack-year history of smoking but no other significant medical history. There is nothing to find on examination, but dipstick testing of his urine shows haematuria ++. There is no proteinuria, and his eGFR and renal US scan are normal.
What is the single best next step in management?

A Obtain a coagulation screen
B Obtain renal CT scan
C Reassure that there is unlikely to be serious pathology
D Refer for cystoscopy
E Refer for renal biopsy

Emergencies

1. A 34-year-old man on haemodialysis for the past 4 years is admitted to the emergency department with breathlessness after missing his dialysis session. His heart rate is 106 bpm, his respiratory rate is 22 breaths/min, his oxygen saturation is 90% on room air, his blood pressure is 167/87 mmHg and his temperature is 36.6°C. On examination, his jugular venous pressure is elevated, he has crackles bilaterally to the mid-zones and pitting oedema of his ankles. Blood tests show sodium concentration, 134 mmol/L; potassium concentration, 6.5 mmol/L; urea concentration, 46 mmol/L; and creatinine concentration, 739 μmol/L. His ECG is normal.

After starting the patient on oxygen, what is the single most appropriate next step?

A IV calcium gluconate
B IV furosemide
C IV insulin and dextrose
D Nebulised salbutamol
E Urgent haemodialysis

2. A 42-year-old man presents to the emergency department with sudden onset of intermittent pain in the right flank. He is distressed and unable to lie still. Observations show a heart rate of 102 bpm, a respiratory rate of 22 breaths/min, oxygen saturation of 100% on room air, a blood pressure of 122/73 mmHg and a temperature of 36.7°C. On examination, he has tenderness in the right flank but otherwise there are no significant findings.
What is the single most appropriate diagnostic test?

A Abdominal radiograph
B Chest radiograph
C CT of the abdomen
D CT of the kidneys, ureters and bladder
E MRI of the abdomen

Integrated care

1. A 93-year-old man is referred to hospital by his GP with abnormal renal function on routine blood tests: sodium concentration, 146 mmol/L; potassium concentration, 5.7 mmol/L; urea concentration, 46.5 mmol/L; and creatinine concentration, 798 µmol/L. He reports fatigue and nausea for the past few weeks but is otherwise well. He has Parkinson's disease and mild depression, but no other medical problems, and he lives in a residential home. He is treated with IV fluids and a catheter is introduced after an US scan of the kidneys, ureters and bladder shows mild hydronephrosis bilaterally. Despite persistent hyperkalaemia, he is adamant that he does not want dialysis and is deemed to have capacity to make this decision.
What is the single most appropriate course of action with respect to his treatment?

A Ask his relatives if they are happy for him to have dialysis against his wishes
B Ensure he fully understands the implications of not having dialysis before making further decisions
C Give dialysis under the Mental Health Act
D Refer to the palliative care team
E Stop all regular medications and repeat renal function 48 h later

2. A 71-year-old woman with stage 4 CKD secondary to diabetes attends a follow-up appointment in the nephrology clinic. Her past medical history also includes hypertension and early Parkinson's disease. She lives alone. Recent blood tests show that her renal function has declined significantly since she was last seen, and her eGFR is now 7 mL/min. She is feeling tired and intermittently nauseous but is otherwise well and is desperate to have more energy.
What is the single most appropriate next step in her management?

A Await a renal transplant
B Palliative care
C Review in 6 months
D Start haemodialysis
E Start peritoneal dialysis

SBA answers

Acute kidney injury

1. C

The history of dysuria and fevers and the finding of pyrexia suggest urinary tract sepsis. She also has AKI, as indicated by the raised urea and creatinine concentrations. In the context of sepsis, AKI is most likely to result from acute tubular injury.

2. E

Given the history of collapse and the possibility of a long time spent on the floor, as well as the clinical findings of dark urine (likely to be due to myoglobin) and AKI, the most likely underlying diagnosis is rhabdomyolysis. The most useful blood test in the diagnosis of rhabdomyolysis is measurement of levels of creatine kinase, an enzyme released when muscle cells are damaged.

The patient's drowsiness and confusion may have been caused by excessive alcohol consumption, head injury, hypothermia or metabolic derangement.

3. C

The patient has taken a large lithium overdose and has signs of toxicity: vomiting, tremulousness, and muscle cramps, and AKI as shown by the increased urea and creatinine concentrations. Because the overdose was several hours ago, neither activated charcoal nor gastric lavage would be effective.

Lithium is excreted renally. IV sodium chloride is given to increase circulating volume and GFR, and thereby increase renal elimination of lithium. In a patient with AKI and signs of toxicity, the most effective means of removing lithium is haemodialysis.

4. B

This patient is showing clinical signs of volume depletion and has mild AKI. The most appropriate next step would be to administer a fluid bolus and assess the response. Neither a bolus of IV glucose nor a 1 L infusion of sodium chloride over 8 h would have an adequate effect on intravascular volume.

In cases such as this sepsis is a possibility. However, the patient is apyrexial so antibiotics are not indicated, at least at this stage. She may have bleeding, but in the absence of cardiovascular compromise or significant blood loss, blood transfusion would not be indicated with a haemoglobin concentration of 91 g/L. Therefore a 250 mL bolus of 0.9% sodium chloride is the best option.

5. C

This patient's symptoms are non-specific, but the combination of back pain, weight loss, anaemia, renal impairment and hypercalcaemia raises the possibility of multiple myeloma. A positive urine test result for Bence Jones protein would support this diagnosis, but renal biopsy would be the gold standard for confirming myeloma as the cause of her renal impairment.

6. C

The combination of gastrointestinal symptoms, AKI, anaemia, thrombocytopenia and schistocytes on the blood film points towards a diagnosis of haemolytic–uraemic syndrome, most likely secondary to a gastrointestinal infection. In this context, evidence for neurological abnormalities should be sought; this would indicate a diagnosis of thrombotic thrombocytopenic purpura instead of haemolytic-uraemic syndrome.

Chronic kidney disease

1. E

This patient has diabetes with renal impairment, proteinuria and hypertension. He will require medication for his diabetes; because he has evidence of end-organ damage, dietary and lifestyle modifications only would be inadequate. Metformin would not be the preferred option in this case, given his renal impairment; however, at this stage an oral agent would probably suffice, so insulin would not be required. Treatment with ramipril is the most appropriate next step, because it has an antihypertensive effect and reduces proteinuria. Bisoprolol may have a small effect on his blood pressure, but it is not a first-line antihypertensive agent and has no renoprotective effect. Gliclazide would be a good choice for glycaemic control.

2. A

This woman has acute arthritis, low-grade fever and borderline tachycardia. In this case, the most important diagnosis to exclude is septic arthritis; this is done by carrying out joint aspiration. However, given the patient's background of CKD, the most likely cause of her symptoms is gout as a consequence of impaired renal excretion of urate.

3. **C**

Anaemia should be investigated and managed in patients with CKD when their haemoglobin concentration decreases below 110 g/dL. This patient has anaemia with a normal value for mean corpuscular volume and a ferritin concentration towards the lower limit of normal. An erythropoiesis-stimulating agent is likely to be required, but this should not be started until iron stores are replete (ferritin > 100 μg/L). This is achieved by giving IV iron. Oral iron supplements would be less effective than IV iron.

This patient is clinically well and haemodynamically stable, so there is no indication for a blood transfusion. Blood transfusions should be avoided in renal patients to minimise the risk of developing antibodies, which could increase the risk of rejection of a kidney transplant.

4. **C**

This patient has a slightly low corrected calcium concentration, a normal phosphate concentration and a PTH concentration towards the upper limit of normal. These results are most likely to be the consequence of a deficiency of active vitamin D, which requires replacement therapy with alfacalcidol. His hypocalcaemia is not severe enough to require IV calcium replacement. To control his phosphate, dietary phosphate restriction, rather than a phosphate binder, should be tried in the first instance. He does not have ESRD, so haemodialysis is not required at this point. He will require repeat blood tests in 3 months; however, intervention is warranted now to try to normalise his bone profile results.

5. **D**

Cloudy peritoneal fluid, abdominal pain and low-grade fever are clinical signs of peritonitis. The essential investigation to confirm this is peritoneal microscopy, culture and sensitivity. The results would be expected to show an increased white cell count (as a result of neutrophilia) and, possibly, growth of an organism. Intraperitoneal antibiotics should be started as soon as possible.

6. **E**

With a history of frequent urinary tract infections in childhood, this patient's renal impairment is most likely to be the result of vesicoureteric reflux. Therefore her hypertension is likely to be the result, rather than the cause, of her renal failure. Use of the contraceptive pill does not cause renal disease, and there is nothing in the history to suggest post-streptococcal glomerulonephritis. Given the patient's high BMI, she may have a degree of insulin resistance ('prediabetes'); however, this would not cause such advanced renal disease.

7. **A**

This patient has diabetes and hypertension, so either could be the cause of his renal impairment; however, diabetes is the commonest cause of CKD, so this is the correct answer. Most patients with IgA nephropathy are diagnosed at a much younger age (16–35 years), and post-streptococcal glomerulonephritis typically affects children. Although metformin should be avoided in renal disease, because it can increase the risk of lactic acidosis, it does not exert a directly nephrotoxic effect.

Primary glomerular disease

1. **D**

The boy appears to have developed the nephrotic syndrome; confirmation requires a low serum albumin concentration in addition to the oedema and proteinuria. The most likely cause in children is minimal change nephropathy; in adults, membranous nephropathy and focal segmental glomerulosclerosis would also be considered. It is rare for either IgA nephropathy or post-infectious glomerulonephritis to present with the nephrotic syndrome, and both would usually also cause haematuria.

2. **A**

This patient has well-preserved renal function and a serum albumin concentration that is only moderately reduced. In such cases, potentially toxic immunosuppressive drugs, for example calcineurin inhibitors or those used in the Ponticelli regimen, are not usually given. Corticosteroids alone are not effective in cases of membranous nephropathy. Anticoagulants may be required, but they are usually given only if the serum albumin concentration is < 20 g/L. An ACE inhibitor will both control blood pressure and reduce proteinuria.

3. **D**

This patient has nephrotic syndrome and probable lung cancer. The likely cause is membranous nephropathy; at his age, this is associated with an underlying malignancy in about 10% of cases. Focal segmental glomerulosclerosis and minimal change disease are possible diagnoses, but they are much less likely to be associated with malignancy. Goodpasture's disease can cause haemoptysis, but its renal presentation is with a rapidly progressive glomerulonephritis. IgA nephropathy rarely presents with nephrotic syndrome.

4. **C**
All these issues are relevant, but the most important point is the likely progression to ESRD. Although immunosuppression may help some patients, it is arguably too late, and not worth the risk with this degree of renal impairment. Losing weight and good control of increased blood pressure are certainly helpful and may slow the progression of the disease, but they are unlikely to change the eventual outcome.

5. **A**
Immunoglobulin A nephropathy typically causes visible haematuria about the same time as an upper respiratory tract infection ('synpharyngitic' haematuria); post-infectious glomerulonephritis occurs 10–14 days later. The joint pains raise the possibility of lupus nephritis, particularly if the patient is African–Caribbean, but this is less likely to cause visible haematuria. Minimal change nephropathy does not usually cause haematuria, and a urinary tract infection does not usually cause significant proteinuria; neither usually causes renal impairment.

6. **B**
This patient has CKD; IgA nephropathy, as the commonest form of primary glomerular disease, is the most likely diagnosis. Minimal change nephropathy does not cause CKD. Membranous nephropathy or small vessel vasculitis could cause CKD, but they are unlikely with no previous relevant history. The patient probably has borderline hypertension, which should be treated if confirmed, but on its own this would be insufficient to cause CKD.

7. **E**
The most likely cause of this woman's nephritic syndrome is post-infectious glomerulonephritis; this would be supported by evidence of complement consumption. Goodpasture's disease and ANCA-associated vasculitis also present with decreased GFR and the finding of blood and protein in the urine, but this is over weeks or months. Lupus is a possibility, but a nephritic presentation would be unusual. C-reactive protein may be increased, but this is a non-specific indicator of inflammation.

8. **D**
The normal C4 concentration, a classical pathway component, suggests that the low C3 concentration is due to activation via the alternative pathway. This complement profile is typical of type 2 mesangiocapillary glomerulonephritis associated with C3 nephritic factor; this would also explain the facial changes, which are caused by the partial lipodystrophy also associated with this factor. The other conditions can all cause renal involvement and complement activation, but this is mainly via the classical pathway, so C4 would be low.

Secondary glomerular disease

1. **C**
The clinical picture is of a rapidly progressive glomerulonephritis, most likely caused by a small vessel ANCA-positive vasculitis. Anti-glomerular basement membrane disease would not cause a rash. Lupus, which is associated with anti-double-stranded DNA antibodies and complement consumption, is unlikely in a man, and at this age. Eosinophilia would suggest eosinophilic granulomatosis with polyangiitis (previously known as Churg–Strauss syndrome), but there is no history of asthma or other allergy.

2. **A**
Systemic lupus erythematosus would explain all aspects of this case, and the most specific investigation is the anti-double-stranded DNA antibody. There may well be complement consumption, but this is not as specific. Similarly, pleural fluid and lymph node analysis are unlikely to be diagnostic. Infective endocarditis could explain some of the clinical picture (not the pleural effusion), and blood cultures would be the crucial investigation in that case.

3. **D**
The chest radiograph is not typical of pulmonary effusion or embolus. Infection is possible, but the patient is apyrexial. Pulmonary oedema is also possible, but in that condition the increased shadowing is usually perihilar and there may be other signs (enlarged cardiac shadow, effusions, Kerley B lines). Pulmonary haemorrhage seems the most likely explanation and would be supported by a decrease in haemoglobin and an increase in carbon monoxide transfer factor.

4. **C**
Most causes of renal impairment, including membranous nephropathy, lead to a low calcium concentration until the development of tertiary hyperparathyroidism. Metastatic

cancer and primary hyperparathyroidism could cause hypercalcaemia and renal impairment, but the latter is usually secondary to salt and water depletion, for which there is no evidence. Obstruction would not cause hypercalcaemia and is unlikely without pelvicalcyceal dilation. Myeloma would explain the back pain, hypercalcaemia and renal impairment.

5. D

The complement profile is typical of type 1 mesangiocapillary glomerulonephritis secondary to type 2 cryoglobulinaemia. A common cause, which is treatable, is hepatitis C infection; this patient's lifestyle puts him at risk for this. HIV and hepatitis B do not usually cause this type of glomerular disease; lupus can, but it is unlikely in a man. There is no history to suggest post-streptococcal glomerulonephritis.

6. E

The patient has increased blood pressure and albumin:creatinine ratio, so an ACE inhibitor is indicated (ramipril in this case). It is reasonable to try lifestyle measures first before adding metformin. Insulin is not indicated at this stage. The results of renal biopsy to investigate the increased albumin:creatinine ratio will almost certainly show diabetic changes and will not change management. However, if proteinuria increases, GFR decreases or both, then renal biopsy might be indicated.

7. B

The patient may have just diabetic nephropathy. However, several features – absence of retinopathy, rapid deterioration in renal function and haematuria – suggest that another, potentially treatable disease is affecting the kidneys. A renal biopsy is required for diagnosis. Blood pressure and glycaemic control are satisfactory, and it is too early to plan for ESRD.

8. B

The haematological picture is of a microangiopathic haemolytic anaemia, which together with the renal impairment is typical of haemolytic–uraemic syndrome. Microangiopathic haemolytic anaemia would not occur with post-infectious glomerulonephritis or prerenal AKI. Accelerated hypertension could cause this picture, but the blood pressure is not high enough for this. There are no additional features, for example neurological involvement, to indicate thrombotic thrombocytopenic purpura, which is also not linked to consumption of undercooked meat.

Electrolyte disorders

1. E

This patient has mild hyponatraemia, which has probably been caused by his bendroflumethiazide. The most appropriate course of action would be to stop this medication and repeat blood tests after a few weeks. If the hyponatraemia is still present, further investigation should be initiated. His blood pressure will need to be monitored, and a different antihypertensive may be required.

2. D

This patient has clinical and biochemical signs of volume and water depletion: cool peripheries, dry mucous membranes, hypernatraemia and increased concentrations of urea and creatinine. Enteral water via a nasogastric tube is unlikely to correct her biochemical abnormality adequately, and rapid volume expansion with a colloid is unnecessary in this case as she is not acutely unwell. Current guidelines recommend using alternating bags of 5% glucose plus 0.18% sodium chloride and 0.9% sodium chloride to correct the water and volume deficit in this context.

3. E

Salbutamol drives potassium into cells and commonly causes hypokalaemia when administered frequently or at sufficiently high doses. Therefore salbutamol nebulisers are sometimes used in the treatment of hyperkalaemia.

4. B

This patient has hyperkalaemia with electrographic changes, so he requires urgent treatment with IV calcium gluconate to stabilise cardiac myocytes and prevent a life-threatening arrhythmia. Insulin-glucose, IV sodium bicarbonate, salbutamol nebulisers and broad-spectrum antibiotics may all be required, but emergency management takes priority.

5. C

This woman has renal impairment and an increased corrected calcium, most likely secondary to her multiple myeloma. The first step in the management of hypercalcaemia (and, indeed, pre-renal AKI) is fluid replacement with IV normal saline. If her calcium concentration fails to normalise with this management, IV bisphosphonate (e.g. pamidronate) should be considered.

6. **B**

High output from a stoma causes loss of electrolytes such as sodium, potassium and magnesium. Therefore hyperkalaemia would be extremely unlikely. Hyponatraemia is possible, but this would not cause ventricular tachycardia. This patient could have valvular or ischaemic heart disease, which could both cause ventricular tachycardia; however, given the clinical context, hypomagnesaemia is the most likely cause of this man's arrhythmia.

7. **B**

This woman has atrial fibrillation in the context of hypocalcaemia and profound hypomagnesaemia. Of the options given, IV magnesium replacement is the most appropriate treatment, because it will help normalise serum magnesium concentration and may terminate her atrial fibrillation. Oral magnesium replacement would not be appropriate given the severity of her magnesium deficiency. Direct current cardioversion is not indicated at this point, because she has a potentially reversible cause of her atrial fibrillation. IV metoprolol and oral digoxin are both used in the management of atrial fibrillation but would not be the first-line treatment in this case.

8. **D**

This patient has CKD, which has resulted in decreased production of active vitamin D and reduction of dietary calcium absorption in consequence. Decreased serum calcium levels stimulate the release of PTH, which in this patient is increased (secondary hyperparathyroidism). Increased phosphate levels as a result of decreased renal excretion can also cause increased PTH secretion, both directly and indirectly as a result of decreased calcium concentration.

If untreated, secondary hyperparathyroidism causes renal bone disease and its associated morbidities of bone pain, increased risk of fractures, and vascular and soft tissue calcification. This patient is already receiving a phosphate binder. To suppress PTH secretion and normalise serum calcium concentration, vitamin D therapy with alfacalcidol should be started.

9. **B**

This woman has an increased calcium concentration and an inappropriately normal PTH concentration, which gives a biochemical picture of unregulated secretion of PTH (in the context of hypercalcaemia, PTH secretion is suppressed, so levels of PTH in the blood should be low.) Multiple myeloma is unlikely at this patient's age, and her history is not typical of thyrotoxico-

sis. Sarcoidosis and vitamin D excess would be possible, but the most likely diagnosis is primary hyperparathyroidism.

10. **D**

This patient has a non-specific constellation of symptoms together with deranged electrolytes and renal function. The most likely diagnosis is tumour lysis syndrome, a condition caused by rapid cell breakdown and the release into the circulation of intracellular contents such as potassium, phosphate and nucleic acids. Acute hyperphosphataemia results in precipitation of calcium phosphate in soft tissues, resulting in hypocalcaemia. Nucleic acid purines are metabolised to uric acid, resulting in hyperuricaemia. AKI is multifactorial but predominantly results from formation of uric acid crystals and their deposition within the renal tubules, as well as nephrocalcinosis from precipitation of calcium phosphate.

Acid–base balance

1. **B**

This man's history of thirst and frequent urination raises the possibility of an underlying diagnosis of diabetes mellitus. With signs of volume depletion, a glucose concentration of 35 mmol/L and marked metabolic acidosis, diabetic ketoacidosis, perhaps precipitated by a chest infection, is likely to have complicated his diabetes.

2. **B**

This patient has shortness of breath associated with clinical signs of volume overload and a metabolic acidosis. He has a history of COPD, but his symptoms do not suggest an exacerbation of this because he has only his usual cough and his sputum is clear. His back injury has prompted him to self-medicate with NSAIDs, which have caused an acute deterioration in his renal function on the background of CKD, resulting in fluid overload and a metabolic acidosis.

3. **D**

This patient has a metabolic alkalosis caused by persistent vomiting resulting in loss of hydrochloric acid from the stomach.

4. **B**

This patient has an acidosis, with increased P_{CO_2}, low P_{O_2}, a negative base excess and a low bicarbonate concentration. This picture is one of a mixed metabolic and respiratory acidosis caused by his gangrene and COPD, respectively.

5. **E**

This woman has an alkalosis with a low P_{CO_2} and a HCO_3^- result within the normal range. The picture is a respiratory alkalosis secondary to hyperventilation (salicylate poisoning results in stimulation of the respiratory centre and therefore a respiratory alkalosis in the earlier stages). The patient's HCO_3^- result is towards the lower limit of normal, which suggests a degree of metabolic compensation; however, this respiratory alkalosis is not fully compensated, because the pH remains in the alkalaemic range.

6. **E**

This woman's kyphoscoliosis has resulted in chronic hypoventilation and chronic type 2 respiratory failure. The blood gases show a picture of partial compensation, because although her bicarbonate is increased, indicating metabolic compensation, her pH is in the acidaemic range. This deterioration in her condition may be because of an intercurrent respiratory tract infection or poor adherence with her noninvasive ventilation.

Hypertension

1. **E**

Apart from the low potassium concentration, none of these features are unexpected in a man of this age with primary (idiopathic or essential) hypertension; most patients will require two antihypertensive agents for optimal blood pressure control. The low potassium suggests hyperaldosteronism; this is one of the more common causes of secondary hypertension, occurring in 5–10% of cases.

2. **E**

All these measures are desirable and should be encouraged. However, the single most potent factor is weight: a decrease of 10 kg will reduce blood pressure, both systolic and diastolic, by 5–10 mmHg. Additional successful lifestyle alterations will add to this and may well mean that drug treatment is not required.

3. **D**

In African–Caribbean patients, hypertension tends not to be as renin-dependent as in white patients, so a calcium channel blocker rather than an ACE inhibitor is the first choice. It would be reasonable to add an ACE inhibitor as the next step, because the the the renin–angiotensin system will have been activated by the vasodilation caused by the calcium channel blocker.

4. **A**

This is a common clinical picture. The absence of urinary abnormalities makes glomerular, and to some extent interstitial, disease unlikely. There is nothing to suggest reflux nephropathy. Myeloma is possible (Bence Jones proteinuria does not register on dipsticks), but atheromatous renovascular disease is much more common.

5. **A**

The clinical picture suggests atheromatous renal artery stenosis (see previous question). However, there is little evidence that intervention (e.g. angioplasty and stenting) is helpful, so angiography is not indicated, at least at this stage. A small decrease in GFR is to be expected when an ACE inhibitor is started and, provided this is not progressive, is not a contraindication to continuing with the drug, which has benefits for cardiovascular prognosis.

6. **B**

The most feared complication is ischaemia of the brain consequent to loss of autoregulation of cerebral perfusion. AKI may occur, but it is treatable and usually reversible. Left ventricular failure may be caused by accelerated hypertension, but treatment will improve this. Digital or hepatic ischaemia, in the absence of other factors, do not occur in this situation.

7. **D**

Methyldopa is the initial antihypertensive drug of choice in pregnancy. Diuretics (e.g. bendroflumethiazide or furosemide) are contraindicated because of potential adverse effects on placental perfusion, and both ACE inhibitors (e.g. ramipril) and angiotensin II receptor blockers (e.g. candesartan) may cause problems with fetal and neonatal blood pressure control and renal function.

Tubulointerstitial disease

1. **E**

This biochemical picture suggests Fanconi's syndrome, a disorder of the proximal renal tubule, which in this case is causing failure to reabsorb glucose and phosphate. Tenofovir is a recognised cause of this; the other drugs are not. Prediabetes is not a well-defined term, but the fasting glucose concentration is in any event within normal limits. HIV-associated nephropathy usually causes a glomerular rather than tubular lesion.

2. **A**

Any form of interstitial disease may be complicated by salt and water wasting, which is the most likely cause in this case. Addison's disease, for which the short Synacthen test is a screen, is much less likely. This patient's renin–aldosterone system is probably already maximally active, so extra mineralocorticoid (fludrocortisone) is unlikely to help. There is no reason to suspect a cardiac or an additional renal problem.

3. **A**

This picture of rash, eosinophilia and renal impairment strongly suggests an allergic acute interstitial nephritis. IgA nephropathy, post-infectious glomerulonephritis and small vessel vasculitis are possible, but they would not explain the rash (usually purpuric if a vasculitis) or the eosinophilia. There is nothing in the history to suggest prerenal AKI.

4. **A**

This patient already has significant renal impairment as a result of reflux-associated chronic interstitial disease. Prophylactic antibiotics and reimplantation of ureters might have had a role in the neonatal period, but it is now too late for these options. Excellent blood pressure control is the best chance of slowing progression of her CKD, but this is still likely to slowly progress.

5. **C**

This patient has acute pyelonephritis. All the organisms are a possible cause, but *E. coli* is by far the commonest. Next most frequent would be *S. saprophyticus*. The others would not normally be detected unless there were other problems, such as previous antibiotic use or urinary tract abnormalities (e.g. renal calculi).

6. **E**

The picture of sterile pyuria with renal calcification and strictures of the collecting system is typical of renal tuberculosis. Schistosomiasis causes problems with the bladder, not the upper tracts. Hyperparathyroidism and sarcoidosis may both be associated with hypercalcaemia and renal calcification, but they would not explain the dilated calyces. Reflux nephropathy is not associated with calcification.

7. **C**

The patient appears to have pyelonephritis, but this would not explain the hydronephrosis. Sickle cell disease can be associated with infarction, but not of the ureter. Ureteric calculi and retroperitoneal fibrosis could explain the findings, but obstruction with a sloughed papilla, a

well-known complication of sickle cell disease, is the most likely cause.

Hereditary renal disease

1. **A**

Bleeding into a cyst is not uncommon in polycystic kidney disease. An infected cyst may give a similar picture, but the patient is usually unwell with a pyrexia; this would also be the case with pyelonephritis. A calculus is possible, but the pain does not radiate to the groin. There is no reason for renal infarction to occur.

2. **A**

Decline in eGFR is usually fairly linear in polycystic kidney disease, so this patient can expect to have an eGFR of 10–15 mL/min (i.e. near end stage) in about 6–7 years. It is too soon to be planning a pre-emptive renal transplant, but this would be the best plan nearer the end stage.

3. **A**

This picture is typical of classic X-linked Alport's syndrome, which is caused by a defect in the α5 chain of type IV collagen. Fabry's disease is also X-linked, but it usually causes characteristic skin changes. Neither Fabry's disease nor the others conditions listed are also associated with deafness.

4. **E**

This picture strongly suggests Fabry's disease, which is caused by X-linked α-galactosidase deficiency. Alport's syndrome (a basement membrane defect) and Dent's disease (a deficiency of the $Cl^-–H^+$ exchanger coded by the *CLCN5* gene) are also X-linked, but they do not cause these skin changes (angiokeratomas) or have nerve involvement. Abnormal transthyretin is associated with amyloidosis causing nerve and renal problems but not the skin lesions. Failure to reabsorb dibasic amino acids is the cause of cystinuria.

5. **A**

This metabolic picture is typical of Bartter's syndrome. Gitleman's syndrome is similar, but it is usually less severe and associated with a low urinary calcium concentration. Prolonged vomiting, and abuse of diuretics, purgatives or both, are essential differential diagnoses to consider but are not suggested by the history.

6. **A**

These crystals are typical of cystinuria, not uric acid (for which allopurinol might be considered) or calcium-containing stones (in which case investigations for hypercalcaemia might be indicated). Given that there is no renal stone burden, increased fluid intake is a reasonable first step. If stones recur, then D-penicillamine could be considered, but this can have toxic effects. Infection can be associated with some calculi, but not in this case.

7. **B**
The skin changes suggest adenoma sebaceum, a finding in tuberous sclerosis. This condition is often complicated by renal angiomyolipomas. These are vascular tumours; large ones confer a significant risk of life-threatening bleeds. Pre-emptive treatment of larger tumours with surgery or interventional radiology may be needed.

Urological nephrology

1. **E**
Thiazide diuretics will reduce this patient's calcium excretion; loop diuretics will have the opposite effect. A low calcium diet will not be helpful, but a low sodium diet may be and should also be suggested. Allopurinol would be useful only for urate stones. A further increase in fluid intake is unlikely to be sustainable.

2. **A**
Benign prostatic hypertrophy is common, and the history suggests this diagnosis. Bladder cancer and urethral stricture are other possibilities, but there is nothing to particularly suggest them. Constipation can precipitate acute retention, but this is a chronic picture. There is nothing else to suggest a nerve lesion, which would be rare.

3. **E**
This clinical presentation is typical of retroperitoneal fibrosis. The condition often responds rapidly to corticosteroids, and it is reasonable to try these first. Biopsy may be required if the condition does not respond, as may some form of drainage procedure. Ureterolysis can be helpful in the long term to avoid prolonged immunosuppression.

4. **B**
There is often a familial occurrence of reflux (as in this case), and this woman's baby is certainly at risk. If diagnosed early, prophylactic antibiotics, or possibly an antireflux procedure, can be considered. Measures aimed at treating the mother are unlikely to have much effect, but she should certainly be monitored for urinary infection.

5. **D**
It is essential to exclude bladder cancer in this case. A renal biopsy, given the normal eGFR and lack of proteinuria, will almost certainly be normal. A renal CT scan may show a bladder tumour but will miss small lesions. Haematuria should not be assumed to be caused by coagulation problems.

Emergencies

1. **E**
Having missed his dialysis session, this patient has signs of fluid overload as well as hyperkalaemia. The most appropriate management step is urgent haemodialysis, which will address both his fluid overload and his hyperkalaemia. With a normal ECG, he does not require IV calcium gluconate at this point and, provided dialysis can be offered immediately, medical management of his hyperkalaemia and fluid overload is not necessary.

2. **D**
This man's symptoms suggest renal colic. The first line investigation for this is a CT scan of the kidneys, ureters and bladder.

Integrated care

1. **B**
This patient is deemed to have mental capacity to make decisions about his treatment. Provided that all the options have been fully explained to him and he fully understands the implications of not having dialysis (i.e. death), his wishes must be respected. The Mental Health Act may not be used to give medical treatment against a patient's wishes, only to detain a patient for assessment and treatment of a mental health problem. If his depression is so severe that his capacity were deemed to be impaired, medical treatment could be given under the Mental Capacity Act.

2. **D**
This patient's renal function has declined to a point at which renal replacement therapy is required. Provided she wishes to be treated, which it seems that she does, then haemodialysis would be the best course of action. In view of her Parkinson's disease, peritoneal dialysis is unlikely to be an option because this requires a certain degree of manual dexterity and mobility. A transplant may be the ideal outcome in this case, but it will take time to assess her suitability and to find a donor and more urgent action is required.

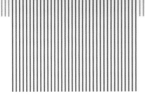
Index

Note: Page numbers in **bold** or *italic* refer to tables or figures, respectively.

WITHDRAWN FROM LIBRARY